I've Just
Seen a Face

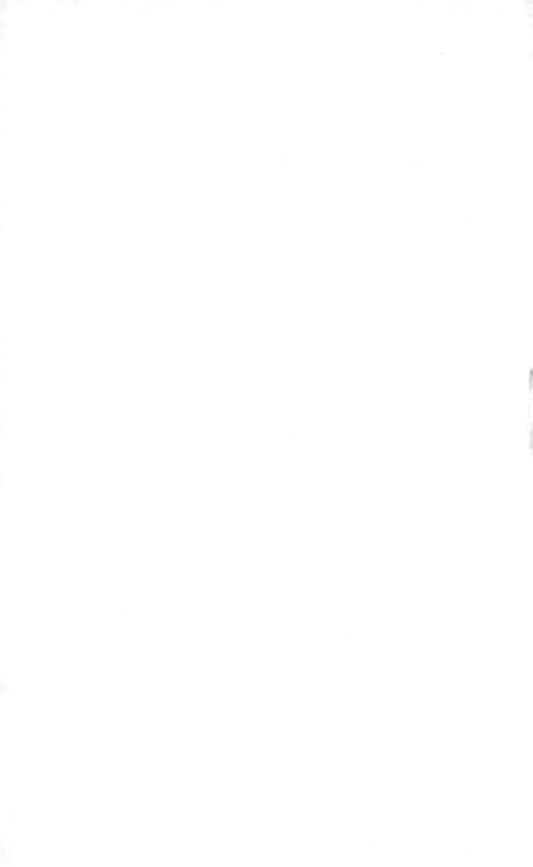

I've Just Seen a Face

A Practical and Emotional Guide for Parents of Children Born with Cleft Lip and Palate

YEAR ONE and BEYOND

Amy Mendillo

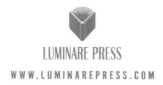

LUMINARE PRESS

WWW.LUMINAREPRESS.COM

Cover design by Jim Cooke

Illustrations by Maria Fong, unless otherwise indicated

Printed in the United States of America

Luminare Press
442 Charnelton St.
Eugene, OR 97401
www.luminarepress.com

LCCN: 2022952027
ISBN: 979-8-88679-080-1

I've just seen a face
I can't forget the time or place
Where we just met
She's just the girl for me
And I want all the world to see
We've met

Had it been another day
I might have looked the other way
And I'd have never been aware
But as it is I'll dream of her
Tonight

—Lennon-McCartney

Contents

FEEDING THE BABY

EARLY DAYS

PRESURGICAL TREATMENT

LIP-REPAIR SURGERY

PALATE-REPAIR SURGERY

BEYOND YEAR ONE

Preface

My Story, Part 1
A Beginning and a Second Beginning

When I think back on learning the news of my daughter's cleft lip and palate (CLP) eight years ago, what comes to mind is eating pasta. It's not that I don't remember the half-dimmed, fluorescent lights of the exam room at the prenatal testing center, or the way my husband and I held our breath as the ultrasound technician glided the exam tool with poised fingers, Ouija-like, across my jelly-covered, pregnant belly, or how she paused here and there to glance up and make clicks on her keyboard.

And of course, I recall how at one point she leaned in close to the screen and stared at the image, then blinked a couple of times and notified us in calm tones that while she was not at liberty to share any medical information (huh?), she would soon leave the room to fetch a doctor who could actually relay the news (what news?). And I remember how my husband and I exchanged glances as a new person entered and picked up where the technician left off, gliding, clicking, and blinking.

Finally, when the dimmed lights and measured motions and even-toned voices had somehow grown loud—and I wanted to stand up and wave my arms if someone didn't share some information already—the doctor informed us that our baby would have a common facial birth defect, likely in its most severe form. He urged us not to worry since there were plenty of resources available. That's when I remember feeling sick.

Pregnancy can cause queasy feelings, sure. But when we learned that our daughter would be born with bilateral-complete CLP, my

1

husband and I saw our family's path shift before our eyes, as if the flippers on a pinball machine had suddenly sent our ball into a strange, dizzying, alternate game space, to the chute located way over on the side of the machine that we didn't see when we were first inserting our quarter—a space with colors and lights and sounds that we had maybe known about but that caught us by surprise nonetheless.

The next thing I remember, we'd left the center and were hurtling down the highway. We weren't hurtling literally. Ever since our ten-month-old son had been born, my husband and I had adopted a style of slow, safe, nearly geriatric driving, with hands perched at ten and two. But as I sat in the passenger seat—my lap covered with shiny, slippery medical pamphlets, in a car traveling at fifty-eight miles per hour—it was my mind that raced. And as I read the information aloud to my husband, we learned that the treatment for CLP would involve a lot more intervention than a simple operation or two on the lip and palate. Like a snowball effect, we found out that the nose can be affected. And the teeth. And hearing (No! Not hearing!). And feeding. And speech. The news kept tumbling in, each piece with its own informational brochure. We found out that our child might need several procedures spanning many years and that she would need a whole team of specialists to handle them. As straightforward as the diagnosis had seemed at first, the treatments and related issues certainly were not.

And then, days later, after a flurry of phone calls, conversations, and several long and only sort-of relaxing walks filled with even more conversation, I went to the kitchen to chop garlic. Not just a dainty clove or two, either—a whole, hulking, southern Italian pile of it, with errant chunks flying wildly under the knife but then gathering into a neater mound that would soon meet with oil. It was a stress-busting exercise, for sure, linguini with garlic and oil. But it also meant that I was feeling hungry.

It marked the beginning of a process—eventually including the first year of our daughter's life—that was indeed stressful and full of worry. The unknowns were everywhere, as I wondered how her operations would go and how she would do in school and whether she'd be happy and how she would respond (and how I could possibly help her) if kids teased her on the playground.

But after getting through that first year with two major operations—and who knows how many pasta sauces—my husband and I realized that the journey had become familiar and circumscribed rather than vague and sprawling. After gathering information and asking lots of questions, we found that our load had lightened. What's more, our daughter's treatment went well. We received excellent care from a kind, capable team of people. And years later, my daughter is thriving. She is well aware of her CLP, but it is not the center of her life. She is beautiful, inside and out. And she is busy going to third grade, playing with friends, eating pasta dinners (still so much pasta), and covering her bedroom walls with pictures of horses.

So, while I certainly recall the details of learning the news, it's the coping during that first year that I most remember, not the crisis. And so I decided to write a book, not only to share practical information that I would have wanted to turn to before and during my daughter's first year, but also to help others explore related feelings and move forward. Most of all, I hope to share with you—parents and expectant parents; biological, adoptive, and foster parents; grandparents, friends, and loved ones; fellow travelers—the good news that you are not alone.

Introduction

About This Book

This book is an insider's guide. When I say *insider,* I define the term broadly. You'll hear my voice throughout as your fellow parent-narrator, the party host who takes your jacket, shows you around the house, and introduces you to some of the other guests. You'll see bits and pieces of my story with my daughter. But you'll also hear from a wide swath of other parents about their experiences with their children.

Are you curious about how others have navigated their baby's early operations? How they dealt with special feeding techniques? How they overcame nervous feelings about what would happen if they ran into a thoughtless stranger—or friend—who made a hurtful comment about their baby? (And how they replied? And whether they actually received such comments in the first place?). These parents, whose voices you'll hear in the following chapters, offer insights and solutions that you may not hear from a professional or discover readily online.

Some of you may want to learn basic nuts and bolts of what to expect for your child. You'll get plenty of that too. While interviews with parents made up a large portion of my research, I also spoke with a full range of experts to gather information and perspectives. I also draw from medical textbooks, the published materials of professional advocacy organizations, and hundreds of peer-reviewed articles. (To view sources and/or pursue further reading, see the references at the end of the book.) This guide covers the basics of cleft care from the prenatal phase through the baby's first year. It starts with a primer on the condition and its treatment and moves forward chronologically to topics such as locating and choosing a cleft team, carrying out presurgical treatments, and ushering a child through surgery and recovery. You will find some of the information that professionals might provide in a consultation or that you might learn in the booklets or fact sheets published by the American Cleft Palate-Craniofacial Association (ACPA).

My goal is to explain the basics in an everyday way and to expose you to words of wisdom from pros on cleft teams across the US. But perhaps more important, in sharing this information I hope to encourage you, fellow parents and caregivers, to feel empowered to become members of the team yourselves—by learning as much as you can about the condition and its treatment, by asking informed questions (I've included many samples), and by speaking up on behalf of your baby.

In short, if you are new to CLP and your mind is racing and you are lying in bed at night staring at the ceiling, please read on. The people and resources included here—this diverse and friendly community of insiders—have considerable information to share. This book is about collected wisdom. It is also designed to be consumed in any way you'd like. You can read it start-to-finish or just as easily jump around.

The voices here are presented anonymously. In the pages that follow, you will notice phrases like, "One parent, Richard, said..." or "According to a nurse on a cleft team...." I have assigned pseudonyms and removed identifying information for all the parents and professionals I interviewed, including names and genders of children, names of hospitals and cleft teams, and cities of origin. I wanted to give interviewees the freedom to be honest and also protect identities, especially of children.

There is one frequent exception: instances where I draw information from publicly available sources such as journal articles, medical textbooks, professional and personal websites, and the like. In these cases, the authors' names are their own (again, you will find these sources listed in the references). Also, while this book offers information, tips, and ideas, I do not endorse a particular surgeon or team. And the material here is certainly not a substitute for medical advice.

I am an introverted person. I write. I avoid social media and avoid talking on the phone (except with my mom). But after my daughter was born, I felt drawn to other parents of cleft-affected babies. The waiting room at the cleft clinic was filled with strangers. But the idea that any one of them could be holding a child like my own made me bubble with excitement. I wanted to talk to these people. I wanted to plop down next to one of them and say, "I see you are holding a Haberman baby bottle. How is your baby doing with it? How are *you* doing? Let's share!"

It felt comforting to find someone going through the same thing I was. Heck, I even felt eager to talk with the professionals on the cleft team. Sure, they were proposing an unsettling, even disturbing course of treatment: they would cut into our baby's face with a scalpel to change an appearance that on some level I didn't want to alter, that I already found beautiful. But when our surgeon suggested that our baby was perfect as she was (What? How did he know?) and reminded us that operating would make her life better and easier, his words felt like a warm blanket. It was reassuring to interact with people—whether in the waiting room or exam room—who understood my unusual constellation of feelings and concerns, people who really *got* it.

The first year of life with CLP can be challenging for parents. But it is my hope that reading this book—in any way you choose—will provide you with information, advice, and encouragement that will make your journey rewarding as well. I hope it will feel like just the conversation you were hoping for.

Cleft Basics

Chapter 1

. . . .

Learning the News

Questions, Answers, and Coping

The road to parenthood usually involves a lot of medical appointments. We have prenatal visits, blood tests, and ultrasounds, followed by more prenatal visits, blood tests, and ultrasounds. Some of us do home studies and wait for adoption updates (and wait and wait). Finally, the baby arrives! At key moments, we wonder: Is everything okay? Is she going to be healthy? In a majority of cases, a medical person tells us, yes. Everything is okay. She's healthy.

Unfortunately, some expectant parents find out, at some point along the way, that something is not quite okay. Cleft lip and/or palate (CLP) is one of the most common and treatable birth defects in the US. Yet for many parents, the moment of learning the news brings a wave of swift and sudden uncertainty. One mother recalled the shaky, shocking minutes after her son's birth when the medical people in the room caught sight of him and lost all animation in their faces. After humming along happily during her labor and delivery, they suddenly went blank—and so did she. "For me, it was traumatic," she said, "a very, very big deal." Another parent described feeling such panic at his wife's prenatal ultrasound, weeks earlier, that he couldn't recall whether he even acknowledged the doctor after learning the news. Overwhelmed and barely comprehending the situation, this expectant father was almost stunned into silence.

Yet every parent's experience is different. While many parents describe a negative reaction to the news, the context and specific feelings vary. This chapter meets parents at that moment, first to explore some common responses, then to describe options for prenatal testing for those who learned the news during pregnancy and want to learn more. The last section offers ideas from social workers, psychologists, researchers, and other parents on ways to help all of us—no matter when or where we learn the news—to make sense of it and cope.

Anxiety? Guilt? Smooth Sailing?

Parents usually learn the news about their child's CLP in one of two ways: at a prenatal ultrasound—typically at around twenty weeks gestation—or at birth. A few feel okay about it. One mother, Carla, recalled the quiet minutes immediately following her daughter's birth when the medical people not only handed her newborn daughter to her, but also relayed the news of her CLP—gently. "The nurse was so nice and so good about it," she said. "I didn't see any panic or hurry. I was holding her, and I was happy." Another mother, Kerry, adopted her son, Willie, from China, where he had already undergone one operation to address his cleft lip. Like some other adoptive parents, Kerry wasn't surprised or daunted to hear of a health issue. "We were fully aware of Willie's condition before we met him," she said. "When you adopt, you get this laundry list of all these things that you are willing to consider. We thought, 'When you are pregnant, you don't get to pick.'" Carla and Kerry learned the news in different contexts, but both took it in stride.

Other parents do not take the news in stride—and mention urgent responses such as anxiety and guilt. "I thought I did it," said one mother about her very first thoughts after her daughter's birth. "I kept asking the nurses what I could have done [to cause it]. I thought my husband would be mad." Another mother felt a whirlwind of confusion, anger, and dismay. "It seemed so unfair," she said. "I took folic acid during pregnancy. I was healthy. I kept wondering, 'Why? What did I do?' Those early weeks, she said, felt like a roller coaster.

Whether we feel anxiety, guilt, anger, denial, shock, numbness, grief—or all or none of the above—our responses are normal and okay. Every person reacts in their own way to the news of CLP, as to any news. And the researchers and professionals who help parents with the emotional aspects of treatment have confirmed that strong feelings are not only common but to be expected.

Aretha M. Miller, a clinical social worker with the cleft team at Miami Children's Hospital, writes that when parents learn that their child has a disorder or craniofacial difference, they frequently respond with the same degree of alarm as if they learned their child is terminally ill. "They often grieve," she explains, "for the child they thought they were going to have." Miller encourages parents not only to give themselves permission to feel these varied, healthy responses but to know that it is common for some of those emotions to recur as time goes on, even after they've largely put them to rest. The grieving process can be messy, and that messiness is all right.

One cleft-team geneticist mentioned the variations that can occur within parent-couples, not only regarding their individual interpretations of the news but also their unique ways of coping. "Neither reaction is more correct than the other," she suggests about these differences. Her advice for a couple, she said, is "to respect each other's process" as it plays out. Mutual tolerance, in other words—or at least a couple's best efforts in that direction—can go a long way in supporting one another as time goes on.

Further Testing

Some expectant parents receive the news of a prenatal diagnosis and wonder: Could there be more? When Callie and her husband learned about their son's CLP at a twenty-week ultrasound, they felt just as destabilized by the possibility of other health issues as they did about his CLP. "The hardest thing, initially," she said, "was the concern that there might be something else going on, something we couldn't see." Callie worried most about potential issues with the baby's heart.

Other parents mention concerns about a possible syndrome. (A *syndrome* is a group of differences that go beyond CLP.) According to geneticists writing in the guide *Comprehensive Cleft Care: Family Edition*, a majority of clefts are isolated, meaning that the baby does not have other health issues. Yet for many parents and expectant parents, the door has opened to the possibility of other problems. "That was very nerve-wracking during the first couple of months," Callie remarked.

Fortunately, prenatal testing has evolved to such an extent over the last several years that expectant parents are not only able to learn the news of CLP during pregnancy but discover further information via follow-up prenatal tests.

PRENATAL TESTING 101

Common Options Following CLP Diagnosis by Ultrasound

If you've received a prenatal diagnosis of CLP by prenatal ultrasound, you may want to learn more. Here are some standard tests you might learn about from your ob-gyn or perinatologist.

Prenatal Ultrasound and Follow-Up Ultrasound. At around eighteen weeks gestation or later, cleft lip can be detected by prenatal ultrasound, a scan of a fetus and placenta using sound waves. Many expectant parents learn about an unborn baby's cleft lip in this way, typically by way of a Level 2 ultrasound, a scan that shows more detailed views of the body parts than a regular ultrasound. Some medical professionals then recommend a follow-up scan, sometimes called a targeted ultrasound, to confirm the diagnosis, examine a cleft lip in detail, take measurements, and possibly look for other birth defects. While ultrasound technology has many benefits, it cannot always detect a cleft palate (see explanation, below).

A **Fetal MRI** is a snapshot of a fetus using Magnetic Resonance Imaging (MRI). This scan, which is noninvasive and takes place inside a large magnetic tube, is sometimes recommended following an ultrasound to learn about the existence of a cleft palate. According to information published in the *Cleft Palate-Craniofacial Journal*, a fetal MRI can show parts of a cleft palate that an ultrasound cannot.

An **Amniocentesis** is performed by drawing and testing a small amount of amniotic fluid (the liquid that surrounds the fetus) to learn genetic information. Analyzing the genes and chromosomes in this fluid can reveal a baby's chances of being born with a syndrome. According to the American Cleft Palate-Craniofacial Association (ACPA), 10-to-15 percent of babies with CLP are also diagnosed with a syndrome. If an amniocentesis indicates that chromosomes are normal, however, the risk of a syndrome is then known to be lower: 8-to-10 percent. An amniocentesis carries a small risk of miscarriage.

A **Fetal Echocardiogram** is an ultrasound of the heart of a fetus. According to a recent literature review published in the journal *Annals of Plastic Surgery*, the presence of a cleft palate increases the odds that a person will have congenital heart disease (CHD; *congenital* means present at birth). The authors state that the risk of CHD is about one percent for the general population, but over seven percent for those with CLP (note that these conclusions refer to patients not diagnosed with a syndrome). Because of the increased risk, some medical professionals recommend undergoing this special ultrasound to take a closer look at the fetal heart.

Prenatal Counseling is an opportunity to work with a professional to look at all available information and learn as much as possible about the health of an unborn baby. After an initial phase of prenatal testing, an ob-gyn or perinatologist may refer parents to the nearest *cleft team*, the group of professionals who work with cleft patients and their families in the prenatal period, through childhood, and sometimes into young adulthood. The cleft team is like a medical family, a hub for all things CLP. Prenatal counseling from the team may include visits with a surgeon, geneticist, otolaryngologist, and/or social worker. These team members will look at all the information available through tests and help make sense of it. They'll explain findings and answer questions. And they may recommend further testing to narrow down (or rule out) other diagnoses.

How Accurate Is an Ultrasound? (Is This for Real?)

Ultrasound technology is an amazing tool, but it has three broad limitations that may be helpful to know about, particularly if you are considering your early test results and wondering if this whole situation might be a big mistake—smoke and mirrors, a false positive. (Disbelief is actually a common response among expectant parents, and I can understand why. It is one thing to see the physical evidence of a cleft lip on a newborn; it is quite another to see an arrangement of confusing, fuzzy blobs on an ultrasound printout.)

The first limitation relates to the skills and techniques of the ultrasound technician—because what we find out depends, in large part, on what the technician notices. In some cases, the person reading the scan overlooks the clefts altogether, as was the case during Barbara's daughter's pregnancy. "My daughter had multiple ultrasounds to monitor [the baby's] growth," Barbara explained, "because she was taking blood pressure medications that had side effects of stunted growth." The ultrasound technician was not looking specifically for CLP—she was, instead, looking for indicators related to growth—and the condition went unnoticed. "My grandson's cleft was a complete surprise," Barbara continued. "It is so weird to look back [at the ultrasound images] and think we never saw his face. It is, of course, obvious now. The tech just missed it. They didn't catch it on eight ultrasounds."

In the case of Barbara's grandson, the technician didn't notice his cleft lip prenatally, even though it was visible on the scan. The technology itself, however, also poses limitations. A cleft lip is possible to detect on an ultrasound, but a cleft palate can be harder to identify, even by the most advanced equipment and the keenest eye. While it is possible to discover a cleft palate using this technology, the shape of the palate and the shadows of the sound waves can make detection difficult. (The fetal MRI, as mentioned above, is sometimes recommended to diagnose CP after diagnosis of cleft lip via ultrasound).

The third and simplest limitation relates to the position of the fetus. In some cases, a cleft can be obscured by another body part, such as a wayward hand covering the mouth. Just at a moment when the ultrasound technician is trying to snap a picture, her efforts are thwarted by an unintentional, prenatal photo bomb.

Given these three limitations in ultrasound technology, the chances of a *false negative* are relatively high while the chances of a *false positive* are not. As the speech pathologist, Helen Sharp, explains on the website of the American Speech-Language-Hearing Association, "the identification of a cleft when no cleft is present— occurs very rarely." Once a technician or other professional spots the clefts prenatally, expectant parents can assume that they will be there at birth.

Coping and the Three Ps

As shocking and overwhelming as the news of CLP may feel—and as varied as our responses may be in the moment or in the days and weeks that follow—it may help to know that pain, loss, and other strong feelings often lessen with time. "This is the crisis time," acknowledged Dr. Ronald P. Strauss about the period after learning the news. "But that is not most of what life is about." In fact, according to a large body of research, one of the hallmarks of recovering from a major setback is the realization that the feeling will not last forever. Psychologist Martin Seligman at the University of Pennsylvania has studied ways in which humans can find hope following a loss. We delay recovery, Seligman found, when we cling to three false beliefs, known as **The Three Ps:**

1. **Personalization**, the belief that an event is our fault;

2. **Pervasiveness**, the belief that an event will affect all aspects of our lives; and

3. **Permanence**, the belief that our feelings will last forever.

Put another way, we are better able to move forward from a setback when we understand that a feeling is not our fault, does not affect every aspect of our lives, and will not last forever. Seligman even links specific brain activity to this process, in an area of the brain he refers to as "the hope circuit."

Many parents have found that everyday steps and information-gathering can help. One mother felt reassured when she found out that her son's CLP was not her fault. "I spent ages researching anything and everything," she said. "I wanted to know why this happened. I felt better when I found out that there isn't really an answer…it just happens." Her realization speaks to the first P, Personalization.

Another parent felt comforted when she learned about the treatment path. When her son was three days old, her doctor showed her a pile of pictures of cleft-affected babies and kids. "I felt more peace after that," she said. One dad felt relieved to get an exact diagnosis from his child's surgeon and team. It took away the mystery, allowed him to plan, and in the larger sense, showed him that the treatment would not take over his child's life. That's the second P, Pervasiveness. "Once we got past the initial feeling of being surprised by it," he said, "we made a game plan."

The third P, Permanence, may seem harder to overcome for this diagnosis because the treatment path for CLP can last a long time. Short-term planning can show us that treatment is containable, but long-term planning isn't really possible. When parents first visit with a cleft surgeon and team, they often learn about the operations and treatments that can happen throughout childhood. It can be helpful to see the big picture; it gives us a sense of the journey and its pace. "This is a marathon, not a sprint," remarked one surgeon about the long view.

Yet these discussions can only go so far. We have to wait and see how our child will do. It will be years before we know how a child feels about their CLP, an awareness that not only emerges slowly as they grow but changes and evolves as the years pass. "The key for us," said one dad, "was when we decided to take it one surgery at a time. One thing at a time." We may have to wait for our own intense feelings of crisis to subside and for our child's feelings—whatever they may be—to emerge.

It can feel scary and deeply unsettling to imagine that our child might have a hard life marked by physical differences and unfair judgments from others. But at some point, we find out that we are not to blame. We learn about treatment and discover that it need not take over our child's life or last forever. We begin to cope and later accept the challenges of a (sometimes) long journey.

These emotional steps may take time and they may be messy. "I felt so awful," admitted one mother in a video by Foundation for the Faces of Children, "that [our daughter] had been brought into the world without the kind of head start that other kids have, and that her future for the next few months would be preparing for surgeries and getting through surgeries, and she wasn't going to be the happy little baby like other kids were." This mother's predictions did not come to pass. "As it turns out," she continued, "[our daughter] *was* the happy little baby like the other kids were. She just looked a little different for a while. It took us a while to recognize that." We can't predict how our child will respond to this condition. But we can take it day by day and plan to seek out the right tools when we need them, even as we, ourselves, cope in the meantime. That's the most any parent can do.

CHAPTER 2

. . . .

Cleft Lip and Palate

Basics

While some parents of cleft-affected children have a family history of CLP or otherwise know about the condition, others have barely heard of it. Many expectant parents wonder: *What is cleft lip and palate? And what does it mean for a child?*

This chapter is a primer on the condition and its treatment. Some aspects are described broadly, others in depth. Feel free to pick and choose your way through the details. If you want to learn some of the anatomy and so forth—wonderful. These sections explain the terms you'll probably hear used by medical people. Otherwise, this information will be here for moments when you want to learn more.

CLP Themes
Treatment for CLP Is Standardized and Excellent

Before we dive into the nuts and bolts of CLP, let's explore a few main ideas described by parents and professionals about the condition and experience. There is a common refrain in cleft care: "Every cleft is different." This phrase makes a lot of sense. Every cleft *is* different; just look at the types and severities discussed below. Even in the absence of complicating factors and additional health concerns, the combinations of CLP can seem endless, especially to an uninitiated parent.

Still, it is important to know three things. First, all the characteristics related to CLP are treatable. Some are treated sooner, some later, and some sooner *and* later (you'll find a sample time line below). Second, the range of cases of CLP is not so wide or varied that medical professionals devise a treatment from scratch each time. The treatment options are usually standardized. A cleft team—the group of specialists who care for a child—will tailor your child's treatment to his or her needs. But as the team members do, they usually draw from a common, established menu of options.

Finally, the outcomes, when delivered by an approved cleft team, can be top-notch. "Because the diagnosis is so common," commented speech-language pathologist Matthew D. Ford in the book *Comprehensive Cleft Care: Family Edition*, "medical specialists have become increasingly knowledgeable in the diagnosis and management of cleft-related conditions." As a result, he writes, patients experience "excellent treatment outcomes and…satisfaction." Cleft care can span years—it's true. But many patients and families say they feel pleased with the results. As one mother remarked, "I have full faith in my son's doctors. I trust them. They have not let us down."

What Is Cleft Lip and Palate?

During the early weeks of pregnancy, around weeks six and seven, the parts of the mouth and face are supposed to join together in the center and fuse. One time in one thousand births—for some reason or a combination of reasons—that process doesn't happen. Nothing is missing, necessarily; there's just a failure of the tissues to come together. The term *cleft* is used to describe the resulting space.

While several kinds of clefts can occur in the areas of the mouth and face, *cleft lip* (a gap in the upper lip) and *cleft palate* (a gap in the roof of the mouth) are the most common. A person can be born with an *isolated* cleft lip (a cleft lip with no cleft palate), an isolated cleft palate (a cleft palate with no cleft lip), or in about 50 percent of cases, both.

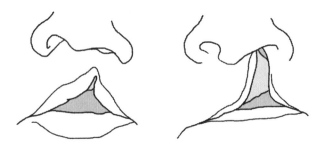

Unilateral cleft lip, incomplete (at left) and complete (at right)

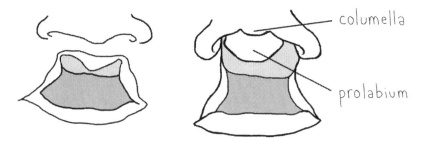

columella

prolabium

Bilateral cleft lip, incomplete (at left) and complete (at right)

Cleft Lip. Let's draw two imaginary lines from the upper lip of a typical face to the base of the nostrils—sort of like a runny nose in reverse. The two most common types of cleft lip, *unilateral* and *bilateral,* occur along these pathways. A unilateral cleft lip occurs on one side of the upper lip; a bilateral cleft lip occurs on both sides. Both forms of cleft lip (unilateral and bilateral) can range in severity. In the least severe form, a cleft could appear as a small notch, sometimes called a *forme fruste* cleft lip. A cleft that does not extend all the way to the nose is called *incomplete*. A *complete* cleft lip extends from the lip all the way to the base of the nose (on one or both sides).

Now, let's consider the *upper lip,* an odd term. In common usage, the upper lip includes the lip itself *and* the area above it, extending all the way up to the base of the nose (technically speaking, the area just under the nose is called the *philtrum*). For a person born with a cleft lip, this whole area—the lip itself and the skin above it—is referred to as the *prolabium*. You may hear professionals use this term during the child's first few months of life.

The anatomy of CLP can be confusing to look at because a baby with a cleft lip may have a very short *columella*, the strip of skin located in between the nostrils at the bottom of the nose, the place that some people pierce with a ring or a bar (i.e., a septum ring). The columella can be short or almost missing for a cleft-affected baby. So, in some cases, a cleft lip can appear to stick straight out of the nose.

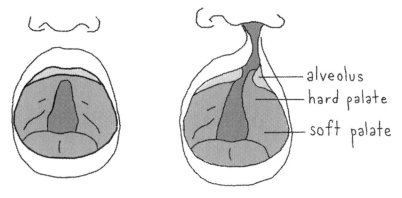

Isolated cleft palate (at left) and cleft palate and cleft lip (at right)

Cleft Palate. The roof of the mouth is made up of two parts, the *hard palate* and the *soft palate*. The hard palate is located at the front of the roof of the mouth, just behind the teeth. It is, in fact, made of hard bone of the upper jaw. The soft palate, located at the back of the roof of the mouth, is fleshier and (you guessed it) softer than the hard palate. A cleft palate can range in size, from a pinhole to a wide-open space. An incomplete cleft palate affects the soft palate only; a complete cleft palate affects the soft and hard palates. In all cases, a cleft palate exposes the cavities of the mouth and nose.

CLEFT TYPES 101

The Mysterious Submucous Cleft Palate

A *submucous cleft palate* is a special type of cleft palate that is characterized by a separation of the muscles located *underneath* the membrane lining of the roof of the mouth. This one is tricky. If you look inside the mouth of a baby with a submucous cleft, the roof of the mouth will probably appear intact. In fact, this kind of cleft shows few noticeable signs and can go undiagnosed at birth.

Some parents learn about a submucous cleft only after they notice that their baby is having trouble bottle-feeding or can't form a proper seal on the breast during breast-feeding. "She couldn't suck," said one mother, Sarah, about the difficulties she experienced with her newborn daughter. Having given birth on a Friday, Sarah did not have immediate access to a full array of specialists in the hospital. And the weekend staff, she added, did not seem to believe her when she observed that the baby was physically unable to form a seal with her mouth. "The staff said, 'Just keep her on the breast, and keep her sucking,'" Sarah said. "I said, 'That is just stupid! She cannot suck!'" All weekend, Sarah felt frustrated and confused as she tried to console her hungry newborn. Come Monday, she learned the baby's diagnosis. But the interim felt frustrating.

Feeding troubles are one of the two common problems caused by a submucous cleft—and as Sarah experienced, they are one of the common ways families and doctors arrive at a diagnosis. The other problem—issues with speech—may surface after the baby grows and begins to speak.

It *is* possible to see the signs of a submucous cleft palate if you know what to look for and the symptoms are actually there. Some babies show no physical markers in the oral cavity. Others have a faint blue or white line down the center of the soft palate, a little nick in the hard palate, or a split *uvula*—a break in the little piece of skin that dangles from the back of the mouth.

Many surgeons take a wait-and-see approach with a submucous cleft. They may not recommend closing it through surgery during infancy, opting instead to wait to see how a child fares with speech, usually later in childhood. In the meantime, feeding issues can be addressed by using a special bottle (see other chapters in this book for details).

Cleft of the Gumline. A baby may be born with a cleft of the *alveolus* (the upper gumline), sometimes called the *alveolar ridge* or *gum ridge*. A cleft in the gumline can affect the teeth. Remember our two imaginary pathways on the upper lip? Let's extend them downward and backward, onto the gums. Any teeth that occupy (or will later occupy) the spaces of those pathways can have problems. The lateral incisors, located on either side of the two front teeth, are usually the unlucky winners. Those baby teeth may be missing, split in two, or located in odd spots on the roof of the mouth. The permanent teeth may or may not exist.

Many children born with a cleft in the alveolar ridge will need to have bone-graft surgery during the school-age years to make that area strong enough to support the eruption of the adult teeth (see the time line below for more information). Children and teenagers may need to undergo various kinds of dental/orthodontic work in that area as well.

If a person is born with a complete cleft on both sides of the gumline, there will be an isolated piece of gum in the middle. That little piece of gumline, which may contain a remnant of the upper lip, is about the width of the two front teeth. It is called the *premaxilla*. Again, you'll hear this term a lot from members of the cleft team, especially during infancy.

The Nose. When a baby is born with CLP, the elements of the nose may not be normally developed, causing a collapsed and/or asymmetrical appearance. Medical professionals have several ways to describe these differences. *Nasal tip deviation* is the term for the asymmetry that happens when, in the case of unilateral clefts, the nose pulls to the left or right side. Also, some people born with CLP have asymmetry inside the nose, when the wall that divides the left and right nostrils, the *septum*, is off-center (called *deviated*). A person may also have a shortened columella, the strip of skin located between the base and the tip of the nose (as mentioned above). A surgeon will likely operate on parts of an infant's nose during primary lip-repair surgery, the early operation to close a cleft lip. Some older children also undergo nose surgery, called *rhinoplasty*, during the teen years when the face has grown.

There's More: Feeding, Hearing, and Speech

Now that we've looked at the anatomy of the cleft differences themselves, let's explore how clefts can cause complications in other areas. Given that the parts of the mouth and face are interconnected, it follows that CLP can affect other bodily functions.

Feeding. A large majority of infants born with cleft palate are physically unable to create the mouth suction necessary to feed from the breast or from a regular baby bottle. From birth until the time of lip-repair surgery, these babies will need to use a special bottle to take in formula or pumped breast milk. During the weeks and months after lip repair, the team may recommend transitioning from a cleft bottle to a special sippy cup or regular cup for liquids (you can read about feeding in Chapters 12–16).

Hearing. Some babies and young children born with cleft palate get fluid in their ears in locations where the air is supposed to be, causing hearing loss and recurring ear infections. These problems are usually temporary and manageable with timely testing and treatment. The audiologist or the ear, nose, and throat (ENT) surgeon on the cleft team may recommend inserting ear tubes, formally called *tympanostomy tubes*. Ear tubes are tiny cylinders, usually made of plastic or metal, which are inserted into the eardrum via a short surgical procedure. Some cleft teams coordinate the timing of this insertion so that it is performed during the same session as another operation (such as the early operation to close a cleft palate).

Speech. A child born with a cleft palate can have problems with speech. If you close your eyes and speak a few words—and in so doing observe how your tongue hits the roof of your mouth—you will notice the connection between the palate and speech. While the *speech-language pathologist* (SLP) on the cleft team may help with a baby's feeding and speech during infancy, an evaluation and treatment of speech, language, and *resonance* (tone of voice) usually occurs during the years that follow. Not every child born with CLP will need speech therapy or other interventions, but the prognosis can be excellent for those who do (for more information on hearing and speech, see Chapter 21).

Treatment Time Line

The following sample time line is a catchall for someone born with CLP. While some children receive every treatment on the list, others skip certain phases or procedures altogether or require special attention in one area. Also, some surgeons/teams perform certain procedures differently than others or at slightly different times; there are variations. Still, this is a standard course of treatment that should give you a sense of the recommendations you may hear from your child's team. It draws in part from the textbook, *Comprehensive Cleft Care: Family Edition.*

SAMPLE TIME LINE FOR A PERSON BORN WITH CLEFT LIP AND CLEFT PALATE

INFANCY

PRESURGICAL ORTHOPEDICS, in coordination with PRIMARY LIP-REPAIR SURGERY

Primary lip repair is a surgical procedure to close a cleft lip and other spaces in the gumline and nose, usually at age three-to-six months (sometimes performed in two stages). Leading up to this procedure, a newborn may undergo orthodontic treatment such as Nasoalveolar Molding (NAM), Latham treatment, or lip taping, to move certain parts of the mouth into place in preparation for surgery.

FEEDING

A majority of infants born with a cleft palate will need to use a special bottle to take in liquids, both before and after lip-repair surgery (as described above).

HEARING

Many babies and young children born with cleft palate have problems with hearing loss due to recurring ear infections and/or fluid in the ears. These problems are usually temporary and manageable with timely testing and treatment. *Ear tubes* are a common treatment, inserted surgically by the ENT on the cleft team.

SPEECH

The speech-language pathologist on the cleft team may help with a baby's feeding (sometimes in coordination with a cleft-team nurse). The SLP will also assess the baby's early development of speech and language.

PRIMARY PALATE-REPAIR SURGERY

Palate-repair surgery is a surgical procedure to close a cleft palate, usually at age nine-to-twelve months. A child with a submucous cleft palate may skip this procedure or delay it until later in childhood if the cleft affects speech.

AGES ONE TO TWELVE

SPEECH EVALUATIONS/SPEECH THERAPY

At age two or three, a child will see the speech-language pathologist on the team for a formal speech evaluation, followed by treatment (if necessary) and subsequent yearly evaluations. According to speech-language professionals, speech therapy during childhood can be very successful.

SECONDARY PALATE-REPAIR SURGERY

At ages four to seven, a child may have a second palate repair, depending on the need, usually to address issues related to speech. Options include *Furlow palatoplasty* (sometimes called "Z-plasty"), *pharyngeal flap pharyngoplasty* (sometimes called "P-Flap"), *sphincter pharyngoplasty*, and others. These procedures address the area at the very back of the soft palate, which if not functioning properly, can affect speech and tone of voice.

LIP-REVISION SURGERY / NOSE-REVISION SURGERY

At ages five to eight, a child may undergo plastic surgery on the lip and/or nose, depending on recommendations from the surgeon and team and the wishes of the child and family. These procedures usually involve small-scale changes related to appearance.

PALATAL EXPANSION/ORTHODONTICS in coordination with ALVEOLAR BONE-GRAFT SURGERY

Somewhere between ages six and twelve, a child may need *alveolar bone graft surgery*, a procedure that involves adding bone to the gumline to support the eruption of teeth. Orthodontic treatment usually takes place beforehand and afterward.

TEEN YEARS

ORTHODONTICS in coordination with ORTHOGNATHIC SURGERY

A child may undergo orthodontic treatment (usually including braces) between ages twelve and eighteen, either alone or in coordination with other treatment, such as implants or false teeth, in the area of the cleft(s). Orthodontics may also be used in coordination with *orthognathic surgery* (if necessary), which corrects the position of the jaw, usually at age sixteen for females and age seventeen or eighteen for males.

RHINOPLASTY

During the late teen years, a child may undergo plastic surgery to change the structure and shape of the nose. This procedure is usually recommended after puberty and also following jaw surgery.

Go, Team!

While the time line for CLP treatment may seem daunting, it is also true that you will have help every step of the way. A cleft team, as mentioned above, is a group of specialists who take care of a child's clefts from prior to birth through young adulthood, usually around age eighteen but sometimes longer. (While there are two types of teams—*cleft-palate teams* and *craniofacial teams*—you'll see the term "cleft team," or simply, "team" in this book to refer to either type.) The cleft team functions as the hub for all things CLP; it is a family's go-to resource for questions, concerns, treatment, and support.

Cleft teams in the US vary somewhat in their makeup. All teams approved by the American Cleft Palate-Craniofacial Association (ACPA) include a surgeon, a speech-language pathologist (SLP), an orthodontist, and a patient care coordinator (we'll discuss approval in Chapter 7). But some teams also include (or may refer patients to) an ear, nose, and throat surgeon (an ENT), a pediatric dentist, a geneticist, a psychologist or social worker, an audiologist, and a pediatrician.

QUICK LINK

Find a Cleft Team near You

The American Cleft Palate-Craniofacial Association (ACPA) Family Services website lists ACPA-approved teams in the US and abroad.

For state-by-state and international listings,
go to the ACPA website:
www.cleftline.org/find-a-team

Given the importance of the cleft team to a child's successful treatment, some parents choose to meet with more than one team, if possible, before deciding on the best fit. See Chapters 7 and 8 for detailed information on team care.

Resources and Support
Many Shapes and Sizes

While the cleft team functions as the central element of a child's treatment, you might be surprised at the number and types of other resources available to individuals and families. The ACPA, for instance, gives clear, thorough explanations of the condition and its treatment, penned by professionals in the field (these are the brochures you'll find in many doctors' offices in the US). Other organizations connect families to support groups, parent networks, annual meetings, summer camps, financial assistance, information, and other forms of help.

**ORGANIZATIONS FOR INDIVIDUALS
AND FAMILIES**
Mission – Location – Website Listed Alphabetically

AboutFace
AboutFace offers education, family events, Camp Trailblazers summer camp, and help in accessing care "for anyone and everyone living with a facial difference."
Canada – www.aboutface.ca

American Cleft Palate-Craniofacial Association (ACPA)

The ACPA is an international society of health professionals who treat and/or research cleft and craniofacial conditions and set standards for team care in the US. The ACPA offers educational publications and videos, referrals to team care, college scholarships, Cleft Courage Bears, and more.

USA – www.ACPAcares.org

AmeriFace / cleftAdvocate

AmeriFace offers information, state resource guides, connections to other families, online networking opportunities, and an annual conference for individuals with facial differences and their families. AmeriFace also partners with cleftAdvocate, a source of social networks, advocacy guidelines, inspiration, and tools for navigating medical care and coverage.

USA – www.ameriface.org – www.cleftadvocate.org

Changing Faces

Changing Faces offers skin camouflage services, counseling support, online communities, and workshops for individuals and families.

United Kingdom – www.changingfaces.org.uk

Children's Craniofacial Association

CCA addresses medical, financial, emotional, and educational concerns related to craniofacial conditions, with services such as an annual retreat, financial assistance, care packages, a newsletter and blog, informational videos, and more.

USA – www.ccakids.com

Cleft Lip and Palate Association (CLAPA)

CLAPA offers volunteer networks, support groups, patient advocates, feeding services, adult services, educational materials, an annual conference, and more, "for all those in the UK affected by cleft lip and/or palate."

United Kingdom – www.clapa.com

Cleft Lip & Palate Foundation of Smiles

Cleft Lip & Palate Foundation of Smiles offers networking opportunities, educational materials, advocacy information, help with funding for cleft bottles, and research materials for individuals and families with cleft lip and/or palate and other craniofacial anomalies.

USA – www.facebook.com/www.cleftsmile.org

Cleftopedia

Cleftopedia is a nonprofit organization and informational website with resources on special feeders, presurgical techniques, cleft teams, and parenting tips.

USA – www.cleftopedia.com

Cuddles for Clefts

Cuddles for Clefts offers customized support packages for anyone with a scheduled, upcoming cleft surgery.

USA – www.cuddlesforclefts.com

FACES: The National Craniofacial Association
Face Equality International

FACES provides financial assistance for medical travel, educational tools to increase public awareness and understanding of facial discrimination, a summer camp for teens and children, and information and support for individuals with craniofacial disorders and their families.

USA – www.faces-cranio.org

Foundation for the Faces of Children

FFC supports the social, psychological/emotional, and educational needs of individuals and families affected by craniofacial differences through educational programming and sessions, instructional videos, scholarship awards, and family gatherings.

USA – www.facesofchildren.org

The Mia Moo Fund

A charitable organization that raises awareness and provides funds for families in the US to obtain treatment for cleft lip and palate.

USA – www.miamoo.org

myFace

myFace offers parent guides, reading materials, support groups and educational webinars for families, newborn craniofacial care kits, housing for patients receiving treatment in New York City, and myFace Wonder Project educational programs in schools.

USA – www.myFace.org

ONLINE SUPPORT GROUPS

FACEBOOK GROUPS

Cleft Lip and Palate Foundation of Smiles

Cleft Lip and Palate Parent Support Group

Cleft Mommies

Cleft Mom Support

Clefty's – Bringing Wide Smiles Open

NAM Support (Nasoalveolar Molding)

OTHER ONLINE GROUPS

BabyCenter Community Group: Cleft Lip/Cleft Palate

Even with so many resources to draw from, many families feel overwhelmed by CLP and all it entails. The details presented in this chapter alone—much less the information we learn from other publications and trusted medical people—can feel surprising and difficult to absorb, especially when we see the secondary issues and treatments that can come into play for children as they grow.

The details of CLP and its treatment, however, are also our tools for success. The more information we have at our fingertips, the more equipped we will be to ask informed questions, make decisions about treatment, talk with other children in the family, share the news with family and friends—and most importantly, support our child through treatment and growth.

Chapter 3

. . . .

Hindsight for New Parents

"That Support Group Turned Me Around"

Did you read the treatment time line for CLP and let out a little gasp? If so, you are not alone. "It was so intense," commented one mother about learning the ins and outs of the condition. The news—the flood of information—can feel overwhelming.

Fortunately, fellow cleft parents have looked back on their experiences—in some cases, years and even decades after their cleft-affected children were born—and shared ways they've thought about this journey and its pacing. While this chapter is officially numbered Chapter 3, I like to think of it more like Chapter 2b, since it includes ideas and advice from parents (and some professionals) on ways to make sense of the flood and, I hope, move toward drier ground.

Expect to Wait and See. A family's early visits with the cleft team will usually involve some discussions about a long-term plan for a child. A surgeon might write out or describe a treatment time line, for example, perhaps along the lines of the one printed in Chapter 2.

I remember jotting down furious notes the first time I met with our team, trying to capture every detail. The particulars, however, were relatively limited, as they often are during such meetings. "One thing I've noticed that frustrates me," said one mother, Jamie, "is that the team is very careful and very vague in the way they talk about the long-term trajectory. They don't discuss details." Other parents have mentioned feeling the same way.

Truth to tell, the professionals *can't* predict the exact nature of a far-off procedure or treatment—or in some cases, whether it will happen at all. Such determinations depend on growth, a child's health, the desires of the child and family, and additional factors that emerge over time. Team members *can* predict weeks or even months of upcoming treatment during the baby's first year. And they usually want us to know general information on the events that might—and often do—occur later on (thus the time lines). But the nature of this condition and its treatment usually involves a lot of "wait and see."

This uncertainty can be hard to live with, especially for those of us who like to plan. "They make an effort not to overwhelm people," Jamie continued. She admitted that it would hardly seem productive to learn the details of a surgical procedure that may or may not take place in, say, eight years. But it took her some time to accept this ambiguity. In the same way that all of us wait to see a child's growth and development in other areas—in schooling, friendships, interests, and even personality—we must allow this process to unfold at its own pace.

Expect to Shift Gears. A child born with CLP can have a very intense first year of life, sometimes including two major surgical procedures, weeks or months of presurgical treatment, several feeding methods, evaluation and treatment for hearing loss, and more. Many parents describe their first year as being in a long, constant state of *cleft mode*. "It was a challenge not letting the cleft world consume me," said one mother. "I was a mama bear on a mission to help my baby." For some of us, cleft mode can feel like a way of life.

While it is true that some babies continue treatments unabated after their first birthday (depending on diagnosis and circumstances), the number of CLP-related appointments and procedures tends to drop off. As strange as it may seem to consider now, many families notice that come year two, things change. The immediate need to buy cleft-related feeding supplies and paraphernalia goes away (Target withdrawal, anyone?). And in the years that follow, operations and treatments may happen—sometimes with intensity—but often with spaces in between. Over the long term, many families experience periods of reprieve.

This shift can be useful to know about, not only during the early days when we may wonder if the intensity will ever end, but also later on, as we help our children learn about the condition and its place in their life. As the advocacy group, AboutFace, says so simply and profoundly in one of its publications, "Having a facial difference is only one aspect of the whole person." Cleft mode may well take over the first year but need not be a way of life—for parent or child.

Consider All Kinds of Support. When I asked parents of cleft-affected kids about their experiences during their baby's first year, they almost always described the people or groups that they leaned on for emotional support. These weren't just casual mentions, either. Many became animated, their voices warming as they explained the ways they found relief and reassurance. The support was just so *helpful*, they said. Perhaps they hadn't anticipated how emotionally taxing their first year would be (I know I didn't). And in some cases, they surprised even themselves with their choices.

One dad, who had been born with CLP himself, never thought he would enjoy an in-person support group. He had always leaned toward shyness, he said, especially concerning his CLP, a topic he had spent many of his early years trying to avoid. But shortly after his son was born with a condition that included CLP, he and his wife learned about a family group in their area that met for casual picnics and playtime in a local park. After chatting with the adults and children, some in each generation born with CLP, he not only relaxed into the experience but came to embrace it. "That support group turned me around," he admitted years later. As he explained how relieved he felt at the time to share his feelings with others—rather than hold them back—his voice brightened. "You start to feel more comfortable dealing with things," he said. "For me, it made all the difference in the world." In-person support groups are usually run by local foundations or small nonprofits—and therefore exist in some areas but not others. Online groups may be an option, however, and/or parenting support groups that go beyond CLP or facial differences.

One-on-one therapy is another popular option. "You can get stuck in a rut, in circular thinking," commented one mother about her decision to start therapy. After a few sessions with a professional, she started to reframe her thoughts, not only regarding her child's condition but to some of the challenges of partnership and parenting during her baby's stressful first year. With time and some work, a weight was lifted. One-on-one therapy and group-based therapy can be costly; health insurance coverage (or lack of it) can be a deciding factor. But parents have emphasized its usefulness.

Other parents mentioned how much they appreciated having even a single friend who understood their situation. One mother asked the coordinator on her son's cleft team for the names of cleft families in the area—and ended up connecting with another mother who was a couple of months ahead of her with her child's treatment. In no time, the two mothers were chatting before and after operations. "She was my mentor and friend the whole time," this mother said. "That made a huge difference for me." Another dad characterized talking to other cleft families as his most helpful source of support. "They know the day-to-day stuff that a team or doctor won't tell you," he said.

Online support groups may be the most popular source of reassurance among new parents, especially private groups on Facebook. These groups allow participants to post pictures and ask questions large and small—all related to CLP. "I love Facebook," commented one parent. "I know it has its pitfalls, but it is a great way to connect. There are so many people who reached out to us." While cleft-team professionals often warn parents not to seek or obtain medical information from these groups (it is always best to direct such questions to the team), they have also mentioned the benefits of such forums in terms of emotional support. Whether you gravitate toward an in-person group, a therapist, a local family, or an online forum, the key is to avoid underestimating your own need for support on this sometimes intense journey.

Expect a Balancing Act. Of all the topics I've discussed with the parents of kids born with CLP, one of the most frequent was the question of how to contextualize this experience. Time and again, parents have wondered, both for themselves and for their children, *How big a deal is it to be born with cleft lip and palate?* On one hand, clefts are treatable, and the treatment is transformative. But, in many cases, that process can take a lot more time and energy than most parents would have imagined or wanted for their children.

Clearly, there is no single answer. Any diagnosis or event that feels momentous to one person can feel less significant, insignificant, or just plain different to another, whether we are a patient or an invested caregiver. But what's emerged from my conversations with parents is a sense that the answers also change over time. Almost all of these parents mention a balancing act—a seesaw—that oscillates between challenging and less challenging moments.

Kathy, mother of Zeke, a seven-year-old born with unilateral CLP, described how the intense periods of cleft treatment could stress everyone in her household, especially at surgery time. "Some days, I feel so sorry for myself and my family," she said. "When Zeke had his recent surgery, his younger brother, who felt abandoned, kept saying, 'Where's Mommy?'" Kathy's heart ached for her younger son, even as she spent days and nights in the hospital, consumed with helping Zeke. When the operation and recovery ended, however, things changed. "Other days, I think, *This is nothing*," she continued. "It is so relative." At certain moments, CLP can feel like a big deal. That feeling is real. Yet the condition need not define a child. The journey can be a balancing act, a seesaw, for the child and caregivers, alike.

Chapter 4

. . . .

Why Did This Happen?

When parents learn the news about their child's cleft lip and palate, often they wonder, "Why did this happen?" And it can be useful to find out *why*. Answers help them come to terms with surprising news. "The search for a reason, for something on which to assign blame," writes cleft parent Kathy Glow on the SheKnows site, "can ease the pain and sorrow parents feel." Answers help us cope.

Yet, when I've asked parents of cleft-affected children, "Why did this happen?" many of their responses are as much spiritual as they are scientific. Unlike other aspects of this journey—such as learning about treatment, finding a cleft team, or helping a child recover from surgery—the discussion of *why* seems most heavily filtered by worldview. Parents often mention empirical facts, like their genetics or prenatal care. Just as often, they talk about God, spirituality, or how they make sense of any kind of surprising news. Many mention guilt.

Now, it is true that some families are more concerned than others in the question of *why*—or in matters related to biology. One adoptive mother laughed as she described her family's very brief visit with the geneticist on the cleft team. "Not an issue for us!" she said. For those of you who *are* concerned, this chapter covers two aspects of the discussion. Part One, "The Science," offers a rundown on the physical causes of cleft lip and palate, including explanations of scientific terms, current research, and genetic tests. Part Two, "Beyond Science," describes the ways some parents interpret the question, "Why?" My hope is that at least some of this discussion helps *you* cope.

The Science

The first time my husband and I met with the geneticist on my daughter's cleft team, my main response was confusion. The conversation started out clearly enough. As she began to explain some basics about heredity and CLP, I was transported pleasantly back to high school science class. *I remember chromosomes!* I thought. About ten seconds later, she had lost me. Each time I took a moment to remember a concept, I would miss her next sentence. The conversation felt like a blur of genes, DNA, and other terms I now realize I never fully understood in the first place. She was remarkably generous, even taking extra time to repeat the parts I didn't get (extra time from a *doctor*!). Still, at that sleep-deprived moment, in a crowded office—with decisions to make about whether to pursue genetic tests—I felt ill-prepared.

That conversation may have felt confusing because the causes of CLP can be hard to understand and explain, even under the best of circumstances. The concepts of genetics, heredity, and scientific research get complicated quickly, sort of like standing on a seashore with a lot of undertow. One minute you're enjoying the sunlight and wiggling your toes in the water, when, *Whoa!* One more step and the undertow takes you down.

The geneticist on your cleft team will help you find specific information and answers; as always, the cleft team should be your primary source of advice. But hopefully, the explanations below, presented in everyday language, will help prepare you for those conversations and serve as a springboard for questions—so when you arrive at your first visit, you will hit the ground running.

The Causes. Not only are the possible causes of CLP hard to explain, but they are also sometimes unknown. Research is moving forward rapidly, but researchers have not yet painted a complete picture of this condition.

The details we do know fall into three broad categories. We know that CLP can be caused by *genetics*, meaning the condition can be passed down in biological families or caused by a spontaneous change in our coding. The condition can also be caused by *environmental factors*, meaning an event during pregnancy or another circumstance unrelated to genetics. And perhaps most often, CLP can be caused by a combination of the two. According to the American Cleft Palate-Craniofacial Association (ACPA), a majority of isolated clefts (those that occur without any other differences) appear to be caused by an interaction between genetics and environmental factors. Let's also remember that sometimes the cause of a person's CLP (or other condition) is unknown.

Passing It Down

First, let's talk about the genetic side. *Genetics* has to do with characteristics that are passed down from biological parents to a child. While the genetic basis of CLP is not fully understood, researchers do know that the chance of having a child born with a cleft is higher than average if one of the parents, or both, was born with a cleft themselves. If one or both of the parents was born with a related syndrome, the chance of recurrence is higher still. (A *syndrome*, as mentioned before, is a condition that includes more than one difference at birth).

To fully explain these statements, we first need to talk about how the chances are calculated. Let's make a brief stop at math class to discuss odds, and then move on to science class to explore more about genetics and available tests.

Math Class: What Are the Chances? According to the ACPA, the chance of having a baby born with CLP is one in six hundred for all parents, or 0.17 percent. So, let's say that two people get together to have babies. Let's name them Pat and Patty. In addition to dealing with confusion and constant questions about their names, Pat and Patty don't know much about their family history. Maybe one of them has a family history of CLP or maybe not. So, let's say that Pat and Patty plan to have a lot of babies—six hundred, to be exact. Now, here is the important part! Patty *may or may not* give birth to one cleft-affected child and 599 children without clefts (though, in any case, P and P will have a lot of other problems on their hands). The key is that while the chances are one in six hundred, they have to roll an imaginary six-hundred-sided die again each time. Of Pat and Patty's six hundred children, any number could be born with CLP, or none for that matter, depending on what happens each time they roll.

There's another wrinkle. These calculations, known as *probability*, deal with the chances for everyone considered together—"One chance in six hundred *for all parents*"—not Pat and Patty, in particular. If one parent—let's say, Pat—later finds out about CLP in his family history or learns about CLP in his genetics through genetic tests, the chances will have been higher that the couple would have a child born with CLP. Their imaginary die will have had *fewer* sides. If they find out later that neither has a family history, their die will have had *more* sides. The more information we know from either biological parent, the more accurately we can determine the chances.

This concept of increased chances is called *genetic predisposition*. People have a genetic predisposition for CLP when there is enough genetic information to presume they have a *higher* chance than average of having offspring born with CLP—that is, that their die has fewer sides. (Note that the term *predisposition* refers to heightened chances in the same way that the word *fever* refers to a heightened temperature. The shorter term, *disposition*, like *temperature*, simply refers to a state of being, falling anywhere on a range.)

The ACPA provides specific figures related to genetic disposition for CLP. Let's remember that if neither biological parent was born with CLP, the chance of giving birth to a person born with the condition is 0.17 percent or one in six hundred. Once a child is born with CLP, however, the chances go up to a 2-to-5 percent chance for a future sibling. And likewise, the 2-to-5 percent probability applies to an affected person's child. Geneticists use the term *recurrence risk* to refer to the chances of a hereditary event happening again in a family. The following pie charts, based on the ACPA informational booklet, "Genetics and You," illustrate the chances.

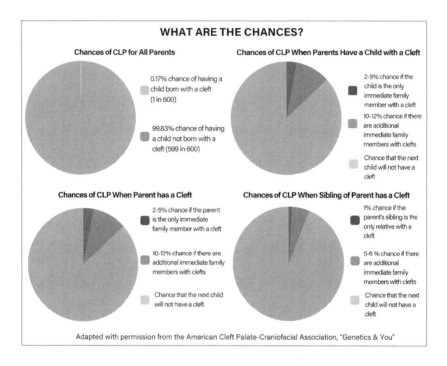

WHAT ARE THE CHANCES?

Chances of CLP for All Parents

0.17% chance of having a child born with a cleft (1 in 600)

99.83% chance of having a child not born with a cleft (599 in 600)

Chances of CLP When Parents Have a Child with a Cleft

2-5% chance if the child is the only immediate family member with a cleft

10-12% chance if there are additional immediate family members with clefts

Chance that the next child will not have a cleft

Chances of CLP When Parent has a Cleft

2-5% chance if the parent is the only immediate family member with a cleft

10-12% chance if there are additional immediate family members with clefts

Chance that the next child will not have a cleft

Chances of CLP When Sibling of Parent has a Cleft

1% chance if the parent's sibling is the only relative with a cleft

5-6 % chance if there are additional immediate family members with clefts

Chance that the next child will not have a cleft

Adapted with permission from the American Cleft Palate-Craniofacial Association, "Genetics & You"

Science Class: What Are the Basics? When the geneticist on the cleft team meets with families, she will usually do a few things: help discover and interpret your family and medical histories, teach you about inheritance, and counsel you on ways to learn more information. Genetic tests are common recommendations. Some genetic tests can be performed during pregnancy, others afterward. The results can provide information about genetic disposition for CLP and whether a child might be born (or has been born) with a syndrome. They allow you to make informed decisions about your child's care. In many cases, the results provide answers as to *why* this happened.

The geneticist on the team will probably mention two terms, in particular—*chromosomes* and *genes*—because problems with each can be associated with cleft lip and palate. Chromosomes and genes are instructions, similar to coding, for how our body is made;

they draw in part from our biological mother and in part from our biological father. Genetics 101, below, explains these terms.

GENETICS 101
Chromosomes, DNA, and Genes
(plus Chromosomal Gumby)

Let's look at our body parts in terms of physical size, starting with one of the largest units of the human body—the organs—and move downward to smaller units.

ORGANS → TISSUES → CELLS →
CHROMOSOMES → DNA → GENES

The human body contains many *organs*, like the stomach, the liver, and the heart. An organ is made up of *tissue*, such as muscle tissue, nerve tissue, and connective tissue (tissues also have different sub-types, but let's forget about that, for now). Tissues are made of *cells*, of which there are many types in the body, including bone cells, red blood cells, and white blood cells. Cells are the building blocks of all living things. We have millions of them in our bodies.

Continuing to even smaller units...every cell in our body has a central core, called a *nucleus*. If you look inside the nucleus, you will see twenty-three X-shaped blobs that, as illustrated in many science textbooks, tend to resemble Gumby, the green Claymation character. Each of the twenty-three Gumby blobs represents a pair of chromosomes. The illustration below shows how the pairs come together. Each pair of chromosomes contains genetic information from our biological mother and biological father (thus the two strand-like components).

Now, let's proceed to even smaller units within chromosomes. DNA, short for deoxyribonucleic acid, is a strand of hereditary material that looks like a twisted ladder. A *gene* is one stretch of that ladder (see the image, at right). The gene is the basic unit of heredity.

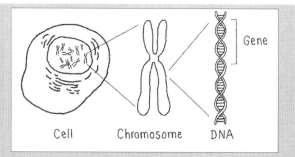

Cell, chromosome, DNA, gene

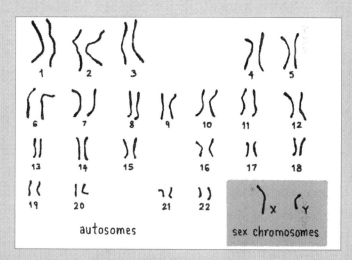

Human chromosomes

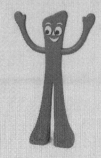

Gumby character (Gumby image, Courtesy Prema Toy, Inc.)

Chromosomes and Genes: What Can We Learn? Let's start by looking at tests that examine our chromosomes. Remember: chromosomes are large units that occur in small numbers (relatively speaking). Just think of twenty-three Gumby characters, each of which actually includes a chromosomal *pair.*

Certain problems with chromosomes are associated with syndromes. A chromosome may be missing (called a *deletion),* for instance, or doubled (called a *duplication).* A *karyotype* test is a traditional test for these conditions. A *FISH* test allows us to look for the presence of a specific chromosomal issue (as one geneticist explained, it "fishes around" for a particular problem). Finally, a *chromosomal microarray,* probably the most common test, looks at all the chromosomes to find out about extra or missing pieces. All of these tests are performed either in pregnancy, on the cells extracted during *chorionic villus sampling* (CVS) or *amniocentesis,* or after birth, by drawing blood.

A positive test result for a chromosomal syndrome indicates, definitively, that a baby will be born with a syndrome (or has been born with one). It also indicates that the particular syndrome was caused by an identified chromosomal problem. There are so many examples of syndromes and such variety among them that I do not cover them in detail here. But some common syndromes related to CLP include trisomy 13 (which relates to a problem with chromosome number 13), Wolf-Hirschhorn syndrome (related to chromosome 4), and 22q11.2 deletion syndrome (which relates to chromosome 22). These syndromes sometimes include cleft lip and/or palate, usually among other physical differences.

It is important to note that while a negative (or "normal") test result for a chromosomal syndrome tells us that a baby will not be born with a particular chromosomal syndrome (or has not been born with one), it does not necessarily eliminate the possibility of another type of syndrome, since some syndromes are caused by problems with genes (rather than chromosomes).

This brings us to genes. While chromosomes are relatively large in size and small in number, genes are just the opposite: tiny and numerous. There are around twenty thousand genes in the human body. To keep them straight, scientists have labeled genes with letters and numbers, kind of like license plates. The entire genome (or parts of it) can be surveyed through tests called *Next Generation Sequencing (NGS)* or *Whole Exome Sequencing (WES)*. But sometimes geneticists recommend testing individual genes for problems (called *genetic mutations*).

Researchers have discovered connections between problems with certain genes and particular conditions. The SUMO1 gene, for example, has been linked with isolated CLP. The IRF6 gene, to give another example, has been linked with isolated CLP in some individuals and, perhaps confusingly, CLP with features of Van der Woude syndrome in other individuals, depending on the circumstances. Likewise, the P63 gene has been discovered to cause either isolated CLP or CLP in the context of a syndrome. A positive test result for one of those mutations confirms conclusively that a child will be born with (or has been born with) CLP (either isolated or syndromic) and that the condition was caused by that particular gene mutation.

As useful as this information may be for some families who pursue genetic testing, it is still true that many genetic mutations have complex, unknown interactions with one another and with environmental factors. If a family receives a positive test result for a genetic mutation, in a majority of cases, they can conclude a child's CLP was probably caused by genetics—that his or her imaginary die had fewer sides. But within that majority of cases, it is also possible that a person's CLP may have been caused by another genetic factor not tested (or even discovered), by an environmental factor, or by some interaction of any or all of the above.

Events during Pregnancy

CLP can also be caused by environmental factors. The term *environmental* refers to anything that happens during a pregnancy that isn't genetic. You may hear the word *teratogen*, as well, to mean more or less the same thing. When an environmental event occurs, it is usually referred to as an *exposure*. For example, *Cally was exposed to a teratogen during pregnancy*. These terms refer to anything besides genetics that can cause a problem with an embryo.

There are many known environmental factors linked with CLP:

- One of the most common environmental factors is a lack of folic acid. According to one study published in the journal *BMJ*, folic acid supplements taken during early pregnancy "seem to reduce the risk of isolated cleft lip (with or without cleft palate) by about a third." Other vitamins and dietary factors, the study continues, "may provide additional benefit." It is important to note, however, that the benefits of folic acid supplements are somewhat controversial since they have been shown to help in some circumstances but not others.
- Smoking during pregnancy has been linked to CLP, according to a recent study published in the *American Journal of Human Genetics*. Another recent study links exposure to the aerosols in e-cigarettes to midline clefts (a rare, centralized cleft).
- Water contamination has been linked to CLP in a study that examined the nitrates sometimes found in private well water.
- Several studies link cleft lip/palate to exposure to certain molds and fungi.
- Medications for seizures have been linked with CLP.
- A recent study published in the journal *Science Signaling* links CLP with fever during pregnancy.
- Current research links obesity to CLP.

But I Took My Vitamins! Environmental factors can be confusing to interpret because all around us we see examples of pregnant women who smoke, for instance, or don't take prenatal vitamins, but then give birth to a child without CLP. Likewise, I spoke with mothers who described doing all they could to have a healthy pregnancy but still gave birth to a cleft-affected child. "I took folic acid," said one mother. "I did all these different things!" Her situation didn't seem to add up. It felt unfair. "I kept asking, *Why?*" she continued. "*What did I do?*"

The answer may have to do with the size and complexity of the scientific puzzle. As extensive as the above list may appear, it is important to note that, in almost all cases, the research indicates "a link," "an association," or an "increased risk" between any given exposure and CLP—not causality. Smoking, for instance, is linked to all kinds of health problems. But current research does not say that it *causes* CLP. Rather, as one geneticist explained, it can play a role when combined with certain genetic factors.

Let's take three imaginary people, all of them pregnant. And let's suppose that person number one smokes during pregnancy but does not also have genetic factors in the picture that raise the chances of CLP. What happens? Her baby will probably not be born with clefts (that is, due to smoking). But now, let's say that person number two *does* have genetic factors that increase the chances of clefts—but doesn't smoke. What happens? Again, clefts are not likely (due to smoking). A cleft *is* increasingly likely to occur—you guessed it—when a person smokes *and* has genetic factors that increase its likelihood.

It can be confusing when we, as pregnant people, hurry to take vitamins, stop smoking, or lose weight—in other words, do all we can to be healthy—and then realize that the situation is not necessarily linear. While the results of genetic tests can give us definitive information on the causes of CLP and the chances of it occurring again, other times we can't know for sure about the cause(s) due to unknowns about genetics, environmental factors, and their interactions. The situation is complicated. What's more, some of us feel responsible for our child's diagnosis when we presume we have more control over it than we actually do.

Beyond Science

Believe it or not, the plot thickens. When I asked parents of cleft-affected kids to share their thoughts on the question of why this happened, many acknowledged scientific unknowns and mentioned their family history of CLP (or lack of it) and other factors. But just as many added another layer to the conversation: their spiritual and cultural beliefs. "My faith plays a large role in it," commented one mother, Marla, about her search for answers. "I believe that God knew every step of [my son's] life before he formed him in my womb." Not only did Marla find this belief reassuring personally, but she also found it helpful as she explained the condition to her eight-year-old son, who, at the time of our conversation, had started asking questions about his CLP. "[My son] knows that God made him special and different for a reason," Marla continued. While she acknowledged that she doesn't yet know what God's reason may be, the possibilities, to her, seemed laudable. "It might be for friendships that he makes in his life, or to encourage others," she continued. "You don't know."

Another mother looked in a slightly different direction; she wondered if her son's CLP had resulted from an action she had taken—a wrongdoing, a sin—that had evoked retribution from God. She recalled scouring her memory after her son was born. "I kept thinking, kept looking back," she said. "I thought, *Did I make fun of somebody?*" This mother, like Marla, evoked scripture to describe her belief in God's higher plan. "He knew what he was doing," she continued. "This [CLP] was not an accident, not a mistake." Both of these parents—and others—found answers, however varied, in their spiritual beliefs.

Other parents feel different. Shana sought scientific information, and that's it. "I spent ages researching anything and everything," she said. Yet after working with specialists on the cleft team, pursuing genetic tests, and searching the Internet for several weeks after the birth of her daughter, she hit a dead end. "I realized that we don't really know why this happened," she continued. "There isn't really an answer." With time, Shana felt okay with that dead end. So did another parent, Cheryl, who turned to her child's cleft team for answers and support. "The surgeon said, 'This happens,'" Cheryl said. "He put me in touch with other parents who had a similar experience. That helped." Toni, a third parent, threw her hands in the air. "We are not religious," she said. "I put everything in one of two boxes: good shit and bad shit. There is good and bad. Oh, well!" Shana, Cheryl, and Toni, like many of the parents I've spoken with, took the scientific information (or lack of it) at face value, without assigning higher meaning or blame.

The question "Why did this happen?" can be challenging to confront, in part because the scientific evidence for CLP is not only incomplete but puzzling. Whether we look for scientific answers, spiritual answers, or both, we all face the challenge of explaining a surprising event in our child's life. These are profound questions that will follow us through cleft treatment, parenthood more generally, and into the longer journeys of our loving relationships, each time we experience an event and wonder, *Why?*

Chapter 5

. . . .

Early News: Gift or Burden?

Twenty Weeks of Waiting and Wondering

When I asked Abby how it felt to learn the news of her son's CLP at a prenatal ultrasound, she sighed. "It was a blessing and a curse," she said. "It was a curse because it robbed me of my pregnancy—it was all I was thinking about. It was a blessing because I was so prepared." A majority of parents I've spoken with echo some of Abby's feelings. Most felt relieved, they said, to have learned the news in advance rather than in the delivery room. "It helped psychologically, to learn early," added another mother. Yet during the remaining weeks of pregnancy, many parents linger on the health unknowns. And some wrestle with a question so sensitive they may not even mention it out loud: "Will I love my baby this way?" How can expectant parents cope with these questions? And move forward?

Relieved? Worried? Both?

During my years of conducting interviews for this book, few conversations occurred on the topic of learning the news in advance—as opposed to later, at birth—that did not involve some kind of whoop, holler, or cheer. Parents, cleft-team professionals, and researchers seem to agree that prenatal diagnosis offers a few amazing advantages. Not only can some expectant parents find out what is a cleft without having to simultaneously care for a newborn, but they can also use the remaining weeks or months of pregnancy to research a cleft team—an important, sometimes time-consuming task. They can learn a little about feeding the baby, and to some extent, plan for treatment during the first year. What a boon! Some of us have up to twenty weeks to get our ducks in a row before the baby shows up. One mother felt relieved to have made a contingency plan with the hospital staff before the birth of her son. "At delivery, the people in the hospital were ready for him," she said. "We didn't know if he wasn't going to be able to feed. We didn't know if he would have cleft palate. So, the doctors notified the NICU in case there was something more." Logistically, learning in advance can be helpful.

Maybe just as importantly, early news gives us time to work through our feelings. "I went into research mode," one mother said, describing the several cleft teams she learned about before her son's birth. The very act of planning helped her wrap her head around the diagnosis and even regain a sense of control. "Slowly, I started to feel better," she said. Another mother talked through the situation with her husband and other close family members... and talked and talked. "By the time the birth day came," she said, "everybody was back to focusing on the baby as a whole and not this one issue." Whether we concentrate on the clefts, move past them, or both, the extra time can give us a chance to work through our emotions about the news.

Yet, as many times as I heard a parent say, "I was soooooooo glad to learn the news in advance," I heard others—in some cases, even the same parent, minutes later—describe feelings of heightened worry or nervousness as they anticipated their baby's birth. One mother, Kristi, felt relieved, initially, to have found a cleft team she trusted, even describing the prenatal meeting in glowing terms. But as her pregnancy wore on, she continued to wonder about palate involvement and other possible health issues that didn't show up on prenatal tests. "We spent the next nineteen weeks worrying if something else might be wrong with [our son]," she writes on the CCA Kids website, "and why we were given this burden to bear." Kristi's extensive planning didn't fully relieve her uncertainties about unanswered medical questions or ease the pain of the news itself.

For Kristi—and others—the early news felt like a mixed bag. And why wouldn't it? Prenatal tests offer an astonishing glimpse into a baby's health. But the idiosyncrasies of these tests can also alert us—or perhaps remind us—of larger, existential uncertainties, not only with health but with parenthood and even the human condition. One parent, Cassandra, realized that it was not her child's cleft that upset her the most. "It was the realization," she writes in the *Cleft Palate-Craniofacial Journal*, "that if the existence of the cleft could not be predicted accurately, then what else could be unknown? I had lost touch with the…wonder that pregnancy evokes." On some level, all expectant parents know that unfortunate things can happen—and probably will happen—to any child. It's just that some of us feel knocked off course when we get a dose of that reality before the child even arrives.

Maybe above all, parents mention fears about bonding, a concern that is difficult to overcome through research and homework. "I kept wondering how I was going to feel when I met my daughter," said one mother. "I was sure I wasn't going to have a bond with her. I would cry every time I thought about it." Another mother described one of her biggest fears during pregnancy as: "How am I going to feel when I see my baby?"

As haunting as these feelings can be—and as difficult as it may be to even articulate them to others—it is also important to acknowledge that they are normal. Some of us were not born with CLP ourselves or never had a close relationship with a person with a facial difference. "If you don't know about clefts at all," commented one dad, "it can really be a shock to you. I had a cleft myself and it was still a shock to see my son come out." It is okay to wonder about our capacity to love a baby who is different from ourselves, different from others, or even just different from what we were expecting.

So, Now What?

Many parents say, in retrospect, that if they had it to do again, they wouldn't have worried so much about meeting their baby. "We all fell in love with him," said one mother about the moments after her son was born. One cleft-team nurse described the glowing faces of the families who arrive in her office. "The parents we see love their baby, regardless," she said. There is even a book for cleft families entitled, *I Wish I'd Known…How Much I'd Love You*. A majority of new parents describe enormous relief when, after months of waiting and wondering, they lay eyes on their baby and love her as is.

Yet as often as this reaction occurs, the feeling of immediate, loving acceptance is not universal. As difficult as it may be to acknowledge, some parents do not describe love at first sight when they meet their baby or even at second sight. As we'll explore later in this book, bonding can be complicated. Some parents bond with their baby immediately, but others don't—cleft or no cleft (even if they do bond later on). There is no fault in that feeling—and no less love, necessarily, over the long term. It's just that we may not hear from the latter group very often because the subject is so personal, and in some cases, not fully understood or accepted socially. As we'll discuss in greater depth in Chapter 11, those who don't bond immediately don't always want to talk about it.

Step by Step

For those who wonder as they wait, there are a few ways to cope in the meantime. One nurse on a cleft team pointed out that as expectant parents grapple with questions of bonding, they are actually mourning a loss. "I see anxiety in parents as they anticipate their baby's appearance," she said. "Because it is an unknown. Because it is considered a birth defect. Because people are alarmed by it and worried about reactions. That is a very difficult milestone to overcome." The way forward, she continued, starts very personally, on the inside. "It is grieving," she said, "and it is a loss of the perfect Gerber baby that everybody hopes is growing inside them." Maybe the first thing to do, then, is to let yourself grieve and to know that that process is normal and okay.

Other small steps can help too. One parent, Jen, felt better when she told people the news about the prenatal diagnosis. By the time her daughter was born, she had already told everyone in her family and everyone on Facebook. "Once they felt comfortable with it," she said, "it made me feel better." Jen even made a point to talk about clefts at her baby shower. "It helped *me* cope," she said. "I started to think that it would be okay, that [my baby] would be beautiful." Another parent, Leticia, made a deliberate decision to set aside her planning before her son was born. "At first, our thoughts about the clefts took over everything," she said. "It was all we were thinking about. We didn't want that to happen when he came into the world. We didn't want to be thinking only about what he looked like." As much as the act of planning eased her mind, initially, Leticia realized that her undivided attention on CLP was causing her to forget the big picture—that is, the myriad aspects of parenting *not* related to CLP.

Perhaps most important is to step back and reflect on your own style of coping. What method has helped you deal with other difficult events in the past? Some people cope through planning or otherwise keeping busy, while others turn to faith, journaling, therapy, or nature. Whether it's sharing the news with others or planning and then *stopping*, as Leticia did, the best route is deliberate and always your own.

Prenatal diagnosis is amazing—almost superhuman. Before my daughter was born, I wondered if the news of the cleft diagnosis might have been a mistake. Had something gone wrong with the crystal ball that day? (There had been no mistake.) Yet, while the test gives us a sneak peak at a diagnosis, the view is clinical and incomplete. That shiny, smudgy ultrasound printout doesn't show the most important part of the picture: a real, whole person.

Some parents love their child despite the clefts, others' clefts and all. Either way, it might help to remember—as you plan and, perhaps, grieve and wait for the baby to arrive—that she will have many more characteristics than a mouth and nose. She will cry. She will burp. Sixteen years from now, she may accidentally drive the car through the garage door. Or love animals or rock-climbing. She will have a personality all her own. These are the delightful, sometimes irritating, fully human characteristics that don't show up on a printout. They go way beyond cleft lip and palate. And they are probably your reasons for wanting to have a child in the first place.

Chapter 6

. . . .

Early News: What's Next?

Preparing for Delivery and the Baby's First Year

When Sarah learned about her daughter's cleft lip and palate at a prenatal ultrasound, she made a swift decision to rethink the rest of her pregnancy. "I stopped reading baby development books and threw myself into researching clefts," she said. Sarah felt reassured to spend the weeks before her daughter's birth learning about the condition and making some treatment decisions. As shocked as she and her husband felt by the news initially, the process of learning and preparing actually helped her cope.

But what did Sarah actually *do* for those twenty weeks? Many expectant parents wonder how to prepare for birth and the early days of infancy. Below are seven tips for a smooth delivery and beyond. Truth to tell, the only essential task is the first on the list—to connect with a care team to treat your child. But the others may make life more comfortable. If there's a sudden hush among doctors and staff in the delivery room, you'll be prepared for it (see Tip 4). If you're wondering how to arrange work schedules and child care to accommodate the busy first year of treatment, check out the table, "How Much Time for Cleft Care?" (Tip 5 and Appendix). Learning the news of CLP prenatally can be stressful for parents, as we've already discussed. The upside—as we'll see again later on through Sarah's story—is a long stretch of time to prepare for the baby's arrival, both logistically and emotionally.

. . . .

TIP No. 1: Connect with a Team. If you have learned about your baby's clefts prenatally, the best thing you can do during the remaining weeks of pregnancy is to sign on with a cleft palate or craniofacial team. The cleft team is the basic, critical element of a child's cleft care—not to mention a primary source of information and support—during the important first year of treatment and, for many cleft-affected children, through childhood, and into young adulthood. While a child will still need to see a regular pediatrician, the cleft team will serve as a hub for all things cleft-related.

Why not connect with a team later on, after birth? On one hand, there's no rush to complete this task, provided you call a team within the first few days after the baby is born. In fact, this scenario happens all the time for families who learn about their baby's CLP (or other craniofacial condition) at birth. And if those families—or you—are fortunate enough to live near a large city, the chances are high that you'll find a team you feel comfortable with regardless of the timing.

On the other hand, not everyone lives near a team. Research published in the *Cleft Palate-Craniofacial Journal* shows that over 25 percent of children in the US do not live within a one-hour drive of an ACPA-approved team. And cleft teams vary. So, it is important, for the sake of your child's health, to find a team that feels right for your family, a group you really trust. Choosing a cleft team is like choosing a place to live. It's a long-term investment with high stakes. It is possible, with luck, to make a successful decision quickly, but a longer, more careful route can feel reassuring.

There are other benefits to starting early. Many cleft teams meet with families prenatally to introduce themselves and lay out a tentative plan for treatment, which in most cases begins shortly after birth. See Chapters 7 and 8 to get started on your search.

. . . .

TIP No. 2: Buy a Special Bottle and Learn—a Little—about Feeding. If a baby is born with an isolated cleft lip (cleft lip with no cleft palate), she may be able to nurse or bottle-feed normally or near normally. A baby with a cleft palate, however (with or without a cleft lip), will likely require the use of a special-needs bottle and some extra attention to feeding during her first year. And in a vast majority of cases, a baby with a cleft palate cannot form enough suction to breast-feed. The news about breast-feeding can be very difficult for some parents, especially mothers, to process (see Chapter 15 for more on this topic). However you cope, you can also take small steps to prepare for the special challenges of bottle-feeding.

<u>**Consult with the Team before Birth**</u>. When it comes to learning to feed a baby with cleft palate, an important first teacher is actually the baby herself, who will give physical cues to show what she needs and when she's done. But some parents describe the feeding specialist on the cleft team—who often serves as a point person for families regarding feeding the baby—as a wellspring of information, a wiz on all things feeding, basically, their guru. Titles and credentials vary among these specialists; the feeding expert might be a nurse, an advanced-practice nurse, such as a nurse practitioner or a clinical nurse specialist, or a speech-language pathologist (I use these titles interchangeably in this book to refer to the same person).

In any case, many of these specialists offer feeding instruction prenatally to give parents a rundown on various special bottles. "When I meet with a family for the first time," explained one such cleft-team pro, "my goal is for them to walk out with some kind of confidence on where to begin with feeding the baby." Not only does the prenatal consultation give you a chance to wrap your head around the idea of bottle-feeding, but it also gives you some hands-on experience (even without the baby in hand). And hopefully, it will reassure you that the cleft team is there to offer help and support.

<u>**Learn in the Hospital (if Possible) after Birth**</u>. It is important to note that many birthing hospitals have feeding specialists on staff to help parents learn how to feed their newborns, including newborns with special feeding needs (like cleft palate), directly after birth. Some cleft parents describe their experiences with these professionals in glowing terms; they recall helpful, hands-on interactions during the very early days with their baby. Other parents, unfortunately, do not have such positive memories. "The person at the hospital gave us a regular baby bottle and told us to just keep trying!" said one mother about her two-day stay in the hospital after her son's birth. It may be helpful, therefore, to prepare for a range of experiences—and to keep the phone number of the cleft team in your back pocket should questions arise immediately after birth (many teams advise calling them directly after birth anyway, as indicated in Chapter 9).

Chapters 12–16 offer more information on feeding a baby with CLP. Remember, though, that preparing for feeding a cleft-affected baby (or any baby) only goes so far without a real, live newborn. While it might be helpful to set the table before a dinner party, the party can't start until the guests arrive—or in this case, a crying, cooing, hungry guest of honor.

. . . .

TIP No. 3: Contact Your Birthing Hospital (if Applicable) and Learn about Resources. Cleft-team professionals sometimes advise expectant parents to contact their birthing hospital in advance of the birth to make sure the staff is aware that the baby will be born with CLP. Situations vary widely, however, in terms of the ways communications take place among practitioners and institutions across the US. One nurse on a cleft team explained that she routinely sends a medical record (also called a *note*) to the birthing hospital, the mother's ob-gyn, and the baby's future pediatrician. But others follow different protocols (*protocols* are detailed medical plans). In any case, it is always a good idea—as recommended by another cleft-team nurse specialist who commented on this topic—to mention the diagnosis upon checking in at the hospital at delivery time and to confirm that the information is in your medical record.

A prenatal orientation session at your birthing hospital can also be helpful, especially for your own peace of mind. Even though many obstetricians advise expectant mothers to anticipate a normal delivery for a baby born with CLP (ask your OB for advice, of course), you can probably expect to use some special hospital resources following birth, such as a feeding specialist and a lactation consultant if you're interested in nursing or pumping milk (as applicable). An orientation session can help you learn about these resources and give you the lay of the land.

Members of the cleft team can also fill in some other blanks about the birth experience. If you meet with members of the team prenatally, don't forget to ask them for information on your birthing hospital. Team members, especially nurses, often know insiders' tips that you won't learn on a hospital tour.

> ## QUESTIONS FOR THE BIRTHING HOSPITAL ABOUT PREPARING FOR BIRTH

- My baby will be born with cleft lip and/or palate. What do I need to do in advance of the birth to make sure this information is in my medical record and to make sure the staff is aware of the diagnosis?
- When and where in the hospital will I be able to find a feeding specialist and special bottles after birth? Do you recommend any particular feeding specialists who have expertise with babies born with cleft palate? How can I get in touch with this person/ people after birth?
- Where can I find a lactation consultant and a hospital-grade breast pump (if applicable)? Can I set up the rental in advance?
- Do you have any additional tips about preparing for birth, given my baby's prenatal diagnosis?

> ### QUESTIONS FOR THE CLEFT TEAM
> ### ABOUT PREPARING FOR BIRTH

- How do you recommend I coordinate medical records among practitioners? Would you be willing to send the medical record of this prenatal consultation, (sometimes referred to as a *note*) to my ob-gyn and the baby's future pediatrician (as applicable)?
- How can I get in touch with the cleft team following birth? On weekends/after business hours? When and under what circumstances should I contact you? Can I expect that the hospital staff will contact you following birth, or is that my job?
- Under what circumstances will a baby with CLP need the services of the NICU? What are some ways to make sure the hospital treats the baby appropriately? (See Chapter 10 for more information on this topic.)
- Do you have any recommendations regarding feeding the baby in the hospital? Do you recommend working with any particular feeding specialist there?
- Do you have any additional tips about preparing for birth and/or for giving birth at Hospital X?

. . . .

TIP No. 4: Anticipate a Crowd. When I asked one cleft-team nurse for tips on the birth experience with a cleft-affected baby, she described a common scenario in the hospital: a delivery room that suddenly fills with people. "Any delivery is dramatic enough," she said. But when the baby actually arrives and the staff members find out about a special issue like CLP, they often direct their attention to that case. "Parents should know that there will be other medical people in the room," she continued. "There might be *a lot* of other people in the room." Even if you've informed the hospital about the baby's clefts in advance, medical people may come running.

A few parents describe another common occurrence: a sudden hush among doctors and staff. "On the one hand, everyone [in the delivery room] was saying, 'This is no big deal,'" said one mother about the quiet-intense moments directly after her son's birth. "But they were certainly not acting like it was no big deal." Another parent described a general downshift in mood. "They stopped talking to me," she said in a video made by the Foundation for the Faces of Children. "They stopped being so positive. All of a sudden, there was this veil that dropped." It is possible, of course, that as soon as the baby is born, professionals will discover health issues beyond CLP. But it is also possible that they are concentrating on the clefts. Since cleft lip and palate occurs one time in six hundred births, obstetricians and other medical people may only come across CLP a few times throughout their careers.

New parents can expect to see a lot of activity later on in the recovery room, as well. Nursing staff may make periodic, recovery-related visits as they would for any birth. Add to that a cleft-related visit from a pediatrician, a feeding specialist, a lactation consultant, and perhaps a member of the cleft team, and the recovery room may start to feel like Grand Central Station. What's the best way to manage visitors amidst the hustle and bustle? Some parents welcome friends and family to the mix. Others prefer to concentrate on the baby, for now. Either way, this may be a decision to consider in advance (see the end of Chapter 9 for more specific ideas).

· ·

TIP No. 5: Take a Good Look at Your Calendar. Learning the news about CLP prenatally gives expectant parents some time—in some cases up to twenty weeks—to plan for the busy first year of treatment. But what are the details of the first year? How much time will CLP require from a caregiver on any given day or night? For how long following birth? How can expectant parents plan for work, child care, and sibling care?

It is difficult to predict how much time and energy to allocate for the care of a cleft-affected baby as compared to an unaffected baby. No two babies are alike, clefts or no clefts, and no two parents make the same decisions in any one situation (just ask my husband). The additional requirements of cleft care depend on many variables as well, including the child's diagnosis, her response to treatment, her ability to feed, the distance/location of the team, the recommended treatment itself, family finances, and more.

It is safe to say, however, that if a child is born with a cleft palate, a caregiver can expect to commit extra time and energy to feeding the baby, bringing her to appointments with the team, and ushering her through surgery and recovery. Child care, too, may be trickier to navigate than it would otherwise be. Some infant-care centers cannot accommodate a baby with special feeding needs or special orthodontics. Even some grandparents find the duties challenging. "My mother tried to help," said one dad about the early days with his son. But at the time, his mother was recovering from wrist surgery; she couldn't quite get the knack of the Haberman bottle. "She will tell you nightmares about not being able to feed him," he continued. "It was an ordeal." The key is *not* to give up on finding logistical support because of these challenges but to know that finding help may involve some legwork, some creativity, and possibly some patience.

The tables, *How Much Time For Cleft Care?* found in the appendix, show what to expect during the baby's first year. Some of the factors listed, such as weekly appointments with the orthodontist on the team, are easy to quantify. Others are harder to predict. Feeding, for instance, can take a lot of time upfront—and a lot of trial and error with special bottles—but should become easier with time.

· ·

TIP No. 6: Share the News, Especially with Your Other Children. One of the perks of learning about a child's cleft lip/palate in advance of the birth is having the time and flexibility to tell others. Sharing the news not only helps you process it yourself (as explored in Chapter 5) but allows you to prepare family members for what is to come.

Siblings in the household may need specific preparation. A new family member will upend any family's routine, cleft or no cleft, as schedules change and parents devote time and attention to the new baby. But the intensity of cleft treatment may place additional stress on a sibling, especially at surgery times. According to the child advocacy group Bright Horizons, young kids fare best with these changes and events when we prepare them in advance. "Children need time to process all of the information that they are exposed to," these experts say. They also emphasize the importance of maintaining routines—with as much daily repetition as possible—to keep kids' stress at bay.

A first step, according to this group, is to tell an older child what is happening and what is to come, almost as if you are narrating a story. You might say to a preschool-age child, "Baby Dylan will be born with a space in his lip called a cleft. He will need to use a special bottle. Do you want to see it?" One mother, Adele, tried to be as truthful as possible with her older son (who was not born with CLP) when she shared information about his younger sister's condition. "It is important to be honest with [a sibling] about what is going on and how you are feeling about it," she said. "The worst thing you can do is pretend that everything is fine when they know perfectly well that everything is not fine. They sense everything."

The pros also suggest telling a child what will happen, materially, in her life, such as which routines will change and, notably, which will *not* change. When the baby is born, for example, will the older sibling spend more time with a grandparent or another person? When, specifically? And where? Knowing the details in advance can help a preschool-age child feel comfortable with a change that, from her perspective, will require a relatively big emotional adjustment.

The next step, according to the experts, is to spend some extra time with an older sibling, one-on-one, especially in the context of play. "During times of change, a little extra attention will go a long way in helping children deal with stress," Bright Horizons advises. The group advises parents to set aside an hour or half-hour each week when an older child has your undivided attention.

As lip-repair surgery approaches, a sibling might appreciate the same kind of advanced preparation. You might say, "On Wednesday, your father and I will take baby Dylan to the hospital so the doctors can close the space in his lip. He will need to stay in the hospital for a few days. You will stay at home with Grandma, and sleep in your own bed, just as usual. She will be here when you wake up and she will give you breakfast, just the way we do. When we come home again with Dylan, his face will look different. Will you help us make a card for him?" The tips excerpted below, from Bright Horizons Family Solutions, are designed to help a child make a smooth transition through any big life change. Cleft-related comments are placed in brackets.

HELPING CHILDREN COPE WITH CHANGE

Give Advanced Warning. Have a discussion, something like, ["Baby Dylan will be born with a space in his lip called a cleft. He will need to use a special bottle. Do you want to see it?"]

Keep as Much the Same as Possible. During a big change, like adding a sibling to the family [or a sibling's surgery], try to keep as much the same as possible. For example, this may not be the best time to also move your child from a crib to a big bed.

Answer all Their Questions. Depending on your child's age, he may have a lot of questions. Do your best to answer them all, even if some are repeated many times. [Pre-school age kids often wonder if a new baby's cleft lip is painful. You can say, "Baby Dylan has a space in his lip. It doesn't hurt! The doctors will close the space when he is older."]

Expect That Some Regression May Happen. At times of change, children may regress to earlier behaviors. For example, a child who was toilet trained may revert back to having accidents. This is normal—strive for patience.

Be Accepting of Grieving. Your child may go through a process that looks a lot like grieving as she navigates new waters with a new sibling. Listen, don't be too quick to distract, and at the end, remind her of all the positives.

Excerpted with Permission from
Bright Horizons Family Solutions

Advanced planning can help ensure the emotional stability of everyone in the family. And these habits will come in handy later in the baby's first year, especially before operations when siblings will not only see their routines change, yet again, but will notice—and react to—the physical changes in their younger sibling's face.

. . . .

TIP No. 7: Sit Tight. Our friend Sarah, as it turns out, did indeed throw herself into clefts during the lead-up to her daughter's birth. She and her husband met with an independent surgeon in their town and then met with an ACPA-approved cleft team located about three hours away, in a large city. They considered their options carefully, ultimately deciding to choose the approved team, despite the distance. They also made contingency plans for child care and both of their jobs. And they had a prenatal consultation with the feeding person on the team. Sarah described the period as a whirlwind of cleft-related activity.

But then, Sarah stopped planning. "It took me a month or more of constant research to say *okay*," she said. "I said, *I am pregnant, I still need to enjoy it.*" For her own emotional well-being, Sarah decided to stop focusing on her daughter's CLP and try her best to enjoy the rest of her pregnancy.

Learning the news of CLP via prenatal testing gives the gift of time to cope with the news, learn about treatment, and plan for birth and beyond.

You can't start the dinner party, however, until the guest of honor arrives. So, however you decide to use your time beforehand—whether you do a lot of research in one burst the way Sarah did or spend your energy in other ways—hopefully, you can find reassurance in the process of setting the table.

Team Care

Chapter 7

. . . .

Team Care

The What and the Why

As parents, when we find out that our baby (or baby on the way) has a cleft lip and/or palate, one of the first things we learn is that we need to contact a local cleft team. But what is a cleft team in the first place? And how important is it for our child's well-being? What if there is no team nearby? Research shows that more than 25 percent of children in the US do not live within a one-hour distance from an approved team. What now?

This chapter covers some ABCs of the cleft team, then offers ideas to consider on why this type of care can be valuable or even critical for a child. If you are in the early stages of looking for someone to treat your baby, you may learn about an independent professional in your area—a local plastic surgeon, for example, who repairs clefts but does not practice with a team. It is common for new and expectant parents, especially those who do not live near a team, to attend an introductory meeting with such a professional during their early research for a provider. While in some cases, an independent surgeon *may* be able to operate with the expertise that you want and need for your baby, it is important to know about the stakes involved; we'll discuss those ideas here. So whether you consult with an independent surgeon, an approved cleft team, or even more than one cleft team—or any combination of the above— you will have enough information to ask informed questions. The goal? To feel comfortable and secure in your decision.

Team Basics

What is a Team? A *cleft team* is a group of medical specialists who care for a child born with cleft lip and/or palate from birth through around age eighteen and, in some cases, into adulthood. The group includes all the specialists you could possibly want or need to treat CLP, working together. Just as the functions of the mouth, nose, ears, and head are interrelated, so are these people who treat them.

Stamp of Approval. Any group of medical professionals can get together and treat CLP and even call themselves a "team." But to be *approved* by the American Cleft Palate-Craniofacial Association (ACPA), the team has participated in a rigorous review process, met certain standards, and earned the ACPA's stamp of approval. The ACPA is a national and international organization that is generally considered the mother ship of cleft support in the US. The group publishes an academic journal, supports cleft specialists, educates patients and families, and sets the standards for team approval. ACPA approval indicates that a team can provide the services necessary for a person born with CLP.

Approved teams are listed in the state-by-state team listings on the ACPA website—at www.ACPAcares.org. If you are interested in reading the standards themselves, which include such criteria as the makeup of a team, the responsibilities of its members, the ways team members communicate with families, and more, they are available at the ACPA website—at www.ACPAcares.org. They are surprisingly user-friendly.

Members of the Team. There are two types of cleft teams: *cleft-palate* teams and *craniofacial* teams. Let's start with the cleft palate team. Every ACPA-approved cleft-palate team must include, at minimum, the following specialists:

- a surgeon
- a speech-language pathologist
- an orthodontist
- a patient care coordinator

Beyond that, this type of team sometimes includes, or refers patients to:

- an ear, nose, and throat surgeon (an ENT)
- a pediatric dentist
- a geneticist
- a psychiatrist
- a psychologist
- a social worker
- an audiologist
- a pediatrician

Cleft versus Craniofacial. What's the difference between a cleft-palate team and a craniofacial team? From the perspective of cleft lip and palate, not much. Both types of teams treat CLP with the highest level of expertise. A cleft-palate team, described above, treats cleft lip and palate, while a craniofacial team treats CLP as well as other conditions of the face and head. If your child was born with a craniofacial condition beyond CLP, of course, the distinction between these two teams might come into play. (As mentioned previously, I use the term *cleft team* throughout this book to refer to either type of team.)

A craniofacial team includes the members listed above, plus the following additions (and/or adjustments):

- A craniofacial team must include a surgeon who has received special training in *transcranial cranio-maxillofacial surgery,* which qualifies them to treat craniofacial conditions beyond CLP.

- The psychologist on the craniofacial team must be qualified to perform certain types of patient assessments.
- The team must have access to other specialists, including a neurosurgeon, an ophthalmologist, a radiologist, and a geneticist.

All at Once? When I first saw a list of the members of a cleft team, I imagined a group of people crowded into an exam room, peering into the mouth of our tiny baby, like a football huddle of white-coated doctors. In reality, a child and family usually visit with the members of the team who are involved in the current stage of treatment—not necessarily everyone at once. And there is no huddle! (At least not at that moment; see more on huddling, below).

These days, cleft teams usually recommend that patients and families meet with members of the team once a year for a long, single visit called a "clinic day." Some teams arrange the consultations sequentially, in separate exam rooms, and others in the same room with several people present at once; the logistics vary. (Chapter 20 describes what the clinic day looks like and how you might prepare for it.)

Approved but Varied. A quick look at team websites will show that some teams have one surgeon on the roster, while others have several. Some teams are made up of many specialists, while others list the core group and only a few others. If you are able to meet with more than one team in person, you'll find that the treatment they describe, such as types of cleft-related surgeries and their timing, will also vary slightly from team to team, depending on a surgeon's training and school of thought (and depending on a child's diagnosis, of course, as well as other factors). Some teams use an orthodontic device during infancy, while others use lip taping or no device. So, even approved teams vary. In Chapter 8, we will explore ways to navigate these differences.

Why a Team?

At this point, it is probably clear that cleft teams have a lot to offer. But you may still be wondering *how much* these teams provide when independent surgeons are practicing all across the US and, in some cases, much closer to home. The parents and professionals who I have spoken with have mentioned the genuine rewards of team care—and unfortunately, some warnings to consider regarding the non-team option.

Many Moving Parts. Cleft lip and palate is a condition that benefits from coordinated care because the functions of the face and head—such as hearing, speaking, eating, breathing, dental health, and mental health—are complex and interconnected. Let's look at one example of how team members might work together (though there are many more) and why those interactions matter.

Let's say a child is having trouble hearing, a common problem related to cleft palate, especially during infancy (note that the problem is usually temporary, solvable, and easy to catch early on if you stay on top of routine appointments). The audiologist or ear, nose, and throat surgeon (ENT) on the team may recommend inserting ear tubes—a short, common surgical procedure. At that point, let's say that the child is scheduled to have another operation—such as palate-repair surgery, which will be performed by the plastic surgeon on the team. The two professionals may work together to determine whether the ear tubes and the palate repair could be performed during the same surgical session. When these procedures are coordinated, a child is exposed to one round of anesthesia rather than two—an important safety measure—because while anesthesia is a necessary component of treatment, it carries risk. And let's not forget that the feeding expert will be part of the picture at this time as well, and perhaps a social worker and/or psychologist. By working together, the specialists ensure that many needs are being met.

At its best, team care involves communication and coordination among professionals to ensure that treatment is as effective as possible while minimizing surgical interventions and risk. This way parents aren't scrambling—and spending a lot more time and money than we otherwise would—to try to coordinate a child's treatment among an array of unconnected providers (a surgeon here, an audiologist there). "The members of the team keep you in contact with the speech pathologist, the social worker, the surgeon…" explained one dad about his experience with his daughter's team. "It makes a world of difference in terms of a parent's comfort level. I can't emphasize that enough."

Dialogue behind the Scenes. While the members of the cleft team will probably not huddle over your baby like football players in an exam room, they do come together at another time to discuss each case and make a plan. Team meetings are one of the essential elements of team care—yet families rarely witness them or probably even know they occur. During my research for this book, I was fortunate to be invited to attend a monthly meeting of a large cleft team. Fifteen or so professionals sat around a conference table reviewing each case one by one. As they discussed options for treatment, the team members questioned one another, challenged each other's reasoning, and parsed details. These people went into the weeds—in the most congenial of ways—to come up with the best possible treatment solution for each child. Their tone was unscripted and direct.

While every team operates differently in terms of internal and external communications, this meeting of the minds is an example of the kind of rigorous, thoughtful debate that is only possible with a team. By discussing cases across disciplines, professionals treat the whole patient—meaning they address a collection of issues taken together rather than single issues in isolation. And by challenging each other's recommendations (such as in the case of the team I visited), team members ensure that each patient receives the smartest, most appropriate solutions. So, not only do members of a cleft team coordinate different aspects of a child's treatment (as mentioned above), but they also do their best to ensure a child receives the highest quality care possible.

High Stakes. Another angle to consider is the potential cost of receiving improper care. "If there is one thing to say about cleft care," commented one clinical nurse specialist, "it is that all kids should get their care from a team and go to people who regularly do this as part of their practice. Not to a plastic surgeon who says, 'Oh sure, I can do that.' There is too much at stake in the long run." Now, is it *possible* that an independent surgeon possesses the necessary expertise and experience to achieve good results? Yes, it is possible, but the chances may be low—and as the nurse mentioned, the stakes are high. At stake is the quality of surgical outcomes early on, but also a child's overall health and well-being over the long term.

Megan and Mark, parents of Liam, described two negative surgical experiences with two different independent surgeons before finding Liam's current cleft team. At each turn, they thought they were making the best possible choice for their son. Unfortunately, the physical, emotional, and monetary expenses were substantial.

FAMILY STORIES
Megan, Mark, and Liam

Three Tries

When Megan learned the news of her son Liam's CLP at his birth, she had never really heard of the condition, other than through ads for cleft-related charities she had seen on TV. "I thought it was cosmetic," she said about her early awareness. Unfortunately, the staff at her small birthing hospital did not dispel that myth. "They told me that he had a little cleft lip and palate and that it could be fixed right up," Megan said about the early comments she heard after Liam's birth. "I had no idea what that meant." As it turned out, she continued, but neither did they.

Megan and her husband, Mark, lived in a rural area, at about a quarter-mile distance from their nearest neighbor. So, the couple was not surprised to learn that the closest plastic surgeon was located a few hours from their home in a medium-sized city. At the time, they thought this independent surgeon seemed well-suited to repair Liam's CLP. While Liam had been born with an extensive cleft palate, his cleft lip appeared relatively minor; it existed on one side and did not extend all the way to his nose. The surgeon seemed friendly and confident, Megan recalled. After speaking with another parent who recommended him, the family signed on.

Unfortunately, Liam's first operation did not go well at all. "The lip repair at age three months was a disaster," Megan said. "The surgeon was horrible." Megan described finding Liam in the recovery room after the procedure and noticing a small notch at the bottom of his upper lip at the site of the cleft. Above the notch, Megan explained, the surgeon seemed to have cut a straight line downward from the nose, without following the contour of the face. His lip looked bumpy, unnatural, and not fully closed.

Megan and Mark were beside themselves. Mark said he thought their son's face looked worse after the operation than it did beforehand. But the couple also felt overwhelmed at the time and naturally, somewhat disoriented. "Everyone told us that the surgery turned out okay," Mark said. "We thought, 'It looks terrible.' But who are we to judge? We are not doctors."

The couple immediately searched for better care for Liam in time for his palate-repair operation. This time, they drove even further from their home to another medium-sized city with a large teaching hospital. "This surgery was even worse," Megan said. "The surgeon was not in pediatric plastics like I thought he was." This surgeon used cadaver bone to repair the cleft palate—a method, as she recalled learning later, that is not the norm among cleft specialists. Eight or nine days after the operation, Liam's repair actually fell apart, leaving not one hole in the roof of his mouth, as before, but two holes (called *fistulae*). To make matters worse, Liam contracted an infection in the hospital that lasted for four months. And as he recovered from the operation and grew into an active toddler with a healthy appetite, the act of eating with two holes in his palate became even more challenging than before. The family ended up spending $500 on an obturator, a dental appliance that blocked the fistulae while he ate.

At wits' end, Megan and Mark engaged in a blizzard of cleft research. They searched online. They read blogs. They spoke with as many cleft families as they could—not just one or two as they had before. "We didn't have a clue until much later," Mark admitted. The couple started to realize that they would likely need to travel a sizeable distance to obtain the care they needed, not only to treat their son's CLP moving forward but to address the problems that had already been created. Thanks to some recommendations from cleft parents they met online, Megan and Mark interviewed members of three cleft teams, mostly communicating by phone. They then decided to travel halfway across the country to visit the third team in person (during a pre-Zoom era). "We were blown away at the difference," Mark said. "The third group was a *team*. The surgeon was a *pediatric* plastic surgeon who had experience with CLP. The whole place—the hospital—was geared toward children." The surgeon on this faraway team eventually refashioned Liam's palate and later his lip and nose, completing those operations by the time he turned three.

Liam is now ten years old and still receiving care from the distant team. As Megan reflected on his early treatment, she mentioned the critical element of the surgeon's qualifications. "I am horrified," she said, "that I ever took my child to a plastic surgeon who does boob jobs one day and cleft repairs the next. I should only have considered surgeons with plenty of experience with cleft lip and palate." She estimated that their family has traveled across the country seven times so far, including a combination of short trips for annual visits and longer stays when Liam has needed surgery. The out-of-pocket costs have been enormous—but the couple is extremely pleased. "Now, I say, money is not important," she said. "The only important thing is quality care for your child. So, what if my car is fifteen years old? So, what if we don't have any days left over for vacation? Our child deserves to have the best care available." In the end, Megan and Mark felt fortunate to have found such excellent care, despite their early trials. "Our son has always been a happy child," Mark said, "and a beautiful child."

Megan and Mark's story is dramatic, even frightening, compared to the early success stories described by other families in other situations. And it raises issues related to costs that can feel daunting to families who do not have the funds or ability to travel for care (find information on this topic in the next chapter). But as Megan and Mark told me later in the conversation, they felt strongly about sharing their experience because they wanted others to know the importance of finding high-quality team care for a child.

Bottom Line: A Match. Given the high stakes involved in cleft treatment, it is important to do some homework before signing on with any provider. But how will you know when you've found a match?

There are several concrete factors to look for; the next chapter includes a detailed list of criteria to consider and questions to ask. But in the end, the cleft parents I spoke with who had positive relationships with their teams tended to circle back to ideas of trust and comfort—not because team members offered flat reassurances, but because they answered questions, large and small, and because they acted as teachers, sounding boards, and partners. One mother, Adele, described the parent-team relationship as the lynchpin of the entire cleft journey. "Your relationship with these people is crucial," she said. "Ultimately, how comfortable your child becomes with them will be a direct outcome of your belief in them and your relationship with them as parents." When parents feel trusting and at ease, a child will notice. And this confidence will not only console her as she prepares for an upcoming operation but perhaps shape her perception of the whole experience—and even her sense of identity.

Postscript: A Parent's Role. As parents, we have the right to be choosy, do homework, and ask questions. In fact, it is *our job.* Adele, the mother who offered advice above, faced troubles similar to Megan and Mark's, switching to a team in a neighboring state during her child's first year when procedures didn't go as planned. In retrospect, she wished she had done more legwork upfront. "To do it over again," she said, "I would have found two or three teams to interview. In the beginning, we just wanted to know what was going to happen, so we didn't take this valuable time. But now, I would say that that is time well spent." It may feel awkward to ask direct questions to a health professional who has spent half her life (or more) attending fancy schools. But when a child's health is on the line, someone's got to do it. And a confident, competent professional should welcome parents' questions.

As important as it is to ask questions and advocate for a child while looking for a team, parents have another crucial role to play later on: as a teammate. Parents may not be members of the cleft team, literally. But no doctor can help a child if a parent doesn't bring her to appointments. Speech therapy only goes so far if a child doesn't practice the exercises at home. A dentist can't come to the house twice a day to brush a child's teeth. Keeping a child healthy is yeoman's work for professionals and parents alike. And as many parents have noticed, the family-team relationships that reflect a spirit of mutual dedication and collaboration—indeed, a spirit of true teamwork—are the ones that feel the most comfortable, trusting, and fruitful for all involved.

Chapter 8

. . . .

Considering a Cleft Team?

Criteria and Questions

Anna knew that deciding on a cleft team for her son would require some research. She didn't predict that the process would feel a little unnerving. "You are making decisions for this person you love more than anything," she said as she anticipated the birth of her son. "And you know that because of the circumstances of his birth, he is going to have challenges." Not only was there a lot at stake, she observed, but her search felt complicated. While Anna was fortunate to have more than one approved cleft team to choose from in her large city, she noticed differences between the ones she visited. Other parents mention similar quandaries. How can this research—and the related decision-making—be made easier?

The cleft professionals I have spoken with have admitted that the topic can be challenging. They say that even ACPA-approved teams vary in terms of size, experience, treatment protocols, and more. But fortunately, these factors can be explored and explained. And many families have found that, with some legwork and perseverance, the process of choosing a team was not only fruitful but reassuring.

Below is a list of factors to consider in your search. Along with each description, you'll find a set of related questions to ask in person, find out online, or just keep in mind. This process is personal. The goal is not for you to go out and get answers to all of these questions. I offer them as a resource, so you can inquire about the factors that resonate with you. And while a lot of this information applies to choosing an ACPA-approved team, the questions can be applied to choosing an independent surgeon, as well. So, if you don't have the option of comparing teams, you'll be able to find the very best independent surgeon possible.

· ·

FACTOR 1. *Team Credentials.* According to experts at the American Cleft Palate-Craniofacial Association (ACPA), the treatment of children born with CLP "is best managed when a team of specialists works with the family to develop and follow a treatment plan." As we've explored in Chapter 7, an ACPA-approved *cleft palate* or *craniofacial* team (I say *cleft team* here to refer to either type of team) can offer excellent care for a child in an area of medicine where the stakes are high physically, emotionally, and financially.

Now let's suppose you are fortunate enough to have two approved teams to choose between, as Anna did. One cleft surgeon suggested that, in such cases, families should rest assured that no matter how they choose, they have already taken a critical first step. This surgeon likened the process of evaluating two ACPA-approved teams to the process of shopping for a midsize Honda or Toyota. If comparing two sedans made by these car manufacturers, she said, of course, there will be differences between the two cars, and in some cases, important differences, depending on your family's needs. "But whichever one you choose," she continued, "you will end up with an excellent car. The same is true for approved teams." So, while it is always important to do your homework and ask questions, in such cases you (and other parents like Anna) can also know that the standards for ACPA approval are rigorous and meaningful.

The ACPA website lists all ACPA-approved teams in the US and Canada, for a total of about two hundred teams. As you look at individual team websites, you may notice that in some cases, certain practitioners on a team may themselves belong to the ACPA. While individual membership offers access to research and opportunities for professional networking, it does not relate in any way to a team's approval. Approval—as a unit—is key.

QUESTION ABOUT CREDENTIALS

Here is a question to ask the team coordinator or to search on the team website or ACPA website:

- Is the team approved by the ACPA?

FACTOR 2. *Qualifications of a Surgeon.* While every member of the cleft team plays an important role in a child's outcomes and well-being—as do parents—the main surgeon is a very important person to consider in your search. The surgeon performs the early operations for an infant born with CLP as well as other procedures later in childhood; this person literally shapes outcomes for a child. "The surgeon we go to has been doing this [work] for fourteen years," commented one mother, Ryley. "He is one of two top guys in our area." Ryley described her process of conducting online research to find the team initially, attending a prenatal visit with several members of the team and then speaking with her child's pediatrician for advice on this particular surgeon. Fortunately, the pediatrician knew of the surgeon's work. "I think it is vitally important to do your research on the surgeon," she continued. "The result, for us, was absolutely worth it."

There are many ways to assess the skills and experience of a surgeon—including asking for references from other medical professionals, as Ryley did, speaking with cleft families who have worked with that surgeon, asking informed questions, and pursuing a second opinion (more on second opinions, below). But the surgeon's credentials—meaning their formal training—are a good place to start your research. Unfortunately, medical job titles can be confusing to interpret. With so many acronyms, post-nominal letters ("MD," "DMD," etc.) and phrases like "cranio-maxillofacial" to wade through, it can be challenging to even identify the main surgeon(s) on the team roster, much less assess his or her qualifications.

The daunting (or at least somewhat confusing) news is that a person could take one of several educational paths to become a surgeon on a cleft team—thus, the profusion of post-nominal letters. The good news is that according to professionals in the field, the key qualification to look for is the *fellowship*, a period of final training that focuses on the operations related to CLP (and sometimes other conditions).

A surgeon on a cleft team has commonly undergone training in one of three areas: plastic surgery, maxillofacial surgery, or ENT surgery. This means that after attending medical or dental school, the surgeon pursued a *residency* in one of those areas of surgery. Then they may or may not have undergone a *fellowship* to receive extra training in cleft-related procedures. See the career time line, below, for an illustration.

According to pros in the field, the additional training of a fellowship determines whether a surgeon has acquired the necessary skills to perform the specialized procedures related to CLP. One surgeon suggested that this education lays a critical foundation for a career in the field. "Most surgeons on a team have done a fellowship," commented another surgeon. "That's important nowadays." Does it matter which field of surgery precedes the fellowship? "Not necessarily," another surgeon said. "It's the fellowship that matters. "That is the big differentiating factor."

CAREER Time Line
Possible Educational Paths of a Cleft Surgeon
College → Medical School and/or Dental School → Residency in Plastic Surgery, Oral-Maxillofacial Surgery, or Ear, Nose, and Throat Surgery (ENT) → [Possible] Fellowship in Craniofacial Surgery or Pediatric Plastic Surgery

Here are some questions to ask the surgeon or to search on the team website:

- In what discipline did you train? What is your title? Did you complete a fellowship? Where? What did the fellowship focus on?
- Which procedures do you perform on a patient born with CLP?

. . . .

FACTOR 3. A Surgeon's Experience/Volume of Patients. Conventional wisdom suggests that surgeons who perform many cleft-related operations each year get the best results. "Volume matters," commented one cleft surgeon on a large team. "It's true for everything done in surgery. High-volume surgeons get better results than low-volume surgeons."

Yet other parents and professionals argue that the matter isn't always black or white. Another cleft surgeon stated that while experience is very important, even crucial, it doesn't necessarily guarantee a good result. Still another argued that the surgeons who treat a high volume of patients may be using "less successful surgical techniques." So, it may be helpful to keep in mind that this factor—like others discussed in this chapter—may not always be straightforward.

Cleft professionals suggest that as parents learn about particular teams, they start by asking questions about the overall number of CLP-related operations a surgeon performs each year. One pro added a twist, suggesting that they also ask about the *regularity* of those operations. "You can get rusty," she explained, referring to the feeling a surgeon gets when being slightly out of practice. "The more you do on a regular basis, the better you are."

So, how many operations and what range of numbers defines "a regular basis"? The consensus among the surgeons I interviewed seems to range between one operation per month and one per week. Another cleft surgeon suggested that if a surgeon performs one cleft-related operation a month, a family can surmise that person is "actively performing cleft operations." But to perform a cleft operation once a week would indicate "very heavy involvement." Another surgeon suggested that the optimal number of procedures is about one every week or two. But many surgeons—most, in fact—perform far fewer.

This matter, again, can be tricky. "You could have a great surgeon who does ten cleft operations a year," commented another surgeon. "You could have a bad surgeon who does twenty-five a year." The key is to ask as many questions as possible about different factors to paint the best, clearest picture you can—and to feel comfortable with the trust and rapport you develop with a surgeon as the discussion plays out.

> ### QUESTIONS ABOUT THE VOLUME OF PATIENTS

Here are questions to ask the surgeon:

- How long have you been practicing?
- How many lip- and palate-repair operations do you perform each year? Each month?

. . . .

FACTOR 4. Life Factors: Cost. Cleft treatment performed in the US is often paid for by group-based insurance (insurance purchased through an employer, Medicaid, or a state-based program like CHIP, or provided through Tricare military insurance). Yet as we all know, costs can have a major impact on our decisions. Recent research shows that out-of-pocket costs for an annual visit with the cleft team can range from $0 to an eye-popping $1,000 for a typical visit. It also shows that high costs can cause families to drop out of care altogether as the years go by.

It may be helpful (and incredibly reassuring), therefore, to find out about coverage, co-pays, and pre-authorizations before you choose a team and start treatment, especially if you are considering a team located out of your network or state. These matters can be complicated and stressful. As the ACPA suggests in a fact sheet for families on this topic, "Health care funding varies from state to state and from one insurance policy to another. It changes constantly."

Pros and parents recommend asking members of the cleft team for help in this area, not only to learn about your coverage for cleft-related visits performed by this team, but to find out how much assistance the team will be able to provide more generally with these matters. Some teams have a designated staff person, sometimes the team coordinator, who helps you understand your insurance coverage and advocates for you if your insurance company denies coverage of a particular service—either by giving you detailed directions for contacting the company or by making those phone calls for you. You could also ask the team whether virtual visits are an option. While your insurance may cover a telehealth appointment as it would an in-person visit, you will save on travel expenses, lost work, etc. if your team is located far from home.

A sticking point that comes up frequently among cleft families relates to payment for cleft-related dental and/or orthodontic treatment. It is important to note that early treatments, such as the NAM or Latham appliance, should usually be filed and covered as *medical* claims rather than *dental* claims with a health insurance company. Again, someone on the team may be able to offer advice. The cleftAdvocate and Patient Advocate Foundation websites are other reliable resources for navigating these waters.

Related Issue: Financial Assistance. If health insurance coverage comes up short or if you lack funds for travel expenses, other forms of financial assistance may be available to fill the gaps. The Children's Craniofacial Association (CCA) offers funds for "ancillary costs of seeking medical care" such as air travel, gas, lodging, and food. The Mia Moo Fund, which offers various forms of assistance, was created by parents of a cleft-affected child who were "living paycheck to paycheck," as mother Missy Robertson writes on the fund's website, when she and her husband opted to "go into debt in order to receive the best care possible for our child." (The couple later created the fund to alleviate that stress for other families.) Other organizations such as the FACES: The National Craniofacial Association and myFace, among others, offer various forms of assistance. Several of the parents I interviewed described these supports as instrumental to securing quality team care for their children.

QUESTIONS ABOUT COST

Here are some questions to ask the team coordinator and/or to ask an insurance representative:

* Does your team participate in my family's insurance plan? Which cleft treatments are covered? What are the co-pays? When are they due?
* Will we need to get pre-authorization for any services? Will we need to confirm with our insurance company that dental and/or orthodontic treatments are covered as medical claims rather than dental claims?

Here are some questions to ask the team coordinator:

* What is your role in helping us navigate insurance coverage?
* (If the team is located at a distance) Are virtual visits an option, to save money on travel expenses?
* Do you have any tips for dealing with insurance plan X? Do you know the best number to call and/or a particular person to speak with about our coverage?
* Can you recommend organizations that offer financial assistance to cover medical expenses and/or ancillary costs?

. . . .

FACTOR 5. Whose Hands? If a cleft team is linked with a teaching hospital, your child's surgeon could be training and mentoring a few surgical residents or a fellow. In most cases, a resident or fellow watches or helps with a procedure but does not actually perform the operation. At other times, the junior and senior surgeons work together, even trading off steps during a procedure. This is how surgeons learn to become specialists—by watching, practicing, and participating.

It is not clear, generally speaking, whether the presence of a fellow in the operating room (OR) is necessarily positive or negative for a patient. No parent wants her child's face to be a practice case for an inexperienced surgeon, nor do they want a senior surgeon who's distracted by teaching duties in the operating room. But it is also true that a fellow may have a fresh perspective on a surgical task. And a senior surgeon continues to learn and grow by teaching. One surgeon mentioned that demonstrating the steps of a given task to a trainee helps him focus (rather than the opposite). And in most cases, the resident assists the surgeon but does not call the shots.

In any case, you have the right to clarify these roles. You also have the right to decide who operates. Another cleft surgeon suggested, "Parents need to demand it: *Are you doing the operation?* If you're not comfortable, don't sign the permission slip. You can say, *I give permission only for Dr. So-and-So to do the operation.*"

On a related note, recent research shows that some surgeons in the US will operate on more than one person at the same time (yes, you read that right!). This means that a surgeon may shuttle back and forth between patients in different operating rooms on any given morning or day. This practice, sometimes referred to as "running two rooms," does indeed occur—in a variety of fields—and is considered highly controversial. So, you have a right to find out whether your child's surgeon will be performing the entire procedure and if they will be present in the room the whole time.

This line of questioning may feel awkward at first (as may the other questions in this chapter). But, asking questions can help you find out as much as possible about what, exactly, happens in the OR and decide on your own comfort levels and what you want for your child.

> ### QUESTIONS ABOUT TEACHING/ MENTORING/OPERATING

Here are some questions to ask the surgeon:

- Is your team linked with a teaching hospital? If so, are you currently training a resident? A fellow?
- Who will operate on my child? Literally, whose hands? Can you tell me how that works?
- Will you be present during my child's operation from start to finish?

FACTOR 6. Treatment Variations and Surgical Technique. When I asked Jim and Lesley about their early research for a cleft team before the birth of their son, they mentioned visiting two teams in their area. "They definitely had different approaches," Jim commented. Not only did each team offer a different method of presurgical infant orthopedics (a topic explored later in this book), but each recommended slightly different timing for lip- and palate-repair operations. The couple found these variations thorny to navigate—as other parents do. Short of going to medical or dental school, how can families tell which treatment or approach is best for a child?

One way to find out more information about treatment variations is to interview more than one cleft team. "Getting a second opinion, if that's an option, and asking a lot of questions can be confusing," offered one surgeon, "but is probably the only way to sort this out." What's more, as you speak with members of different teams, you can ask each team about the *other* opinion—that is, you can ask Team B about the treatment plan described by Team A (and vice versa). "Each time we spoke to the doctors," said another parent who was concerned with variations in presurgical orthopedics, "we always asked them what they thought about the other team's device." Not only will this line of questioning offer more opinions about the method in question, but it can also clarify the choices and values of both teams—a win-win.

You can also keep in mind that as you ask team members to explain treatment variations, you are gathering information that goes beyond the answers themselves. Most of us can't know which technique is best. We can learn, however, how carefully the team members think about each case and with what priorities.

One cleft surgeon proposed that families go one or two steps further. First, he suggested that families inquire with a surgeon about their *surgical methods* for a child's early cleft operations. What are the names, for instance, of the surgical techniques they would use when performing lip repair and palate repair? And has research shown these techniques to be successful? (See Chapter 26 for basics on surgical techniques).

This surgeon also suggested that families might try to get a sense of a surgeon's willingness to acknowledge variations in viable methods. "In cleft surgery, there are things that are agreed upon [by many surgeons in the field] in terms of general timing and technique," he said. Most surgeons in the US agree, for example, that a cleft lip should not be repaired during the first week of life. According to the ACPA, outcomes are improved when an infant undergoes this operation after she has grown to be at least ten weeks old. But within certain parameters—say, if one surgeon would suggest operating at age four months and another at age six months—there can be acceptable variations. "Some [surgical] techniques may be better than others," he explained, "but you can get the same good outcomes with different techniques if they are done well." The key, he said, is for a team to acknowledge those differences to families. "It is important for a surgeon to admit that there are lots of good ways to do it. If you hear, 'This is the best or only way to do it,' it could be a red flag."

Does the idea of pursuing a second opinion make you feel nervous? When my husband and I were finishing up our introductory prenatal visit with members of our daughter's team, we mentioned to the surgeon that we were considering pursuing a second opinion with another cleft team in a nearby city. I remember holding my breath, wondering if the conversation would end awkwardly or somehow turn sour. As it turns out, his response surprised me. "The one thing that is better than a second opinion," he said, "is a third opinion." Other cleft professionals have praised this type of attitude. "A good provider and a good team should not be defensive about facilitating second opinions," commented another cleft-team pro, "either within the team or outside of the team."

> ### QUESTIONS ABOUT TREATMENT VARIATIONS AND SURGICAL TECHNIQUE

Here are some questions to ask the surgeon:

- Could you talk us through the technique you would use for our child's lip-repair surgery? Palate repair? Can you show us examples of research that shows outcomes with those techniques?
- What is your reasoning for using presurgical device X (NAM, Latham, lip taping, etc.)?
- At what age do you perform lip-repair surgery? Palate repair? What is your reasoning for that timing?
- What is your take on treatment X recommended by cleft team/surgeon X?

* *

FACTOR 7. Complications. If it feels nerve-wracking to bring up the topic of pursuing a second opinion when speaking with members of a potential cleft team, the idea of discussing surgical complications—that is, the things that can go wrong during or after a procedure—might feel like a doozy. But the cleft professionals I spoke with on this topic were actually eager to inform families about related issues and offered some possible questions to ask while searching for a surgeon/team.

It may be useful, first, to know where to direct these inquiries. One cleft surgeon explained how some hospitals—or units within hospitals—keep statistics on the complications that arise after patients undergo operations. A cardiac center, for instance, may report its outcomes publicly. "This is what true transparency should look like," he said. An issue that can arise with CLP-related reporting, unfortunately, is that the classifications are not always cut and dried. A lip repair that "is not esthetically ideal," as this surgeon explained—meaning that "it leaves a visible secondary cleft deformity"—may not get counted as a complication by the hospital. The key, then, is for families to ask a surgeon directly how often complications have occurred among her patients.

Another surgeon suggested that as families ask a surgeon about complications related to lip-repair surgery, they might phrase their questions in terms of follow-up procedures. For instance, you might ask: "How many of your patients have undergone follow-up operations on the lip?" And more importantly: "Were they minor or major revisions?" The best circumstance, of course, is for a child to undergo no further operations on the lip. But this surgeon explained that follow-up procedures do, indeed, happen from time to time. Some are quite minor, he said, and can be considered "acceptable." A scar may not heal properly, for example. Or a surgeon performs "very nice work" initially on the lip and/or nose, but it "needs a very minor tweak" later on because of the way a child grows. (It is important to note that some patients and families opt to undergo these types of minor revisions, while others take a pass. See the end of this chapter for more discussion.) A major revision, on the other hand—one that requires a substantial second repair to get it right—should raise a red flag.

Complications can occur after palate-repair surgery as well. A few cleft surgeons suggested that families ask about two complications in particular: the likelihood that a child will have abnormal speech later in childhood and the chances that they will have a postsurgical hole in the palate called a *fistula*. Abnormal speech, called *velopharyngeal insufficiency* or *VPI* (and sometimes referred to as *cleft palate speech)* happens when the back of the soft palate doesn't function the way it should when a young person speaks, even after having undergone surgery during infancy. Both VPI and a fistula can require further surgical intervention to correct.

While these two palate-related complications are undesirable, they do happen and, in some cases, are common (for a variety of reasons, including a child's normal growth); the details go beyond the scope of this book. But given that further surgical intervention is taxing for all involved—and given that these complications, like the outcomes of lip repair, may not be reported accurately by hospitals—it might be useful to ask a potential team about these issues upfront.

QUESTIONS ABOUT COMPLICATIONS

Here are some questions to ask the surgeon:

- [About lip repair] How many of your patients require a major revision following lip-repair surgery? Minor revisions? Can you describe the circumstances?
- [About palate repair] How many of your patients require a second operation to manage cleft-palate speech (VPI)?
- [About palate repair] What is your rate of postoperative palatal openings (fistulae)?

. . . .

FACTOR 8. *Contributions to the Field.* Some cleft specialists write academic articles about their work. "A surgeon has an obligation to learn and teach, to study and write," commented one cleft surgeon about his commitment to performing research. Many team members list "publications" or "research" alongside their credentials on the team website.

Truthfully, a person's writing, or lack of it, may or may not influence your opinion of their work in the exam room or operating room. One cleft surgeon commented, in fact, that a surgeon's articles or leadership positions do not indicate much of anything—for better or for worse—about surgical skills or outcomes.

At the same time, another pro suggested that a quick look at someone's work might give an impression of their dedication to the field. When looking at a professional's articles (see online search tips, below), consider asking: Do the topics relate to cleft lip and palate? Or, as this surgeon asked, is the person writing about something unrelated?

> ### QUESTIONS ABOUT ACADEMIC ARTICLES

Here are some questions to search online:

- Do the surgeon and team members write academic articles? What topics are represented?

Online Search Tips:

- Look at the team website for articles listed with team bios
- Search PubMed, a free database of biomedical literature
- Do a simple web search for surgeon "Dr. So-and So, MD," speech-language pathologist "So-and-So, SLP-CCC," and others on the team.

. . . .

FACTOR 9. Manner. Cleft parents have expressed a range of opinions about the bedside manner of the professionals on the team and in particular, the manner of their child's main surgeon. Some parents don't mind if their child's surgeon has a gruff or indifferent style in the office as long as he or she does a wonderful job in the operating room. "Our surgeon is not warm and fuzzy," commented one mother. "I've realized that you need to decide what you are looking for. Some people want more bedside manner and don't care so much about reputation and experience." For other parents, a surgeon's manner makes or breaks their confidence in his or her work. "I think it's important that a parent can ask any question and get a respectful response," said another parent, Joelle. She described her son's surgeon as "old and crusty"—in an affectionate way. "He was great," she said. "He took the time and drew the diagrams. I had a lot of faith in him." Joelle's trust in her child's surgeon related directly to his willingness to listen, answer questions, and teach.

Most of us would probably agree that the ideal surgeon would have both qualities: a warm, respectful manner paired with exceptional surgical skill. But in cases where bedside manner and surgical skill don't coincide, the questions that arise can be disorienting. If a surgeon doesn't treat a patient (and family) respectfully, is there reason to lose trust? And will that manner affect how productively the surgeon works with other members of the team?

These questions are challenging—and the answers may be individualized and highly subjective. But one way to resolve them may be to evaluate your own response as clearly as possible. Do you have a funny feeling about the manner of a surgeon or team? If so, you might consider analyzing that feeling. Parents tend to talk about two broad issues related to manner: Do you detect a language barrier or a social barrier? Or is your response related to kindness and respect? Some parents are willing to accept a language/social barrier or a certain amount of grumpiness, for instance, but chafe at a lack of respect. One surgeon on a cleft team suggested that, as a rule, team members should always be willing to listen. And in so doing, they should *always* acknowledge and address families' concerns—even if those concerns do not warrant any special actions or intervention.

As you consider different aspects of a surgeon's manner, you may also want to think about the long-term nature of the relationship. The process of searching for a team usually takes place when the patient—a child—is very young or not even born. At that point, the patient-team relationship is effectively a *parent-team* relationship. But over time, the child will participate more in conversations and decisions about his or her care. Consider, if possible, how your child's growth may affect your thoughts about bedside manner, both in terms of kindness/respect and communication/teaching. Some parents don't care if a surgeon treats them brusquely, but they care deeply—or differently—when the surgeon interacts directly with their child.

QUESTIONS ABOUT MANNER

Here are some questions to consider, personally:

- How do you feel about the manner of the surgeon and team?
- If you find the manner of the surgeon/team off-putting, is the situation a sign of a language barrier or social barrier? Or is it a matter of kindness and respect? Are these issues surmountable?

. . . .

FACTOR 10. Teamwork. Does the team seem to get along? Do they relay information in an organized way? Do they use similar language? These questions relate to how well the team members work together.

Team cohesiveness may not seem as pressing a factor early on as some of the others mentioned on this list, but some parents have suggested that it can become more important over time. As treatment evolves from the very first surgical stages into possible areas of speech, orthodontics, bone grafting, and beyond, the team will work together in different ways and configurations, often more intensively than before. "We really needed a cohesive team later on," said one parent about her school-age son. "Early on, the surgeon and the feeding method mattered most for us. But by age two or three, we needed a *team,* especially for speech and dealing with tubes in the ears." By the time her son reached nine or ten, she said, the dental professionals played a central role. Other parents have echoed these words, saying that as treatments progress and change—especially for school-age children and older—intra-team communication and coordination feel more important than before.

The cohesiveness of the team can also affect a parent's overall impression of its work. One mother recalled meeting twice with a surgeon on a local team, once before her daughter was born and then afterward. "We just didn't leave with a good feeling," she said, "and honestly, it took his staff two weeks to return a phone call or email." In theory, the mishaps of a single administrator—who fails to return phone calls, for instance—may not relate whatsoever to the skills or outcomes of the other team members. In reality, these factors can affect a family's confidence in the whole operation.

One way to find out how well the team works together is to talk with families who are currently in that team's care, especially those undergoing orthodontic treatment. Another approach is to ask the team members directly what their interactions look like. Cleft teams tend to function in different ways—some members working strictly within their own area of expertise, with others weighing in more freely across disciplines. The specifics may not matter as much as your impression of how thoroughly and carefully they exchange information and ideas.

Related Issue: Teamwork outside the Team. While intra-team interactions can play an important role in a patient's experience with cleft treatment, occasionally some families—particularly those who travel great distances for care—have mentioned instances in which team members also cooperate and coordinate with practitioners outside the team. Laurel, for example, described traveling halfway across the country for her daughter's cleft care. During the several months when her eight-year-old daughter was wearing a palate expander before her bone-graft surgery (a common treatment path during the school-age years), the cleft team coordinated this presurgical treatment with an orthodontist located in the family's hometown. That way, the patient and family could attend weekly visits with the local orthodontist instead of having to fly across the country each time. The sense of teamwork was "awesome," Laurel said.

But some teams are less willing to cooperate with others. One surgeon suggested that parents should beware of teams that "aren't willing to work with others or don't even entertain the idea of working with others." This unwillingness could be a sign of insecurity, he said, or worse. "In my experience," he continued, "[this unwillingness] is a high predictor of mediocrity." While most families do not travel great distances for cleft care, there may be other instances—for example, in areas of speech—in which a cleft team may be called upon to work with others outside the team.

QUESTIONS ABOUT TEAMWORK

Here are some questions to ask members of the cleft team:

- How do you function as a team?
- Does the team get together to discuss each case? How often? What does that meeting look like?
- Are there instances when you work with practitioners outside the team? How does that work?

Here are some questions to ask another parent:

- In your experience, do the team members work well together? Do they seem to get along? Do they communicate well with one another and with you? How has that experience gone for you?

* Do you have experience with team members working with practitioners outside the team? How has that experience gone for you?

. . . .

FACTOR 11. Outcomes. The factor of *outcomes* may seem like the single best measure of a cleft team, the one factor that outweighs the rest. But measuring the results of treatment can be difficult, in part because there is currently no standardized measure of outcomes across cleft teams in the US (though these measurements are standardized in the UK). So, as parents, we are left to assess a surgeon or team's outcomes on our own, a tricky prospect given how widely circumstances vary from one patient to another. Simply looking at another child's postoperative appearance, listening to their speech or tone of voice, or finding out about their hearing or teeth may or may not provide an accurate sense of possible outcomes for your own child. Also, as we explore elsewhere in this book, a family's or affected person's *perceptions* of outcomes can be colored by all kinds of factors (understandably) and, therefore, can be difficult to parse. Still, there are a few ways to learn more.

Fellow parents offer a wealth of information. As always, it can be very helpful to ask other families working with the team how they have felt about their experience and whether the results, so far, have met their expectations. You might take the additional step of simply asking the surgeon and team, directly, what to expect from treatment.

One mother, Gina, realized quickly that the first cleft team she visited would not be a good match for her son, Dylan. "The surgeon was very negative and told us that Dylan had a very severe cleft," she said, "and that on a scale of one to ten, Dylan was a twelve." The surgeon actually told the family that Dylan would not have a good outcome. Gina and her husband went into "panic mode," she said, scrambling to research surgeons/teams who were skilled with bilateral CLP. They asked other parents for suggestions, including families they had met via online support groups. "We were not terribly impressed," Gina continued, "until we contacted Dr. X," who displayed a positive outlook on the situation. He informed the couple that their son had been born with a typical bilateral cleft with a severity of five on a scale from one to ten and reassured them that Dylan "would look great." Gina knew immediately that she wanted this surgeon to perform Dylan's operations. "He spent a lot of time talking to me and making me feel comfortable," she said. In this case, Gina and her husband drew from both resources—parents and the pros themselves. They also asked bold questions and trusted their instincts.

Before-and-after pictures can show the results of lip-repair surgery and/or broad change and growth over time. One cleft professional suggested that families ask to see such photos of patients who are old enough to be nearing the end of their treatment path (or are as far along as possible). Some teams even facilitate in-person introductions between new families and young-adult patients who have "graduated" from treatment. "It gives them a sense of where it is all going," explained a member of one such team.

Still, it is important to know that before-and-after pictures (and perhaps even in-person introductions) will only be helpful with a lot of background information since the factors of diagnosis, presurgical treatment, and other variables can vary widely from one person to another. "A single picture is not representative," suggested one surgeon. A cleft-team orthodontist also noted that cleft surgeons, however well-intentioned, may be inclined to show families examples of *best* outcomes rather than typical outcomes. Another commented that it can be surprisingly difficult for a surgeon to obtain pictures at all (or be allowed to show them) because of privacy protocols. In any case, the images can be helpful with some informed caution on our part. What's more, in asking to see these pictures, we can learn information that goes beyond the answer itself. "Any team that is unwilling to show pictures, good and bad, is usually hiding something or doesn't believe in their own ability," suggested one surgeon.

> QUESTIONS ABOUT OUTCOMES

Here are some questions to ask the surgeon or team member:

- What can we expect in terms of outcomes over the long term? What will my child look like? How will she sound and speak?
- In your opinion, how severe is this case?
- Can we see before-and-after pictures? About the pictures: What was this patient's diagnosis before surgery? What kind of presurgical treatment was used and how diligently? Who performed the operation? When was this picture taken? Is this result typical?

Here are some questions to ask another parent:

- How was your experience with this surgeon and team?
- Are you pleased with the outcomes for your child? Has the experience matched your expectations?
- If you had it to do over again, would you make the same choices? Why?

FACTOR 12. Approach to Appearance-Related Decisions. As early as age four or five, some children born with CLP undergo a follow-up operation to change aspects of appearance, such as symmetry or fullness of the lip or nose. One surgeon described how a baby's postoperative appearance can change with growth. "Even though the lip tissue might look nice and full right now," he said, referring to the period directly after lip-repair surgery, "it tends to get thin. Thirty-to-forty percent of my patients need a revision at some point during childhood. They need more tissue in the lip."

The key word in his sentence? *"Need."* While some surgeons take a firm stance on whether a child should change aspects of her appearance, as this one did, others approach the decision collaboratively—by presenting treatment options to a patient and family and then inviting a discussion among all parties before making a plan. Still others introduce these options later when a child is old enough to weigh in.

Families vary, too, of course, not only regarding issues of appearance, but to decisions of when, why, and whether to make changes to a child's face. So, it may be useful to find out how a surgeon approaches these matters. Is the surgeon's philosophy more or less in line with yours? As abstract as these questions may feel to an expectant parent or a parent of a newborn, they may come into play just a few years down the line.

QUESTIONS ABOUT ISSUES OF APPEARANCE

Here are some questions to ask a surgeon on the team:

- How do you approach decision-making about procedures relating to appearance rather than function (for example, a lip revision)?
- How do you approach discussions with older children regarding matters of appearance?

Final Factor. Is It a Match? For many parents, the process of researching a cleft team (or an independent surgeon, if no team is available) is no small task. "It was very intense," commented one mother, Jane, about her experience. "But my husband and I were just so happy to find a place we were really happy with."

Jane described a sense of achievement once she finished her research and made a final decision.

Every family has different priorities—and the process of clarifying those priorities can feel confusing at times. But the goal for every family, as Jane intimated, should be to find a good match, to find people you trust. One cleft professional described these ideas in a slightly different way. A family's aim, she suggested, should be to make a meaningful connection. "Not all connections are the same for all people," she said, "but everyone knows when they've made a good one. It may not be the first person you meet, and it may not be the first team you meet."

Fortunately, there are many cleft teams in the US, Canada, and elsewhere that dedicate their practice to helping children born with CLP. "There are a lot of doctors that are doing it really well," added another mother. Whatever team or individual you choose, the goal is to feel comfortable, trusting, and secure.

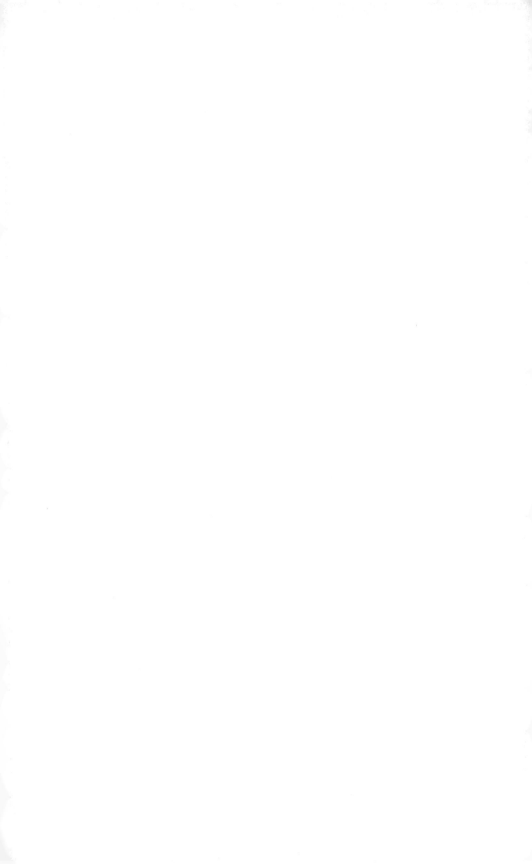

Birth

Chapter 9

. . . .

Birth! What's Next?

A Hospital Reference

*"After You Catch the Baby,
You Need to Call Us"*

The baby has arrived! Congratulations! A medical professional has probably said, "Your baby was born with a cleft lip and palate." Some parents heard this phrase weeks or months ago at a prenatal ultrasound. Others learned the news minutes or hours ago, at birth. Yet, here you are, in the hospital, baby in hand. Now, what? What do you do first? What do you do *right now*? Parents and professionals offer the following suggestions.

This is the time to triage, just as the hospitals do. A few tasks can be done now, while you still have hospital resources at your fingertips. Others can safely wait until later. Below, you will find a discussion of three hospital tasks. First, if you have been able to find a cleft team ahead of the birth, you should call them now. If not, this is the time to make initial contact. One cleft-team nurse put it this way: "If the father, partner, or coach is with the mom at the time for the birth, we give them a job. After you catch the baby, you need to call us." Next, get some help feeding the baby. Then find a lactation consultant, if applicable. You will also find a bonus tip about not learning the news in advance (it's okay).

HOSPITAL TASK 1
Pick Up the Phone: Call a Team

Here is a five-minute task that will do a world of good. Parents need to get in touch with a cleft team, a group of specialists who work together to treat a child's cleft lip and/or palate starting at birth (or in some cases, before birth). According to professionals in the field, patients who are treated by teams have better outcomes than those who go to independent providers.

> **Find a Cleft Team in Your Area**
>
> If you go to only one website, go to the Family Services arm of the American Cleft Palate-Craniofacial Association (ACPA). ACPA Family Services offers reliable information on cleft care and a state-by-state listing of approved cleft teams:
>
> www.cleftline.org/find-a-team

Why contact these folks now? Many parents and professionals have noticed an information gap between the staff at a birthing hospital and the specialists on a cleft team. Since cleft lip and/or palate occurs in about one in six hundred births, a large birthing hospital may see many cleft-affected babies each year. Some of its staff may know the ins and outs of feeding a cleft-affected newborn and finding the appropriate level of care for her. Wonderful!

A smaller hospital may lack this experience, however, simply from a lack of exposure. One cleft-team nurse in a large city described getting frequent phone calls from birthing hospitals after a baby is born. "Pediatricians call me from outlying hospitals one hundred miles away," she said. Those doctors, she explained, don't always know how to care for a cleft-affected baby in the short term. "I say to them, 'Send me a picture.'" A cleft team can relay information quickly, she continued, to help hospital staff with details on feeding and determining the appropriate level of care in the hospital. If the baby needs the Neonatal Intensive Care Unit

(NICU), the team will confirm it (see more on the NICU in Chapter 10). If the baby belongs in your room, they will confirm that too.

If you didn't know about the clefts in advance of the birth, this is fine. Right now, you need to find and contact a cleft team. The team you contact today may not be the team you choose for your child's long-term care. What matters now is closing the information gap in the hospital. Researching and choosing a team—one that will care for your child over the long term—is a larger task that may be better left for the days and weeks after you get home from the hospital. Then, you can devote some time and careful consideration to making the right choice for you, your baby, and your family (see Chapters 7 and 8 for more information).

Don't want to make the call yourself? One cleft-team nurse suggested that if parents have not connected with a team prenatally, that responsibility could be placed on the staff at the delivery hospital. It is perfectly fine, she said, to ask a staff member: "Could you call the nearest craniofacial center and talk to them?" The key is to ensure that help is on the way in the short term, no matter who makes the call.

One more thing. If you happen to live close to your cleft team, and you contact them right away after the birth, and the timing and logistics (the stars?) are perfectly aligned, you may receive a hospital visit from a person on the team. With a personal visit, the team members can tell you their first impressions of your child's needs. They can connect you with hospital resources, remind you of what to do in the upcoming days, and hopefully, reassure you that you are on the right track. My husband and I received this kind of visit in the hospital, and I'll tell you it made a challenging few days much better.

HOSPITAL TASK 2
Get Some Help Feeding the Baby

A parent's first task in caring for any baby is to feed her. As you may already know, a cleft-affected baby may require special care with feeding because of her unique anatomy. A baby born with cleft lip only—with no involvement of the palate—may be able to breast-feed and bottle-feed normally or near normally. A baby born with cleft palate, however, cannot make a perfect seal between the mouth and the nose and, therefore, cannot create suction. Unfortunately, in almost all cases, the presence of cleft palate rules out breast-feeding or sucking from a regular baby bottle.

Some mothers feel sadness and loss at not being able to nurse (see Chapter 15 for more discussion on this topic). Many parents also feel overwhelmed with the task of feeding, including handling a special bottle and reading a baby's physical cues. But don't worry—you will have time to process your feelings, absorb this information, and hone your skills in the upcoming weeks and months. In the meantime, it may be helpful to take advantage of the resources available in the hospital.

Find an Expert. While you are still in the hospital, the best way to get started is to seek help from a feeding specialist, and if your baby was born with a cleft palate, get your hands on a special bottle. A feeding specialist at a hospital can usually supply you with such a bottle (if you don't have one already) and give hands-on instruction on how to get started with it. Job titles vary; this person may be referred to as an occupational therapist (or "OT") or a speech-language pathologist (SLP), may work on a newborn feeding team or may be linked with the NICU. Title aside, this specialist offers expertise in feeding newborns with special needs. They can help you learn to feed your baby *right now*—that is, during the time directly following birth, until you meet with the specialist on your child's cleft team. (Note that while many cleft parents said that CLP did not affect the type of formula they used, it is always best to consult with your baby's pediatrician about this choice.)

Find a Bottle. Special baby bottles, sometimes referred to as special-needs bottles or cleft-palate feeders, allow a caregiver to feed a baby born with cleft palate. They can also be useful for babies born with isolated cleft lip (cleft lip only—with no cleft palate), depending on specific anatomy. There are four such bottles currently on the market: the Enfamil Cleft Lip/Palate Nurser by Mead Johnson; the Medela Special Needs Feeder by Medela (formerly called the Haberman Feeder); the Pigeon Bottle by Respironics; and the Dr. Brown's Specialty Feeding System by Dr. Brown's. Each of these bottles has different features and characteristics—and can be purchased online or obtained from a feeding specialist in the hospital (as mentioned). In any case, it is worth repeating: a baby born with cleft palate will not be able to draw milk from a regular baby bottle. (For more information on feeding, see Chapters 12 through 16.)

Find Even More Help. Once you've gotten started with a special bottle and had an instructional session with an OT or other feeding specialist in the birthing hospital, don't hesitate to ask for a repeat visit. The key is to get as much help as possible during your stay in the hospital—from an OT you have already met or, perhaps just as useful, from another OT starting a new shift. Remember, some specialists in birthing hospitals have more experience with CLP than others. What's more, each specialist offers a slightly different method, feel, or way of explaining things. For a hands-on technique like feeding a baby, the right explanation can make all the difference.

Lean on the Team. If you don't find a groove with any of the OTs at the hospital or with feeding your baby in general, fear not. The feeding specialist on the cleft team, typically a nurse, clinical nurse specialist, or speech-language pathologist, will not only serve as a family's point person for feeding during the baby's first year, but according to many cleft parents, will act as a teacher, troubleshooter, and a wonderful source of support and encouragement. Expert help is at the ready, regardless of what you learn—or don't learn—in the hospital. (This is another reason to pick up the phone and call a team.)

Remember: feeding a cleft-affected baby requires special equipment and assistance. But it often requires trial and error, time, and patience as well. Feeding can be a specialized affair. If you don't get the hang of a particular bottle or feeding system right away, keep at it. Specialists on cleft teams will assure you: these bottles can do the job. You can do the job! This task is doable.

HOSPITAL TASK 3
Pumping Milk? Find a Lactation Consultant

Nursing and pumping breast milk can pose all sorts of unforeseen challenges to a mother. Clefts may add a few more. If you plan to breast-feed your baby (for a baby with an isolated cleft lip) or pump breast milk, it may be helpful to find a lactation consultant at your hospital.

Learn about Breast-Feeding (Isolated Cleft Lip). A lactation consultant in the hospital will be able to show you special ways to position the breast tissue to accommodate the wide opening of the baby's upper lip. She may also make recommendations on suitable accessories or techniques to help minimize the leakage of air, a common problem for babies with isolated CL.

Learn about Exclusive Pumping. A lactation consultant can also offer practical instruction related to *exclusive pumping,* the act of squeezing (or *expressing)* milk from the breast to deliver to the baby through another means (usually a bottle). She may give advice on techniques and accessories and provide information on how to rent a hospital-grade breast pump, a must-have if you plan to pump milk.

It is important to note that *exclusive* pumping is different from the more common practice of *supplemental* pumping. With exclusive pumping, the baby never feeds directly from the breast—in this case, because they are unable to draw milk. And because a single person may or may not be able to pump milk and bottle-feed at the same time (depending on a few factors), the mothers (and families) who take on this extraordinary endeavor will nearly double their time commitment to feeding the baby. So, while exclusive pumping requires time and special equipment to start, it also requires determination and, as many parents have mentioned, logistical and emotional support.

If you make a meaningful connection with a particular lactation consultant, don't forget to ask if they accept calls after you return home. These specialists rotate shifts and may not be in the hospital from one day to the next. Does this person have a direct number? Would it be possible to return to the hospital in the upcoming days and weeks for another in-person consultation if necessary? Many hospitals also have 24–7 hotlines for feeding specialists and/or lactation consultants who can help with the critical few days following your return home.

BONUS TIP
For Parents Who Learn the News of CLP at Birth

It's okay to feel overwhelmed at not learning this news in advance. Parents who found out about their baby's clefts prenatally have had some time to prepare for birth, logistically and emotionally. Those who learned at birth are still processing the news. Many feel shocked. "I was so traumatized in the hospital," said one mother about the few days after learning the news of her son's CLP. "We had all these friends who wanted to visit, and we were such a mess."

As upsetting as the news may feel, it is important to know that medical professionals, particularly those on the cleft team, are ready to help—whenever you happen to contact them. You have not missed the bus. One mother, Amanda, recalled receiving questions from friends and family about how she felt to have learned the news of her son's condition at birth rather than via prenatal ultrasound. "A lot of people say to me, 'I bet you were mad that you didn't know the news in advance,'" she said. Despite those comments—and despite her rush to learn about cleft care following her son's birth—Amanda felt okay about the situation and the way she learned the news. "You know what?" she continued. "After the birth, we found out what we needed to know." There is time.

The act of giving birth itself can feel momentous and over-whelming, clefts and other news aside. And the hustle and bustle of a birthing unit or NICU can heighten those feelings. Whether you learned the news in advance or are just finding out now, the key is to do your best to get the help you need—whenever that may happen—so you will also have time to rest, recover, and get to know your newest family member.

Chapter 10

. . . .

Birth and the NICU

Speaking Up for Appropriate Care

The Neonatal Intensive Care Unit, or NICU, is an area in a hospital where some babies go directly after birth for help with extraordinary health needs. A NICU (often pronounced "NICK-you") provides sophisticated equipment and specially trained staff who can help babies born with low birth weight, breathing problems, infections, and other special medical concerns.

Many expectant parents wonder whether a baby born with cleft lip and palate will need to go to the NICU after birth. The short answer? Probably not. The longer answer? Maybe—it depends on several factors. We'll explore some of those factors here. The most important advice from professionals on cleft teams, however, is for parents to know about the notion of *appropriate care* in the hospital—the concept of seeking just the right amount of medical intervention—and to speak up and ask questions on behalf of your baby to make sure that happens.

Why the NICU?

The professionals I spoke with on cleft teams have explained that, in most cases, babies born with CLP will not need to go to the NICU. "I tell parents that if there are no other issues, they should expect normal everything," commented one clinical nurse specialist. "For a cleft only, most of the time, you would not end up in the NICU."

Indeed, cleft parents have described just this situation—one in which their newborn did not go to the NICU and, in fact, received "normal everything."

Still, there are a few reasons why a delivery team may order a stay in this unit. For one, the baby may have problems beyond CLP. "If the baby comes early, or there is another birth defect or another issue," remarked another cleft-team nurse, "those are the indicators for the NICU. Those are the things that we may not know about at the time of a mom's prenatal visit." Two other cleft team feeding experts, Patricia D. Chibbaro and Mary Breen, suggest in the medical textbook, *Comprehensive Cleft Care,* that the unit may also be needed for a cleft-affected baby with a problem with the heart, an unstable airway, or Pierre Robin sequence. In other words, the NICU may be necessary for an extra medical reason, the likelihood of which may be associated with CLP, but the nature of which does not necessarily relate to the clefts themselves.

The NICU might also be used to perform certain tests. Michelle described a preplanned visit to the unit for her daughter Riley, after learning the news of her CLP prenatally. The hospital staff referred to the stay as a "drive-by" visit, Michelle recalled. "Before she was born, they said to us, 'We will take her up to the NICU to make sure there are no extra issues with the clefts, do a check, and then release her.'" As the visit played out, Riley was held in the unit for several days because of a problem with her heart. But the original purpose for the stay had to do with an effort to rule out related health issues from cleft lip and palate.

Most often, parents mention visiting the NICU to get help with feeding, an activity that requires special know-how but rarely any fancy equipment (besides a special bottle, as described elsewhere in this book). In these cases, the reasons for a NICU visit often relate more to geography and logistics than anything else. According to the previously mentioned cleft pros, birthing hospitals vary in terms of where (in the hospital) they offer special help with feeding. While some hospitals ask feeding specialists and/or occupational therapists to visit babies and families in their individual recovery rooms—let's call it the "they come to you" model—other hospitals do it the other way around, asking staff members to stay in one place—the NICU—so the babies and parents go to them.

All of these examples are common scenarios in which a delivery team might order a baby with CLP to go to the NICU—a health issue beyond CLP, an evaluation to rule out other medical issues, or a feeding-related visit to get help from specially trained staff.

Issues to Know About

While it is true that the NICU offers many resources—some of which may be useful or even essential for a baby's health, as mentioned above—cleft specialists often advise parents to keep an eye out for instances when hospital staff attempt to overtreat a cleft-affected baby. There are drawbacks, they say, to using certain resources or equipment of the NICU when not strictly necessary. If an otherwise healthy baby is sent to the NICU for feeding purposes, for instance, she should probably need only two resources: a special bottle and a special person to help with the feeding (and even then, as one cleft-team nurse commented, the parents should also participate in the feeding itself, if possible). In most cases, a baby should *not* need other kinds of special treatment.

The superfluous use of a *feeding tube*, for instance, can interfere with a baby's normal process of learning to bottle-feed. According to Chibbaro and Breen, a feeding tube such as an *orogastric* (OG), *nasogastric* (NG), or *gastrostomy* (G) tube should *not* be used to feed a baby with CLP until caregivers have undergone an "adequate trial" with a cleft-palate bottle. "Babies with any type of palatal cleft can usually tolerate oral (by mouth) feedings," they explain. A feeding tube can actually cause an infant to become *orally defensive*, these pros warn. Oral defensiveness is an aversion to having something placed in the mouth, sometimes caused by the unnecessary use of a tube. It can make bottle-feeding very difficult later on.

The key to avoiding this issue is to try to find the appropriate level of care—not too much, not too little. In some cases, a feeding tube or another special treatment is necessary for a baby's health. But ideally, a baby should get the help she needs with the least amount of intervention possible.

Now, What?

Not only is this a time to be aware of overtreatment, but it is also a time to speak up about it if necessary. If you're not sure you understand a certain intervention in the hospital or NICU, don't be afraid to find out the reasoning behind a doctor's order. If the birthing team says that a tube is needed, for example, it is okay to ask for a meeting to learn more. Another cleft-team nurse went so far as to say that in some cases, especially in small birthing hospitals, parents may know more about cleft treatment than the hospital staff themselves. "If something seems strange," she said, "if [the staff] are being overly cautious or medical, or if you are scared about what is going on, we encourage parents to call us immediately, even if they are at a distance."

Chibbaro and Breen (mentioned above) offered a slight variation, suggesting that parents connect the hospital pros with the experts on the team. "Parents who have already met with a cleft team should share their team's contact information with the doctors and nurses," they write. "Parents should ask them to consult with the cleft team for advice." No matter how you access the cleft team, they are there to help. Are you unable to reach the team right away? The American Cleft Palate-Craniofacial Association (ACPA) offers a factsheet on CLP that is written specifically for the staff at newborn nurseries (see the references for details).

Unsure? Ask questions. And when in doubt, pick up the phone to contact the nearest team—even if you don't end up working with them long-term.

The period following the birth of a baby can be exhausting and emotional for all involved, in part because two people—the mother and child—are recovering from birth and may need medical attention—and in some cases, very special attention. The challenge in this context is to find the energy and courage to advocate for the baby, a skill that will be necessary throughout parenthood, for cleft treatment, and in other settings alike.

Chapter 11

. . . .

Birth and Bonding

Bundle of Joy? Or Just a Bundle?

My conversation with Mandy was bouncing along. As she described the ups and downs of her son's first year of treatment for CLP, she marveled at his fun-loving personality. Despite some early challenges, she said, he always seemed to smile. His resilience made her proud. Yet when I asked Mandy about her early experiences with mother-son bonding, she grew quiet. The conversation hung in place for a moment. She took a breath. And then she told a courageous story of parental love—and of her own resilience—that did not start the way she had hoped or anticipated.

When Mandy's son was born, she didn't fall in love with him right away. In fact, she didn't even want to hold him. The unusual look of his face took her by such surprise that she felt taken aback, shocked. "I was expecting this cute little baby—this cute little nose," she said. "He came out of the womb, and I thought, *This is not my baby. I didn't carry this for nine months*." A few minutes later, someone informed her that her son had been born with cleft lip and palate. "I started crying," she said. "I said to the nurse, 'I can't hold him right now.'"

Mandy's response to meeting her baby is relatively unusual compared to the reactions typically recounted by other new parents. Many adore their baby's unique, wide smile, describing their early parent-baby interactions with tenderness and joy. "We fell in love," is a common response. But Mandy is not alone. Others also lose their breath as the topic of bonding comes up, searching for words or fighting tears as they share memories of similar feelings. According to research, a delay in bonding is normal for any parent and baby, for all kinds of reasons. With time, parents do bond with their babies, the research shows, maybe even more in the context of a health issue (like clefts) than they would with an unaffected baby. The challenge, however, occurs in the meantime, when some parents feel ashamed, guilty, or silenced by expectations about how bonding is supposed to play out. How can these parents cope?

Myths and Hurdles

It is hard to walk into a shopping mall, attend a baby shower, or even turn on the TV without seeing messages about how parents are supposed to feel about a new baby. Popular culture and gender norms direct us—and especially women—blatantly toward joy. (Who has ever heard of a "bundle of anxiety?") But many parents don't feel joy at first, nor should they necessarily expect to. Anthropologist Sarah Blaffer Hrdy suggests that the mothering "instinct" can occur right away, or just as reasonably, following a series of events after birth. "It is not true that women instinctively love their babies," she writes in *Mother Nature: Maternal Instincts and How They Shape the Human Species*. "There is probably no mammal in which maternal commitment does not emerge piecemeal and chronically sensitive to external cues. Nurturing has to be teased out, reinforced, maintained. Nurturing itself needs to be nurtured." Immediate feelings of affection, in other words—perhaps like the love at first sight of an adult romance—may indeed arise for some parents. But the feelings that develop with time and energy can be equally meaningful and healthy.

Hrdy's research may be particularly helpful for parents of cleft-affected babies who don't feel an immediate connection. If bonding is a delicate process that needs to be cultivated, as she suggests, it might be reassuring to know that it is normal and reasonable—perhaps even more than reasonable—that the stress of a health issue could hamper it. Learning the news about a birth defect can feel jarring and frightening. Parents find out that treatment can be more complicated than they may have known. "We were so overwhelmed by the diagnosis," said one mother about learning the news. "It pulled the rug out from under us." Others describe similar roller coasters of emotions involving distress, helplessness, and guilt. Of course, bonding might be difficult in this context! How can we possibly "nurture a sense of nurturing" while feeling so stressed out? Ironically, it seems that some parents may be sidetracked from bonding due to their enormous concern for their child's well-being.

The writer Andrew Solomon suggests another reason why bonding may not play out in fairy-tale fashion—general unfamiliarity with something new. Parents may be slow to connect with their cleft-affected baby because they've never seen a cleft before or have only seen the condition in pictures. "To be honest," admitted one mother about her first interactions with her daughter at her birth, "it took me a while to get used to looking at her." She started to cry. "I didn't feel that instant love," she continued, "that instant connection." According to Solomon, the more any of us learn about a difference in another person, the easier it becomes to accept it. "Intimacy with difference fosters its accommodation," he suggests in *Far From the Tree: Parents, Children, and the Search for Identity*. It is reassuring to know that the more time we spend getting to know our baby—our whole baby—the better equipped we'll feel to bond.

Good News

Given this profusion of challenges, you would think none of us would bond with our babies. But research shows just the opposite—that parents and babies do bond—some sooner, some later. Prenatal diagnosis may offer a leg up on the process. "We learned about our son's clefts during pregnancy," said one mother. "During the rest of the pregnancy, my husband, especially, had a lot of worries about bonding. But the minute we saw Danny, all of those fears just went away." Medical professionals see a pattern here. "With prenatal diagnosis, parents can plan," commented one cleft-team nurse specialist. "They can find out about feeding. They can prepare for the birth." The key advantage may come from the extra time before the baby is born, during which parents can familiarize themselves with the idea of their child's difference—just as Solomon suggests.

Also, the long-term prognosis for bonding is hopeful. A recent multicenter research study performed in France indicates that the rate of parental depression is higher among cleft parents than in the general population during the weeks and months after birth. But the parent-baby relationships—described by researchers here in terms of "withdrawal behaviors"—were no different from those found in the general population, regardless of the timing of lip-repair surgery. "The resilience of both children and parent is remarkable," the authors commented. What's more, another study published in the journal, *Infants & Young Children,* suggests that babies born with clefts and their mothers may actually bond *more* than their unaffected peers. It's an underdog theory, as mentioned later in this book. "Infants with a cleft may be perceived by their mothers to be particularly vulnerable," researchers say, "heightening maternal responsiveness and resulting in stronger attachment characteristics." Mothers (the study didn't include fathers) may be inclined to bond with their child over the long term because they're rooting for her, hoping she will overcome big obstacles. Both pieces of research offer the good news that even if bonding does not occur immediately, there is no reason to fear that it won't happen at all.

Baby Steps

So, what can you do if you meet your baby and do not bond right away? A first step might be to examine your feelings and—especially—your expectations. As another mother, Kate, anticipated the birth of her son, she had heard a lot of advice from other parents and professionals. "Everyone told me that once I saw him I'd instantly fall in love with that tiny wide smile," she writes in a post on the CDC website. "But that's not the way it happened." As Kate puzzled over why she didn't bond with her son immediately, she considered that she didn't get to hold him for his first two days of life and didn't breast-feed. "Whatever the real reason I had trouble bonding with [him]," she continued, "I felt it must be because he was different and that I was a horrible person for not being able to love him."

It can be disorienting to make a profound investment in becoming a parent only to feel so-so—or worse—when the baby arrives, whether we're a parent of a baby born with a birth difference, a mother with postpartum depression, or any parent, for that matter, who feels exhausted and overwhelmed by a new child. But the situation worsens when we also blame ourselves, as Kate said, for not meeting certain expectations. Perhaps the bonding process would unfold more easily if we could first let go of the notion of love at first sight—however disappointing that idea may feel—and enjoy the anticipation of a bundle of joy while accepting that it's perfectly okay to start with just a bundle.

In the short term, we can also take steps to foster a connection. "I think that parents' feelings about bonding are expressed primarily in private," observed one nurse specialist on a cleft team. "People put on their best face." Realizing that parents may not be forthcoming about such a sensitive topic during an office visit, she and other members of her cleft team encourage all new parents to engage in skin-to-skin contact with their babies—and for mothers to put the baby to the breast, even if they are not breast-feeding—to help their relationships along. "It is so important," she continued, "for the baby, the mom, and the dad."

Mandy, whose son was taken to the NICU after her tumultuous birth experience, engaged in exactly that activity. "I tried, sincerely, to bond with him," she explained, describing times when she held him on her bare chest during his stay in the hospital. But at that point, her efforts stemmed more from perseverance than from pleasure. "It was hard," she continued. Hours, days, and weeks passed, during which time Mandy alternated between practicing skin-to-skin contact and pumping breast milk for her son. "Even though I didn't want to be there, and I didn't want to hold him, and I didn't want to feed him," she said, "I still did it because he was my baby and that was not going to change." Mandy did not feel inclined to bond with her baby, but she kept at it, doing all she could to spend time with him and take care of him in the hope that her efforts would eventually pay off.

Experts from Harvard Medical School HelpGuide Collaborative advise taking even more specific actions. In order to improve the parent-baby bond, the group advises, parents should work on two fronts—reducing stress and then "tuning in" to their own feelings and those of their infant through repeated, one-on-one interactions. "This process of mutual discovery can only take place when you and your baby are relaxed enough to focus intently on one another," suggests psychologist Jeanne Segal, PhD, in *Creating a Secure Infant Attachment*. At the same time, as this psychologist suggests, you can actually practice looking into your baby's eyes. Segal recommends following a baby's cues, by looking at her directly and then looking away for a moment when she's had enough. The steps themselves may seem small. But the key is to take them over days and weeks— and to try to be easy on yourself in the process.

Relaxation can be a tall order, especially for a new parent. And the small steps described by the experts may feel frustrating at first. But this process is doable. What's more, further help is available. Whether the intense personal feelings relate to CLP, to the baby more generally, or to other concerns, it might be useful to speak with a therapist, have honest conversations with members of the cleft team (particularly those who specialize in mental health), practice mindful meditation, talk with a faith leader or trusted friend, or search out some other method that feels right.

Some Sooner, Some Later

After a very long month, something changed for Mandy. "Finally, we brought him home from the hospital," she said, "and I had this moment." She described sitting in a rocking chair by a window, with her son propped up on a Boppy pillow. They were having skin-to-skin contact, she said, to keep up her milk supply. "He moved his hand up onto my neck," she continued, "and he looked up at me. And that was it. It hit me: *I can do this. I can handle this.*" Mandy reflected on the environment of the NICU, where her son had been wrapped in a big swaddle and fed through tubes in his throat and stomach. "That stuff freaked me out," she continued. "At home, all that stuff was gone. At home, all I had was my baby. We could give him a bath. He became cute. I thought, *I don't care that you don't look normal. I don't care that you don't look like your sister. You're my baby.*"

Most new parents do bond with their cleft-affected babies. Just look at the chorus of loving, shout-it-from-the-rooftops social media posts on cleft-related Facebook pages every day, not to mention the exuberant messages of the #cleftstrong movement—all affirmations from families who not only bonded with their infants but couldn't wait to share their joy with others. But all the examples in the world may not console the expectant parents who wonder how the most immediate example—their own—will play out. The key—whether we embrace our baby right away or sometime later on as Mandy did—is to remember that both scenarios are healthy and okay. The act of waiting for something to happen doesn't mean that it will not happen at all, or that the feeling will be diminished for arriving late. The second, longer path may start with just a bundle but need not end that way. The meantime requires patience, persistence, courage, and self-forgiveness.

Feeding the Baby

Chapter 12

. . . .

My Story, Part 2

The Baby, the Process, and the Dance

The first time I fed my newborn daughter, I did a clunky job of it. A few hours after her birth, as my husband and I waited in our recovery room with our shiny, new Haberman baby bottle in hand, we sat up straight, craning our necks, listening for the approaching footsteps of the feeding specialist in the ward. While the imminent visit would involve feeding our baby for the first time, it would actually be our second consultation with a feeding expert. We had already learned a few things about this particular cleft-palate bottle from Nurse Margaret, the specialist on our daughter's cleft team, during a prenatal visit, weeks earlier. She'd shown us how to assemble the contraption, deftly demonstrating the placement of a paper-thin rubber valve inside an extra-long, squeezable nipple, and reassuring us that as convoluted as this task may seem and as many bottle parts as there were to align, she was sure we'd get the hang of it once the baby arrived. We'd left that prenatal visit feeling excited, even jazzed. She'd promised that we would get hands-on help from a nurse in the hospital, after birth. And the bottle seemed fancy. We filled it a few times with water at home, to test it out, and chuckled as we mock-squeezed it into our own mouths. *Come on out, baby*! We felt nervous about our daughter's arrival, but more or less up for the task of feeding her.

Yet now, in the hospital, with an actual newborn in hand—a newborn with a sizeable hole in the roof of her mouth—my husband

and I were realizing with growing urgency that while we had learned how to assemble this special bottle, we didn't really know how to use it. And our daughter was starting to whimper. Until then, she had been resting contentedly, looking adorable with her strawberry-button cleft lip and gentle tufts of dark hair. But now she was wiggling her tiny arms and legs and starting to spring free from her swaddle. When would the specialist arrive? Should we fill the bottle with formula and just give it a go? Our baby was clearly hungry. I sat up even straighter. My husband started to pace.

Finally, the feeding specialist entered the room and time slowed down. She smiled. Had there been any problem, any rush? This woman was a Mr. Rogers of a nurse, moving calmly as she laid out the bottle parts on the lip of a nearby sink and explained how to mix the formula and position the baby. And as soon as she started to demonstrate the feeding itself, cradling our sweet daughter for a moment, the activity once again seemed doable. She instructed us to squeeze the nipple repeatedly and to coordinate our compressions with the baby's suckling motions. She even suggested a little trick to determine the correct rhythm: we should sing "Row, Row, Row Your Boat" as we squeezed. When we arrived at the word *boat,* we were supposed to rest for a moment. Great! *I've got this!* I thought. *Yes.*

Yet as soon as the nurse handed me the baby and the Haberman, I wasn't so sure. The bottle felt awkward and imbalanced in my hand as if I could no longer tell whether I was left- or right-handed. I chose what seemed like a reasonable spot on the long nipple, looked at the baby's motions, and pinched three times, gently releasing the milk into her mouth, but it wasn't clear whether my daughter actually swallowed any of it. She continued to mumble and fuss, shaking her head tentatively from side to side as the liquid dribbled onto her chin. The nurse smiled, leaned in, and encouraged me to try again—and to focus more intently this time on the "Row, Row, Row Your Boat" rhythm. I took a breath and gave the nipple a few more squeezes, but the baby's complaints grew louder. While her physical motions seemed to indicate that she was eager to eat, I couldn't see how the row-row-rowing could possibly relate to her cues. And the milk seemed to be flowing in the wrong direction. It was as if I had mistakenly decided to feed a doll rather than a person (*whoops!*), a baby with a mouth but no innards. I tried again, squeezing more firmly than before on the nipple. This time, my daughter let out an abrupt cough snort. The formula that had first traveled to her chin was now making its way into the crevices of her tiny, newborn hat.

I continued to squeeze. I started to sweat. My husband and the nurse both leaned in, now hovering like flies, puzzling over my missteps. My husband wondered aloud if I had been squeezing too quickly. Or too hard? I kept trying. But by now, our baby's sounds had crescendoed beyond cries into full-on, repeated shrieks that went echoing out into the hallway, like some kind of new-born-powered fire alarm. Time sped up. My daughter's face, once serene, now looked as if it might explode. Without hesitation, Mrs. Rogers upped her game, still as kind as could be, but now making grand gestures, waving her arms in wild, sweeping motions to help me understand the proper pacing, as if she were conducting a full symphony orchestra in a rousing rendition of "Row, Row, Row Your Boat." And believe it or not, I was a person who should have known how to follow a conductor. At the time, I was actually a professional classical musician. I had spent more than twenty years—tens of thousands of hours—honing my sense of rhythm. Yet I could not get the hang of "Row, Row, Row Your Boat" and could not feed my baby. I wanted to cry.

Eventually, someone had the very good idea to let my husband take a turn. Sweet relief! At least for a moment, I would have a chance to gather my thoughts as my husband took the wheel. But as I slid our red-faced bundle into his arms, I could tell almost immediately that he was going to do an A-plus job with it. And he did! He was like Fred Astaire with the Haberman bottle, squeezing smoothly and easily, with a feather-light touch. After a few tries, he was actually able to feed our baby, who by then had started to calm down and swallow the liquid. The nurse stepped back, beaming. *How can this be happening?* I thought. *My husband can't even sing! He's a Russian historian!* But he had grasped the nurse's ideas in full as if the two of them had been speaking some sort of secret language.

Finally, a tiny ray of sunshine peeked through the clouds. Nothing changed physically; my husband continued to feed the baby as the nurse and I looked on. But for a brief moment, he looked up, eyes sparkling, and shot me a little smile. Now at that point, Ethan and I had been married for about seven years and had been together for a little while longer. I don't know how adeptly other couples communicate, but he and I certainly did *not* have any sort of secret, silent language of our own or a third-base coach type of lovers' lingo. No. Most of the time, if I were to look at him from across a crowded room and raise my eyebrows as if to say, "How about let's leave this party now," he would probably smile at me affectionately, miss my point entirely, and make his way to the buffet table to fill another plate. But this time was different. This time I was sure that he was looking at me encouragingly, as if to say, "It's okay. Don't worry about it. Don't worry about the bottle or the boat."

It turns out that I was right, and he was right: I needn't have fretted. Things got better. We practiced using the Haberman in the quiet privacy of our hospital room and later at home. We had subsequent visits with wonderful Nurse Margaret on the cleft team, who examined the situation more specifically—now that we had our baby with us—and offered tips on how to adjust the bottle and manage the squeezing. I worked on my timing. And I realized that learning to feed our baby would be a process. While my husband took to the task right away, I found out later that many other parents don't figure it out immediately—and that's okay. Every baby's cleft anatomy is different. Every caregiver is different. Every feeding specialist, whether on the cleft team or in the birthing hospital, has a slightly different way of explaining things. The four cleft-palate bottles currently on the market are varied and newfangled, with bells, whistles, and other features that often require adjustments. The process is naturally one of experimentation and discovery.

What's more, I realized that the act of feeding a baby with a cleft palate actually does—and should—resemble a classic scene with Fred and Ginger: it's a dance. Feeding experts from cleft teams mention again and again how important it is for parents to learn to read a baby's signals, an essential activity for the two so-called assisted-delivery bottles (where the caregivers do some of the work for the baby by squeezing the liquid into her mouth) but also a necessary concept for the two other cleft bottles on the market, which require caregivers to make mid-course adjustments based on how the baby is doing. "The big thing is to focus on your baby," commented one cleft-team nurse specialist, "instead of the cleft, the bottle, or the gear." The baby is leading. As important as it is to have the proper equipment—because without a special bottle, the dance cannot even begin—the act of reading a baby's signals is usually the best way to choose a bottle, learn to use it, *and* adjust it to work as well as possible.

Truth to tell, I never became a superstar baby-feeder. I often lingered too long in a single feeding session, squeezing cautiously on the nipple for fear of flooding the baby and causing her to choke. I held back. (As you'll read in Chapter 14, I broke the rule called, "After Thirty Minutes, It's All Celery.") But I learned how to get the job done—and more calmly and efficiently than my first few tries in the hospital.

The process of learning to feed a cleft-affected baby may take some work. It often requires trial and error, not only with adjusting our equipment but with developing a sense of patient curiosity to read our baby's cues. And oftentimes, the help we get from the cleft team can make all the difference. But then again, there's that dance. Dancing can be a pretty intimate activity. And now we get to do it with our baby.

Chapter 13

. . . .

The Bottles

A Tour of Cleft-Palate Feeders

When Daphne learned during a prenatal ultrasound that her son would be born with CLP, she did some research into the four baby bottles designed for infants with cleft palate. In fact, she did a *lot* of research. "We bought them all!" she exclaimed, describing her desire at the time to cover her bases before giving birth. "Then we crossed our fingers. We were just hoping that one of them would work." Daphne's son ended up using three of the four bottles—and several combinations of differently sized nipples that went along with them—during his first few weeks of life as Daphne and her husband experimented to see which setup would make the best match. It was a bottle extravaganza, they said. But the new parents ultimately settled on a bottle (the Pigeon) that worked well for their baby—and for them—until the time of his lip-repair surgery.

If, like Daphne, you are preparing to purchase a baby bottle (you won't need to buy all four!) for your newborn or your baby-on-the-way—or if you are making midcourse adjustments during your baby's first year—you have come to the right place. This chapter is a guide for the four special bottles currently on the market for babies born with a cleft palate: the Mead Johnson, the Haberman, the Pigeon, and the Dr. Brown's. Here you will find basic information on each bottle, such as how it works and how much it costs, followed by loads of tips, tricks, and opinions from fellow parents and cleft-team feeding specialists. At the end of the chapter, you will find descriptions of a few "alternate" vessels that parents and professionals have mentioned beyond the traditional four cleft bottles.

Which one of these bottles is the best of the bunch? Unfortunately, you will not find that answer here—because no one bottle works for every baby and family. Not only is the matter personal, but it may also require some time and trial-and-error to find the best fit. Ready to dig in? Here we go.

. . . .

The Enfamil Cleft Lip/Palate Nurser by Mead Johnson

Common Nicknames: "The Mead Johnson Cleft Palate Nurser" or "The Mead Johnson"

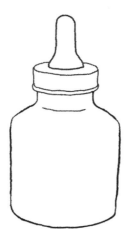

How It Works. The Mead Johnson bottle is one of the oldest cleft-palate bottles on the market. It is considered an *assisted delivery bottle*, meaning that the caregiver is responsible for delivering the liquid into the baby's mouth—in this case, by gently and rhythmically squeezing the body of the bottle itself. While a baby with a cleft palate will make repeated biting motions with her mouth and swallow the liquid (just like any other baby), the recurring compressions of this soft-walled bottle will help her receive the liquid that she is unable to draw through suckling.

Like other cleft-palate bottles, the Mead Johnson features a long nipple with an x-shaped crosscut at the tip that allows the milk to flow freely—a critical component of feeding a baby who cannot form suction with the palate. Also, since the neck of this bottle is universally sized, a caregiver can attach a different type of nipple to the body of the bottle (more on substitutions, below).

The MJ is the simplest specialty bottle on the market in terms of design and construction. You'll find no bells and whistles here. Because of the basic setup, it is up to the caregiver to determine how hard to squeeze the walls of the bottle and how and when to coordinate the pulses with the baby's feeding rhythms. According to the ACPA, the Mead Johnson "takes a little bit of practice." An upside to this bottle, according to many parents and professionals, is that the caregiver has a lot of control over the flow of liquid. A downside, they say, is that the flow can feel unwieldy and difficult to master.

Where to Get It and Cost. The Mead Johnson is available at Amazon for about $4 per bottle or less if you buy in bulk. Many hospitals and cleft clinics keep this bottle on hand because it works well for a wide range of feeding issues (beyond those caused by CLP). Occasionally, parents mention receiving an MJ for free from the staff at their birthing hospital.

Experts' Tip for Making It Work: Open the Crosscut. Many parents discover that the Mead Johnson bottle works best when it's been modified a bit. "If you leave it as is, it can be very difficult to squeeze," commented one clinical nurse specialist, who added that she always cuts open the crosscut on the nipple of this bottle to help a cleft baby drink easily. Another nurse noted that Mead Johnson nipples can be inconsistent from one to another in terms of stiffness. She advised filling the bottle with liquid (milk or formula) and turning it upside down. "If it doesn't drip once every three seconds, the nipple hole is not big enough," she said. "It needs to be able to have milk flow through it freely."

To open the crosscut on a Mead Johnson, you'll need to use a very sharp knife to slowly (*slowly!*) increase the size of the X at the tip of the nipple. Then you can test it by turning the bottle upside down. According to the ACPA, "If it flows rapidly, but you can still see individual drops," you have probably got it right. The ultimate test, of course, is to see how well the flow of milk suits the baby—and to read her cues and make adjustments accordingly.

If you feel twinges of concern about the idea of cutting into a perfectly good piece of medical equipment with something as crude as a knife, you are not alone. The concept can feel strange and unorthodox. Most of us probably don't purchase objects to immediately damage them, especially when a baby is involved. This practice, however, is commonplace and normal among cleft-team professionals. You might think of the Mead Johnson bottle (and others) as a tool delivered in unfinished form. Once you buy it and bring it home, you will need to finish its setup to make it work best. That said, I would advise that you read on before you make your first cuts to find out about another option. Hold up. Please. PUT DOWN THE KNIFE!

Experts' Tip for Making It Work: Add a Vent. While the most common recommendation from cleft-team nurses/feeding specialists regarding the Mead Johnson bottle is to cut into the crosscut of the nipple, a few have described a curious alternative. "Do not cut the X bigger," advised another nurse about the tip of the nipple. "Don't even touch the X." Instead, this nurse advised clipping a hole near the *base* of the nipple, so that when you fill the nipple and flip it upside down, it is no longer able to hold back the milk.

The idea, in other words, is to add a tiny vent to the nipple. Here is a metaphor to consider (warning: a middle-aged person has entered the building). Do you remember when fruit juice used to come packaged in a can, as opposed to a glass jar or a plastic bottle? If you ever felt thirsty for tomato juice in the 1980s or earlier decades and wished for the liquid to actually pour out of the can instead of remaining mysteriously trapped inside, you needed to know to pierce the lid of the can *twice*: first to make a large, primary cut at the spot where you wanted to pour and then to add a smaller hole for ventilation on the other side of the lid. The same concept applies here. "You need to have a fine pair of scissors," continued the nurse. One parent had better luck with a brand-new pair of nail clippers. The key, if you decide to try this method, is to create a small, second hole somewhere near the base of the nipple to allow air to displace the liquid. As always, start small.

Making It Work: Ways to Prevent Leaks. According to several parents, the caps that secure the Mead Johnson nipple tend to crack and leak, making a mess and driving them crazy. One suggested a generic replacement—the caps that come with cheap Gerber bottles sold at Walmart. Another parent proposed storing water or breast milk in a completely different container, then transferring it to the Mead Johnson bottle at feeding time to forestall leaks.

Another solution doesn't involve replacing the cap at all. Cleft-team nurses have observed that the cap of the Mead Johnson may leak if the nipple is too stiff. As pressure builds up from a too-stiff nipple, they say, the cap may strain and crack. The solution is to loosen up the nipple, either by increasing the size of the crosscut or by adding a vent (as described above).

Parents Say: This Bottle Works...but Oww! Parents offer mixed reviews overall for the Mead Johnson bottle. While one mother acknowledged that the bottle was adequate, she didn't enjoy using it. "It was horrible squeezing the milk for eight or nine feedings a day," she said. "It took so long. And it would hurt. You could get carpal tunnel with this bottle, from the squeezing!" This mother experimented constantly with this bottle, not only by making adjustments to the vessel itself and switching up the components but also by modifying her own squeezing technique—yet she never found a sweet spot. "If the hole was too big, he would choke," she continued. "If the hole was too small, he would get too tired trying to eat." Another parent admitted to actually developing carpal tunnel syndrome from using this bottle. Still others can get the hang of it. "As a technician by profession, I enjoy figuring things out," said one dad. "I remember I kind of liked figuring out how to use that bottle." While some caregivers find a groove with the Mead Johnson, others find it crude and frustrating to modify.

Nurses agree that the Mead Johnson can be tricky for a lot of parents. "With the Mead Johnson, you have to have a very tuned-in caregiver," said one nurse. "You have to watch the baby's face. They eat in bursts. They go, *eat, eat, eat, breathe*. You can't be exhausted—you can't be tending to other kids—or you could squeeze while they are breathing and choke the baby."

Bottom Line. While the Mead Johnson can be appealing for its simplicity and rock-bottom cost—and while after years on the market this bottle remains a strong option for many babies—parents and professionals agree that it often requires experimentation and patience.

The Medela Special Needs Feeder
by Medela

*Formerly Called: **The Haberman Feeder***
*Common Nickname: **"The Haberman"***

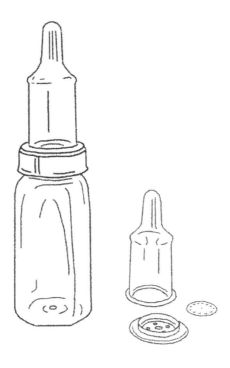

How It Works. The Medela Special Needs bottle is another example of an *assisted delivery bottle* that requires a caregiver to release liquid into the baby's mouth by compressing some part of the bottle—in this case, a soft, elongated nipple with a crosscut at the tip. Unlike the bare-bones Mead Johnson bottle, however, the Haberman (to use its common nickname) is brimming with features. The bottle, which is available in standard and preemie sizes, is made up of five parts: a nipple, a disc, a rubber valve, a collar, and a standard plastic bottle. The long nipple of the Haberman is the star of the show, acting as a small holding chamber for the milk. As you squeeze the nipple in coordination with the baby's rhythms, liquid is released from the main body of the bottle through a small, rubber valve (the underappreciated genius sidekick).

The Haberman nipple offers three "speeds"—slow, medium, and fast. You can control the flow of the milk by rotating the nipple in the baby's mouth to speed up or slow down the release of liquid.

Where to Get It and Cost. The Haberman is available at standard online outlets for somewhere between $22–$33 per bottle. Yes, you read that figure right. A few lucky parents can get this bottle for free from hospitals and cleft clinics that keep the Haberman on hand for babies with special feeding needs. Insurance companies may cover costs for this bottle, as well; they may classify it as "durable medical equipment." (See additional tips from parents on circumventing costs, below.)

Experts Ask: Do You Need a Rolls-Royce? One characteristic of the Haberman bottle is its overall ease of use. "The Haberman is very precisely made," commented one nurse specialist on a cleft team. "You don't have to apply a great deal of pressure to pulse the nipple," she said, as she compared it to the much more labor-intensive Mead Johnson. With this bottle, the caregiver can usually control the flow easily and predictably, similar to driving a fancy car.

A logical question that arises with this bottle, then, is whether a baby and caregiver actually need its full range of features. On one hand, the bottle offers a lot of flexibility. One cleft-team nurse described three or four distinct phases of cleft treatment during a baby's first year when conditions in the mouth change and/or can become sensitive to the touch. While other cleft bottles may work well for one period but not another, she said, the Haberman usually works for them all. "You can get the baby started in the beginning," she explained. "Then, when the NAM is in place, you have options to adjust the way you use the bottle." Even after lip-repair surgery, the Haberman is adaptable. "It gives you options," she said. "I like that." Other specialists echo her words, praising the design of the bottle and its adaptability over time.

This flexibility, on the other hand, comes at a cost—literally. "It is expensive," said another nurse. "I will be blunt: it is a captive audience. It is hard to believe that bottles cost that much to make." Some feeding specialists advise using the Haberman only for special feeding needs that go beyond typical CLP. Others mention its usefulness before, during, and after NAM treatment. "The Haberman has a place," said another nurse. "It can be useful for certain, specific situations." While some parents find relief in knowing that this bottle can accommodate a range of needs, others find it just too much, both in terms of capacity and expense.

Experts' Tip for Making it Work: Be Mindful of Timing. One of the advantages of a Haberman bottle, according to parents and professionals, is its capacity to be rotated in the baby's mouth to align the nipple to a slow, medium, or fast setting. Caregivers usually do *not* find a need to adjust the speed of the Haberman many times during a feeding session—perhaps only once toward the end of each session to speed up the flow of liquid as the baby tires. Yet one nurse on a cleft team advises parents to be mindful of timing as we do so. "If the baby is in an active suck mode, do not pull the nipple out to rotate it," she said. "The baby gets very tired very quickly," she explained. If you pull out the nipple repeatedly, you can disrupt her rhythms, leading to frustration and worse. "The baby finally says, 'I am done,'" she warned. A simple and easy solution is to delay this rotation until the baby rests to swallow or until you reach a burping session.

Parents' Tip for Making It Work: Protect Your Investment. One of the drawbacks to using a bottle that operates with small, beautifully designed working parts is that they will need to be washed, supposedly in or near a kitchen sink—creating a possible problem with runaway components. A simple remedy, unfortunately, would require action at the corporate level. If the Medela company were to repackage its bottles to include a spare rubber valve—a pennies-on-the-dollar investment on their part—it would save exhausted, bleary-eyed, pajama-clad parents from getting down on hands and knees on the kitchen floor at 2:00 a.m. to recover a contact lens-size rubber valve—or from inserting a bare hand into the garbage disposal and risk bloody catastrophe to feed their baby. Please, Medela. How about a spare part or two?

Meanwhile, a cheap mesh drain cover will go a long way. So will a dark-colored kitchen towel spread on the countertop to store the clean bottle parts securely and visibly. No one wants to lose the valve for an expensive Haberman bottle, as brilliant as its design may be. If you lose the valve, you lose the bottle.

Parents' Tip for Making it Work: Pack It for Travel. For on-the-go feeding, several parents recommend a quick trick: storing the Haberman nipple setup inside the bottle itself. Simply turn the nipple upside down and insert it into a bottle—filled with liquid if you like. Place the disc/valve onto the top of the bottle, upside down. Now, screw the collar onto the top of the bottle. Voila. You can toss the unit into a bag and leave the house.

Parents' Tip for Making It Work: Cut Costs Creatively. Many parents mention the cost of the Haberman as a major sticking point for choosing this bottle, yet some have been able to circumvent the problem, at least in part. The most common solution is to purchase replacement nipples, which are sold separately at around $20 each, instead of buying entirely new bottles. Another option is to seek low-cost options for the whole kit and caboodle. One mother made repeated phone calls to her insurance company to inquire about coverage, a time-consuming, frustrating, but ultimately fruitful process that led to a nearly overflowing mailbox full of Haberman bottles (she eventually donated the unused bottles to local cleft families). The key, she reported, was to refer to the bottle as "durable medical equipment" when speaking with insurance people.

Another parent discovered that her cleft team's hospital pharmacy offered the Haberman bottles at $18 a pop, a price that exceeded the cost for regular baby bottles but undercut the $27 she had previously been paying online. In my case, my husband and I found that while the Haberman bottle was expensive (and one of only two cleft bottles available at the time), we only needed to purchase two or three bottles and only a few replacement nipples during our baby's entire first year. Our daughter, we discovered, actually took in more volume of formula and seemed happier with worn-out Haberman nipples, which had cracked and widened, rather than new ones. Finally, another parent had good luck purchasing near-new bottles from other cleft parents on Facebook support groups—at steep bargains compared to the retail price. She used that method as her primary way to buy bottles.

Parents Say: Thumbs-Up. Clara described feeding as the most challenging issue she faced with her son shortly after his birth—in part due to a lack of education from the staff at her local birthing hospital. "The hospital sent him home with a regular bottle and said that he would get the hang of it!" she exclaimed. Unsurprisingly, he did not get the hang of it. After about four weeks, Clara's son had lost a lot of weight and become dehydrated, prompting a warning from his pediatrician that he might need to return to the hospital. "We were already so frustrated," Clara said. "We had an eighteen-month-old at home and this new baby that would not stop crying." Finally, the pediatrician put in a special call to the plastic surgeon on the family's cleft team who had not planned to meet with the family until the baby was six weeks old. The family visited the team the next day. "We got our first Haberman and learned how to feed him," Clara said. "Then, he was a different child."

While this transformation might have occurred with another available cleft bottle, Clara found the Haberman easy to use. She also appreciated knowing that it had come recommended by the team and would be adaptable over time and during different stages of her son's cleft treatment. Many other parents feel the same way. While some admit that they can't get the knack of reading a baby's cues and have difficulties teaching secondary caregivers to do so as well, others find it relatively straightforward to use and even enjoyable. "At first I thought, 'Our hands are going to be tired if we use this bottle!'" commented another parent. But she also appreciated the element of caregiver participation. "I liked doing the squeezing myself," she continued. "Holding him and looking at him and feeding him…[the experience] didn't feel all that different than it had with my older son, whom I nursed." Some of these criteria are personal—one person's frustration may be another person's pleasure. But to this mother, the assisted delivery element of the Haberman felt special, even helping her bond with her baby.

Bottom Line. The Haberman bottle is expensive. It may offer features that babies do not need. It requires training for caregivers. Still, many parents and professionals find this bottle easy to use and extremely convenient to adapt as a baby undergoes various stages of treatment and growth during her first year.

. . . .

The Pigeon Bottle
by Respironics

Common Nickname: "The Pigeon"

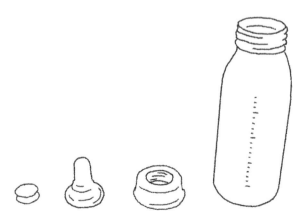

How It Works. Unlike the Mead Johnson and Haberman bottles, the Pigeon Bottle is *infant-directed.* There is no squeezing to do here, tired caregivers! The baby brings the milk into her mouth herself by compressing the nipple of the bottle—offering parents, grandparents, babysitters, older siblings, day-care providers, and others an opportunity to feed the baby with ease.

The Pigeon Bottle has four parts: a nipple (which comes in two sizes), a one-way valve, a collar, and a standard-size bottle. While the nipple of the Pigeon does not appear elongated and New Agey like the nipple of the Haberman, it has a unique design that includes a special Y-cut at the tip, an air vent, and weighted walls. The heavy, hard side of the nipple goes on top when you insert it into the baby's mouth, just under her nose. The lighter, soft side, which allows for easy compression, goes on the bottom. The caregiver can control how fast the milk flows from this bottle by tightening or loosening the collar at the base of the nipple; the looser the collar, the faster the flow.

Where to Get It and Cost. Pigeon bottles are available through major online vendors for somewhere between $13 and $25 per bottle. The larger (standard size) of the two Pigeon nipples can be ordered separately online as well for about $11. According to the Cleftopedia site, a wonderful resource for cleft products and information, the Pigeon nipple is available in a clear-colored silicone version or in a gold-colored latex version. Many parents prefer the clear version, the site authors report, because "it is more durable and collapses less" than the other nipple. This bottle, like other cleft-palate feeders, is sometimes covered by insurance companies as "durable medical equipment."

If you are hoping to acquire a Pigeon Bottle or two for free from your birthing hospital, you may be out of luck. Parents and cleft-team nurses have noticed that hospitals tend to carry the Mead Johnson and Haberman bottles instead of the newer cleft bottles (such as the Pigeon and Dr. Brown's) because the assisted-delivery options tend to work for a range of special feeding needs beyond CLP. Still, it can never hurt to ask the hospital staff whether they carry it. One mother received three free Pigeon nipples this way.

Parents and Experts Say: Leakage Aside, It Works. A majority of parents of cleft-affected babies offer positive reviews for the Pigeon Bottle. "My son loved the Pigeon," said one mother. "The nipple leaked a little bit," she added, but the issue was surmountable (see below for solutions). Feeding specialists on cleft teams have also praised this bottle. "It has a nice-sized nipple," commented one nurse. "The valve means you don't get as much air. The bottle is normal-looking. It works." Another especially liked the flexible, baby-friendly design of the weighted nipple. "The babies are in charge," she commented. Still another said that the infant-directed design of this bottle (and the Dr. Brown's) has been a game-changer for cleft babies and families, taking the stress away from feeding a child with a cleft.

Making It Work: Troubleshooting with the Pigeon. Parents and pros have mentioned a few ways to solve common problems with the Pigeon Bottle:

* **Initial Use:** While the Pigeon should not require physical adjustments to the bottle itself (the way the Mead Johnson does), this bottle may require an initial cut at first use to ensure the air vent and Y-cut are fully open.
* **Collapsed Nipple:** According to the ACPA, if the Pigeon nipple appears to collapse during use, the collar on the bottle is probably too tight. The caregiver should loosen the ring until the nipple decompresses, then resume feeding.
* **Lack of Control:** The ACPA (and many parents) suggest combining the infant-directed Pigeon nipple with the squeezable Mead Johnson bottle, so the caregiver can assist the baby if needed or desired.
* **Leakage:** To address the common issue of leakage, the Cleftopedia site (and many cleft parents) suggests combining

the Pigeon nipple with any regular bottle, including the Dr. Brown's (this option seems especially popular), the Playtex Ventaire, the Gerber, or the Parent's Choice. Other parents specifically recommend sticking with the Pigeon Bottle to prevent leaks.

- **Lack of Flow Midway through Feeding:** Clog alert! According to parents, the valve on the Pigeon Bottle can get clogged or fall out during feeding. Keep an eye out for obstructions and clean the valve, if necessary, to resume normal flow.

- **Too Much Air Intake:** The ACPA suggests combining the Pigeon nipple and valve with a vented bottle such as the Dr. Brown's bottle.

Parents and Experts Advise: Watch for Fit. While parents and cleft-team feeding specialists praise the Pigeon Bottle overall, they mention two major issues that can come up. The first relates to the size of its nipple and its adaptability—or lack thereof—over time and, in some cases, over certain forms of treatment. One mother, Kayla, had problems finding a suitable bottle for her son shortly after he was born. Her son's cleft was so wide, she explained, that a variety of special nipples didn't work—until she found the Pigeon. "He took to it like a champ," she said. To Kayla's relief, her son ate adequately within moments after trying it. A few weeks later, however, the same gloriously wide nipple that fit her son's mouth overwhelmed him in the presence of his new NAM device. "The Pigeon nipple was too big to fit into the smaller space," she said.

Other parents and cleft-team feeding specialists have described variations on Kayla's story. The Pigeon nipple (and bottle) often work wonderfully for children during early infancy, even solving initial problems with feeding. When NAM treatment begins, however, in many cases the nipples no longer fit inside their mouths. "The Pigeon nipple is great, but it is giant," commented one mother. And unfortunately, the smaller of the two Pigeon nipples doesn't always solve the problem. "The smaller one is very, very slow," explained a cleft-team nurse. In certain cases, a change in bottle is in order. So, while the Pigeon has advantages, some say it offers limited options for making adjustments to suit the baby's needs over time.

Parents and Experts Ask: Too Much Work for the Baby? Another major issue that arises for babies using the Pigeon Bottle relates to inertia. In order to draw milk from this bottle, the baby needs to compress the nipple. While the bottle does *not* require suction to pull the liquid—after all, it is designed for babies born with CLP who cannot suckle—it requires physical actions from the baby to initiate the flow. Unlike the Dr. Brown's bottle (described below), the Pigeon will not drip milk if you simply turn it upside down.

One parent switched away from the Pigeon Bottle for precisely this reason. "Sometimes my daughter gets lazy," she said. "She doesn't want to work that hard." A cleft-team nurse echoed this concern. "The Pigeon Bottle tends to work well for robust babies," she said. This bottle can be a good match, she said, if an infant is an energetic, adaptable eater and does not have physical issues beyond CLP. As she reiterated later in the conversation, the choice of bottle really depends on the particular needs and preferences of the baby.

Experts Warn: Check for Availability. Cleft-team professionals have described availability issues with the Pigeon bottle over the years and consistency problems of the product itself. "The Pigeon can be hard to get," commented one cleft-team nurse, who noted that Amazon has suspended sales, which originate from Japan, a few times within the last few years. Another pro suggested that the company has stopped distributing the bottle in the US. But families have also reported quality control problems with this bottle. "You don't always know what you are going to get in the package," commented the first cleft-team pro.

Bottom Line. While parents and professionals extol many features of the Pigeon Bottle, such as its wide nipple, weighted walls, relatively reasonable price, and in particular, its infant-directed design, they have also run into issues with leakage, lack of adaptability over time, too much work for the baby, lack of availability, and the inconsistency of the product itself.

. . . .

The Dr. Brown's Specialty Feeding System by Dr. Brown's

Common Nicknames: "The Dr. Brown's" or "The Dr. Brown"

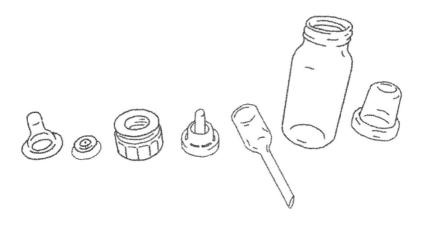

How It Works. The Dr. Brown's Specialty Feeding System, like the Pigeon Bottle, is *infant-directed*, meaning that babies can draw milk from the bottle themselves by compressing the nipple. Again, in this case, a caregiver is not required to squeeze the bottle or nipple to deliver milk into the baby's mouth.

The Dr. Brown's, to use its common nickname, offers a three-ring circus of features. In fact, to call this item a *bottle* is almost a misnomer. Technically speaking, the Dr. Brown's is labeled a *system*—and families have found that the device lives up to its name.

The bottle includes six parts: a silicone nipple (which looks like any other standard nipple); a stiff, disc-shaped infant-paced feeding valve (which fits into the nipple); a two-part internal vent system; a collar to hold it all in place; and a standard-size baby bottle. The valve, one of the costars in this show, allows a baby with a cleft palate to draw milk effortlessly—with no need to compress (or form suction). The two-piece ventilation system, which looks like a long straw inside the bottle, is designed to reduce air intake, thereby reducing problems with colic, spit-up, gas, etc.

Where to Get It and Cost. The Dr. Brown's Specialty Feeding System is sold on Amazon either as a package of two complete bottles, currently priced at around $13, or as a large starter kit that includes five full-bottle setups, travel caps/discs, wire cleaning brushes, and more, all for about $31. The starter kit is also available online through Walmart.

The Dr. Brown's starter kit includes the most commonly used nipple sizes (Level 1 and Level 2 for slow and fast flow, respectively), though the nipples themselves are available for separate purchase as Levels 1–4 and in two preemie sizes.

Parents and Experts Say: It's Easy. Parents have offered overwhelmingly positive reviews for the Dr. Brown's bottle, starting with the most common observation that this system, with its infant-directed design, is straightforward to use. "The Dr. Brown is even better than the Haberman," commented one mother about her early decision to switch her son from one bottle to the other, "because he can self-pace. He gets more enjoyment that way. It is less stressful for me too." Another mother recalled that of the four cleft-palate feeders she brought to the hospital at her daughter's birth, the Dr. Brown's seemed like the best fit for both baby and caregiver. "She took to it right away," she said. This mother described subsequent trial-and-error to determine the best-size nipple, and it turned out that her daughter needed a faster flow than she would have guessed. But before this mother knew it, her daughter was feeding with no problems.

Cleft-team nurses echo these sentiments. "You just put it together and go," commented one feeding specialist about this bottle. While she noted that the Pigeon Bottle works largely the same way as the Dr. Brown's since that bottle is also infant-directed, she praised the Dr. Brown's for being relatively cost-effective—and with the all-in-one starter kit easy to procure.

Parents and Experts Advise: Wait and See for NAM, Lip Repair. A question that comes up for any cleft-palate bottle is its adaptability over time as a baby grows and undergoes various types of treatment. NAM treatment, in particular, can change the equation with bottles and feeding. A Nasoalveolar Molding (NAM) device, as discussed later in this book (and mentioned above), is a retainer-like appliance that fits inside a baby's mouth to manipulate the segments of the upper lip, gumline, and nose before lip-repair surgery. The device is usually worn 24/7, including during feeding sessions.

Since the NAM device takes up some room physically inside the baby's mouth, it reduces the size of that space overall. The treatment itself, too, can cause discomfort. "Some babies are very sensitive to the changes in the NAM," explained one cleft-team nurse about the weekly adjustments. In some cases, a baby may refuse to eat afterward. The Haberman bottle, she noted, allows parents to adjust the flow of liquid as needed—a characteristic not readily available in infant-directed cleft bottles like the Pigeon or Dr. Brown's. "With the Haberman, you have much more control," she said. "I sometimes [recommend] it for kids who use the NAM."

The same issue can occur at the time of lip-repair surgery. One mother recalled that her son thrived with the Dr. Brown's during early infancy but then refused to use it following that operation. The infant-directed design that worked so well initially became too demanding and even appeared painful following this procedure, she explained. At that point, this mother switched her son to the

Haberman. Other babies, on the other hand, do wonderfully with the Dr. Brown's over time and through various types of treatment, some even preferring it to other bottles.

It is clear that the Dr. Brown's bottle works well for some babies over time—but does not work for everyone. If your baby is sensitive to physical changes in general, it might be helpful to keep more than one type of bottle on hand and to be flexible with feeding methods as time goes on.

Making It Work: Troubleshooting with the Dr. Brown's. Parents and pros have mentioned a few ways to solve common problems with the Dr. Brown's bottle:

- **Leakage:** While the instructions for the Dr. Brown's system indicate that the bottle should not leak if assembled properly, some parents have found the bottle finicky. One mother admitted that, technically speaking, the bottle did not leak—but only if it was assembled absolutely perfectly. The company advises caregivers to loosen the collar to stop leaks. Parents recommend making repeated adjustments (and having patience) to get the cap just right.

- **Lack of Control:** One parent praised the infant-directed nipple of the Dr. Brown's bottle but wanted to give her infant more assistance. She had good luck assembling the Dr. Brown's nipple with the Mead Johnson bottle and keeping the parts in place with a simple, generic Gerber cap (from a regular, commercially available baby bottle).

- **Slowdowns with Breast Milk:** Perhaps the most pressing complaint with the Dr. Brown's comes from mothers who pump breast milk. "Every person's milk has different fat content," explained one such mother, Lisa. When she filled the Dr. Brown's bottle with breast milk, its long, straw-like ventilation peg would get clogged with milk fat. "My daughter would be drinking and drinking, and the level wouldn't be changing," she said. Eventually, Lisa realized that she needed to open the bottle mid-feed to clean it out—every time she fed the baby. While she praised the Dr. Brown's overall and was pleased to find this solution, she described the constant interruptions as bothersome.

Parents' Tip for Making It Work: Experiment with Auto Drip. One of the major distinctions between the Pigeon and Dr. Brown's bottles is the amount of work required to draw milk from the nipple. If you were to fill both bottles with liquid and turn them upside down, the Pigeon would not leak—since its Y-cut nipple requires compression to draw liquid. The Dr. Brown's, on the other hand, would dribble milk all over the place. Now according to parents and professionals, this auto-drip feature can be either a bother *or* a boon to babies, based on personal preference (as discussed above). Some infants find the trickly flow of milk annoying or overwhelming when it hits the back of their throats, while others seem to find it easy to adapt to. One mother described the Dr. Brown's as a perfect match for her son following lip-repair surgery, in particular, when his mouth was sore and sensitive. The liquid dripped out readily, she recalled, just at a moment when he needed all the help he could get.

If you are curious about experimenting with these two types of flow, you do not need to switch bottles to do so. The website Cleftopedia has offered a cool tip. The Dr. Brown's company, the site authors explain, offers a Y-cut nipple that does not emit milk unless compressed—just like the Y-cut Pigeon nipple. This nipple is not marketed for cleft babies and is sold separately from the Specialty System (you can find it on Amazon), but the nipple is standard size and compatible.

Parents Say: It Doesn't Look Like a Spaceship. The appearance of the Dr. Brown's bottle has not gone unnoticed by parents, many of whom appreciate its typical, "just like any other baby bottle" design. One mother actually doubted the effectiveness of this bottle, at first, because as she watched her son drink from it, the activity looked so subtle that she couldn't tell whether he was consuming any liquid. Soon thereafter, when she turned the bottle the other way up to measure the contents, she realized that he had taken in quite a bit of formula. "I cried when that happened," she said. "I realized that my baby could use a normal-looking bottle! Now we won't get stared at when we're in a doctor's office." While some parents find the Mead Johnson and Haberman bottles fun and funky-looking, others don't want to stand out in a crowd. As parents and nurses have noted, the Dr. Brown's (like the Pigeon) looks like many other commercially available options.

Bottom Line. While parents and nurses most often praise the Dr. Brown's for being easy to use—particularly as a result of its infant-directed design—they also give it high marks for being reasonably priced, a cinch to find and purchase, typical-looking, easy to teach to others, and effective for issues with gas, reflux, and colic. Complaints relate to clogged components for babies who drink pumped breast milk as well as general issues with leakage. While some sensitive babies prefer the easy-to-control Haberman during NAM treatment or the periods following operations, the Dr. Brown's receives high praise overall from parents and professionals alike.

Other Feeding Options

The Comotomo Baby Bottle. The Comotomo Baby Bottle is a commercially available bottle that is not marketed as a cleft-palate specialty bottle but has been praised by some cleft parents as a modern update to the Mead Johnson. "These bottles answered our prayers," said one mother who had a child born with cleft palate and other physical issues that affected feeding. This very soft, squeezable, silicone bottle, which functions as an assisted-delivery bottle, is available from Amazon for about $23 for two bottles.

A NUK Nipple with a Mead Johnson Bottle. Was your baby born with a particularly wide cleft? The Pigeon Bottle is a common solution. But the cleftAdvocate site—and some cleft-team nurses—also recommend looking for a NUK brand nipple that is wide and flat, sometimes referred to as an "orthodontic" nipple, and assembling it with a Mead Johnson bottle. "We sometimes recommend this combination for kids born with wider clefts, to fill the space," explained one such nurse. This setup can also be useful for a bilateral cleft, she continued, if the middle segment is flipped forward. "It depends on the anatomy," she added. It is important to note that for this option to work, caregivers will need to add a crosscut to the nipple to release the flow of milk.

The Squeezable Nuby Bottle. According to another cleft-team feeding specialist, Nuby makes a bottle that resembles the Mead Johnson but is sold commercially and marketed for non-cleft babies. "It is a squeezable bottle that doesn't have a crosscut in the nipple," she explained. She emphasized that parents would need to add a crosscut to make this option viable for a baby with cleft palate.

The TenderCare™ Feeder and the Common Syringe. Syringe feeders, such as the TenderCare™ Feeder and the common syringe, are devices that enable a caregiver to deliver very small amounts of milk into a baby's mouth. Syringe feeders do not have anywhere near the capacity to supply a baby with liquid for everyday use. They can be extremely useful to have on hand following a baby's surgery, however, depending on the instructions from your child's surgeon (as discussed elsewhere in this book). The TenderCare™ Feeder includes a long, thin tube that attaches to a squeezable bottle; it is available in a pack of five bottles for $20 from the website Pediatric Medical Solutions. Common straw-and-plunger syringes are widely available for less than $1 each.

The Dance

Feeding a cleft-affected baby can require give-and-take. It may change over time and with different forms of treatment. The baby *will* cry. But hopefully, these tips and tricks, not to mention the input from feeding professionals and fellow parents, will come in handy for key moments—thus helping you to rest assured that your baby is eating happily and well.

Chapter 14

. . . .

Lunch Is On

How to Feed This Baby

Just as every cleft is different, so is feeding every cleft-affected baby. For some parents and babies, feeding is simply not much of an issue, logistically or emotionally. Some babies, especially those born with an isolated cleft lip, will take to the breast or the bottle and that is that. Even infants with a cleft palate may respond to a particular feeding method without much fuss. Technological advances with special bottles have come amazingly far in the last decade, enabling some lucky babies to eat relatively easily. Wonderful. Boom. Some parents are off to the races.

For others, feeding a cleft-affected baby can be a challenge—for a slew of reasons. "Feeding our son felt like trial-and-error the whole time," said one mother, describing her struggles with various bottles and nipples. "Feeding is our main job! I felt like I was messing up my main duty." Several other parents described feeding as the biggest hurdle of their first year. The task *can* be overwhelming, especially when it's two in the morning, the baby is screaming and cough-sneezing, and instead of feeling patient, alert, and optimistic about the experimentation that is sometimes necessary when addressing problems with feeding, we are steaming, desperate, and flabbergasted that the seemingly simple task of delivering food from Point A to Point B can be so elusive. I have been there myself. I surely uttered a few choice words.

Fortunately, help is available for those who need it. This chapter offers detailed instructions on how to feed a cleft-affected baby—first for those born with an isolated cleft lip and then for those with a cleft palate. It also includes tips on the ever-important issue of positioning the baby (and ourselves) and a primer on dealing with reflux. But it is important to remember that other resources abound. The feeding specialist on the cleft team, usually a clinical nurse or speech pathologist, functions largely as a teacher—and sometimes a lifesaver—by offering hands-on (and sometimes even virtual) advice. Fellow parents, too, can offer in-the-moment information via social media groups.

Feeding a Baby with an Isolated Cleft Lip

When Noelle's son, Ashton, was born in the late 1980s, she was surprised to learn the news of his isolated cleft lip. "For me it was devastating," she said, "because I had put it to rest." Having been born with CLP herself, Noelle had requested a full array of prenatal ultrasounds to find out whether she would pass on the condition to her unborn child—only to discover at her son's birth that his cleft lip had, indeed, existed but had not shown up on the scans.

The news felt like a blow. And subsequent moments only felt shakier when the medical professionals in the room somehow avoided her questions. "No one would talk to me," she said. "They didn't seem confident in their knowledge of the subject. No one seemed to know what they were talking about." As a result, the first hours of Ashton's life felt chaotic and lonely. It was only when Noelle started to breastfeed that her outlook brightened. "Feeding was actually pretty easy," she said. While Noelle felt flummoxed by the news of her son's cleft lip, she described nursing as almost a nonissue.

While any baby can have challenges with feeding—clefts or no clefts—the prognosis for a baby born with an isolated CL generally resembles that for a baby born without clefts, as was the case with baby Ashton. According to the ACPA, an infant with an isolated cleft lip will usually be able to nurse and bottle-feed normally or near normally. With the palate intact, the group explains, a baby should be able to create suction inside the mouth.

Leakage and Feel. As near typical as the feeding process may be for a baby born with an isolated cleft lip (but no cleft palate), a few challenges may arise, the most common of which relates to the leakage of air. According to one nurse specialist on a cleft team—and other professionals and parents—the physical gap of a cleft lip can cause a baby to pull in air while feeding, whether she is breast-feeding or drinking from a bottle. "Mothers should know that a baby born with cleft lip may not have a very good feel," she said. "If [feeding] seems to take too long or you hear a hissing noise, it is possible that the baby is taking in too much air."

One solution to the problem of leakage is to breast-feed, if possible. According to another clinical nurse specialist, not only is direct breast-feeding possible for a baby with a cleft lip, but it can also be advantageous as compared to bottle-feeding. "The breast will fill in the cleft," she explained. "The bottle doesn't have all that tissue and will not make as good a seal." If the baby is still leaking air while breast-feeding, a nipple shield may help. A nipple shield is a thin, silicone breast-feeding accessory that can help some babies form a better seal.

A second possible solution to the issue of air leakage, according to another cleft-team pro, is for the caregiver to use a finger or hand to gently close the baby's cleft while she is eating to seal it off—whether she is feeding from the breast or from a bottle. Finally, cleft-team nurses have recommended that breast-feeding mothers hold the baby face-up in a so-called "football hold" to see the baby as clearly as possible. (See the text box, below, for a full description-summary of tips.)

Special Bottles? If a baby with an isolated cleft lip can make a perfect seal around the nipple of a bottle and is able to create suction with the palate, she will probably be eligible to use any number of regular, commercially available baby bottles. If the cleft somehow prevents her from forming that perfect seal, however, she may benefit from a special cleft-palate bottle.

While cleft-palate bottles are plentiful and excellent these days, the choice of a suitable bottle for a baby with isolated CL will usually depend on her specific physical features. An in-person visit with the feeding specialist on the cleft team, therefore, can be very helpful (as is true for any baby born with clefts). One clinical nurse specialist described conducting frequent office visits with infants and caregivers to determine the best possible feeding solutions, noting that for babies with isolated CL, the most common issues usually relate, again, to air leakage and general inefficiency. "The anatomy of the cleft would dictate which nipple is best," she explained. Several other feeding experts mentioned the Dr. Brown's bottle as their first recommendation in such cases. According to others, a so-called *assisted delivery* bottle might be another good option (such as the Mead Johnson bottle or the Haberman). See Chapter 13 for descriptions of these special bottles.

FEEDING TIPS
For a Baby with an Isolated Cleft Lip

For Direct Breast-Feeding

Use Your Hands. According to one clinical nurse specialist on a cleft team, it can be helpful or even critical to mold the breast tissue as you breast-feed a baby with an isolated CL. "The tissue needs to fill the space of the cleft," she said.

Use Your Fingers. A well-placed finger on top of the baby's cleft may help form a seal with the breast.

Consider Using a Nipple Shield. Some lactation consultants and cleft-team feeding specialists recommend that nursing mothers use a breast or nipple shield during nursing. These soft, thin, funnel-shaped products are made of silicone or rubber and can help some babies form a good seal. (Ask a professional if this option might be helpful in your case.)

<u>Remember Peyton Manning: Consider a Football Hold.</u>
Feeding experts suggest trying a football hold for breast-feeding a baby born with a CL (the quarterback extraordinaire is rumored to have been born with a cleft lip). "A football hold is sometimes easiest for moms, at least initially, during breast-feeding," commented one nurse specialist. "They can watch the babies a bit better and fit them in a bit better." Hold the baby under your armpit, face-up.

For Bottle-Feeding

<u>Use Your Fingers.</u> A well-placed finger on top of the baby's cleft may help her form a seal with the bottle.

<u>Consider a Special-Needs Bottle.</u> If air leakage is an issue, consider using a special-needs bottle. While suction is not usually a problem for a baby born with an isolated CL, the soft nipples of these special bottles may help reduce leakage. A feeding specialist on the cleft team may be able to help.

For Direct Breast-Feeding and Bottle-Feeding

For additional advice on how to feed a cleft-affected baby, see the step-by-step instructions later in this chapter on how to bottle-feed a baby with a cleft palate. While infants with an isolated cleft lip may not face the same issues as their CLP peers, the tips from parents and pros on positioning the baby (and yourself) may come in handy.

Feeding a Baby with a Cleft Palate

The baby has arrived and she is hungry! Below is a ten-step guide to feeding a baby with a cleft palate, followed by a summary, *Feeding, In Brief*. Please don't be daunted by the number of steps; several of these activities go by quickly and will soon feel like second nature. The goal with bottle-feeding, according to the ACPA, is "to get the right amount of food, in the right amount of time, without taking in too much air." Ready to do it? Here we go.

Time to Eat

How to Bottle-Feed a Baby with Cleft Palate
STEP-BY-STEP

. . . .

STEP 1. Fill the Bottle. Is your baby waving her arms and legs all around, sucking on her fingers, sighing, cooing, or starting to cry? If so, she is probably hungry. It is time to fill a bottle. If you are using formula, the process goes as follows: measure the powder; dump it into a clean, empty bottle; add the appropriate amount of water; put on the cap; and mix. Several cleft parents have recommended swishing the bottle side-to-side as you mix rather than up and down, to avoid clogging the nipple mechanism (especially true for cleft bottles) and to keep air bubbles to a minimum.

If you are using pumped breast milk, you will need to pour some milk into the bottle—either after expressing the milk or after removing it and/or defrosting it from storage in the refrigerator or freezer. Exclusive pumpers have recommended doling out relatively small amounts at a time, reasoning that it's better to refill the bottle mid-feed than throw away hard-won milk.

How Much Formula? Be sure to ask your child's pediatrician for information on how much formula to give your baby. The usual rule, according to numerous sources, is to feed a newborn two-to-four ounces of formula per feeding session. A more specific suggestion, according to one clinical nurse specialist on a cleft team, is to calculate how many ounces of formula the baby will need to consume in one day—and then aim for that volume as you proceed through any twenty-four-hour period. The baby should take in two-and-a-half ounces of formula for every pound of body weight, the nurse said. So, if she weighs eight pounds, for example, her target consumption should be twenty ounces per day. If she weighs ten pounds, the nurse continued, she should take in twenty-five ounces per day (and so on).

Take Note! Some cleft-team pros recommend keeping a simple log to keep track of a baby's daily intake. The information will come in handy each time the baby is weighed, as the baby's pediatrician (or member of the cleft team) assesses whether she is taking in enough calories for optimal weight gain. "Some infants with clefts may need additional calories for a variety of reasons," commented the above-mentioned feeding expert, "including increased effort required for feeding." This nurse said if a baby is meeting daily goals for intake but still not gaining adequate weight, it is important to ask for extra help with nutrition and/or seek a medical or pediatric evaluation.

. . . .

STEP 2. Wrap Up and Pat Down. After you've prepped a bottle, it is important to take a minute or so to help the baby relax and prepare for the experience ahead. One clinical nurse specialist on a cleft team recommended two quick steps.

First, you'll want to wrap the baby tightly. "When infants are hungry, their arms are flailing, and they want to grab on to your breast or the bottle," this specialist explained. Swaddling calms a baby down and prevents her from feeling frustrated. As another feeding expert, Allyson Goodwyn-Craine, suggests in an article on this topic, this creates "trunk stability," making breathing easier for the baby while she eats. Swaddling also allows a caretaker to concentrate on the task at hand, without the baby's hands getting in the way. In order to swaddle, you'll need to wrap the baby with a soft blanket or sheet, like a burrito, with her head sticking out of the top.

Then, it's time for a little burp—also to calm the baby. A mini-burping session can go any number of ways, but this nurse specialist suggested pressing a middle finger or thumb down the length of the baby's back. "If you run your finger just below the rib cage," she continued, "you can feel the baby's stomach. If it feels full, give it a little massage to get rid of the air." A gentle pat on the back may also do the trick. The key is for the baby to get rid of any excess air before eating—and for a caregiver to remember to pay attention to air and gas more generally during the feeding session.

. . . .

STEP 3. Get Comfortable. As easy and logical as it may feel to focus on the baby before and during a feeding session, it is important for us, as caretakers, to attend to ourselves during this time too—and specifically, to do things to stay calm. One nurse specialist advised sitting on a comfortable chair or couch. Have lots of pillows, she advised. Take some deep breaths. "Just as with any baby, you want it to be a relaxed time. The baby will feel that." Fellow parents mention the same idea. "It is only stressful if you make it stressful," commented one mother. "If you learn to relax, they relax. They read your feelings." As convenient as it may feel to skip this step— especially if the baby is crying and eager to eat—it is also true that the more we can do to feel calm ourselves the easier it will be for the baby to follow suit.

. . . .

STEP 4. Position the Baby. Next, you'll want to situate the baby and yourself. Physical positioning is one of the keys to success in feeding a baby with a cleft palate. The goal is to minimize milk coming out of her nose (called *nasal regurgitation*). Regurgitation is usually not painful for the baby, but specialists often recommend minimizing it for the sake of efficiency and general comfort.

While there are many options for positioning a cleft-affected baby during feeding—we'll cover some specific positions below— the most common rule is to keep her upright. "You need the gravity to get the milk to go down instead of out the nose," explained one cleft-team nurse. Another professional suggested thinking of the upright position in terms of how and where the milk will land inside the baby's mouth. "The milk should go into the baby's mouth as a series of squirts—not a stream," she said. "It should land at the back of the mouth, where it can be directly swallowed." Still another expert advises parents to position the baby upright—but not too upright. The baby's head and shoulders should not be positioned directly over the hips and legs (as if she is somehow standing up) until she is about four months old, this expert writes.

Don't worry if it takes some time to find the best arrangement. Specific positioning will depend on the baby and caregiver. As mentioned elsewhere in this book, learning to feed a baby is a process.

Bonus Prep! Another feeding specialist added a final trick to ready the baby. "Sometimes just before putting the bottle in the mouth at the beginning of the session," she said, "I give them a knuckle to suck on, to get him started." The knuckle acts as a jumpstart, of sorts.

. . . .

STEP 5. *Prime the Nipple and Position It.* Before you insert any nipple into the baby's mouth, it should be full of milk (not air). You'll want to prime it by giving it a small squeeze and turning the bottle upside down. When you let go and return the bottle to an upright position, milk should fill the nipple.

It is also important to consider the position of the nipple inside the baby's mouth. Ready for a mini-lesson on the mechanics of feeding? One feeding specialist on a cleft team suggested that all babies use three mechanisms to feed: *suction, compression*, and *tongue movements*. Suction (the ability to form a seal in the mouth) is almost always compromised or eliminated when a baby is born with a cleft palate, as previously discussed. Compression (the way a baby presses on a nipple when feeding) can be altered when a baby has a cleft palate, on account of her unique anatomy.

This brings us to tongue movement. Some new parents may be surprised to learn that a newborn's tongue will "naturally cup the nipple," as the nurse specialist (above) commented. So, you'll want to help the baby along by placing the nipple of the bottle in the center of the tongue (as medical people sometimes say, on its "midline.") At the very least, you'll want to position the nipple downward, toward the tongue, and *away* from the space of the cleft palate, if possible. "Often the nipple will want to shift into the region of the cleft and off to the side," the nurse commented. "A parent will need to actively ensure the nipple remains midline and does not sit in the clefted area."

. . . .

STEP 6. *Feed for Fifteen Minutes.* Now it is time to feed the baby for fifteen minutes, more or less, with the baby in an upright position. You'll want to put the nipple in the baby's mouth, as described above, and either squeeze it rhythmically to release milk (for the Mead Johnson or Haberman bottles) or allow the baby to compress the nipple at her own pace (for the Pigeon or Dr. Brown's bottles). The ACPA advises keeping any bottle tilted so the nipple is always filled with milk. As you feed her, watch for her cues. Are you following her *suck-swallow-breathe* rhythms? Is she getting just the right amount of milk?

Suck-Swallow-Breathe: "Suck, Swallow, Breathe" is a baby's feeding reflex; it is sometimes referred to by feeding specialists as "Suck-Swallow." Take a look at your baby's physical motions when she eats. The motions usually look like this: *suck, suck, pause.* These are the behaviors to notice and follow when feeding her, in particular when using a so-called *assisted delivery* bottle like the Mead Johnson or Haberman. (The other cleft-palate bottles do not require you to pay such close attention to the baby's suck-swallow because they are designed to allow the baby to feed at her own pace). Remember: this activity is a dance. If you are using the Mead Johnson or the Haberman, you should squeeze the bottle (or nipple) in a rhythmic way to match the baby's cues. When she stops, you should stop, too.

Heads Up! It is important to note that a baby may follow a slightly different suckling pattern during the first few days of life. According to the ACPA, many babies omit the resting stage at first. "Most babies will figure this out within a few days and develop their own rhythm of sucking, swallowing, and resting," the group states.

Too Much Milk: If the baby is getting too much milk, she will let you know by coughing, spitting, choking, gulping, gasping, or showing "stress cues," as one cleft nurse mentioned, such as getting watery eyes or a pulling away from the nipple. If you are using an assisted-delivery bottle like the Mead Johnson or Haberman, you are probably squeezing too hard or not fully letting go of the bottle in between squeezes. If you're using an infant-directed bottle like the Pigeon or Dr. Brown's, you'll need to adjust the mechanism of the bottle to release less milk or switch to a slower nipple.

Not Enough Milk: If the baby is not getting enough milk, she may look strained or frustrated. Squeeze a little harder or adjust the bottle to increase the flow. You don't want the baby to eat too slowly because she'll run out of energy before she takes in enough calories (more on this topic below). Also, keep in mind that increasing the flow of milk often comes with the added benefit of reducing the amount of air a baby swallows—provided you don't go too far and give her too much (see above). As cleft-team pros have commented, the amount of milk—not too much, not too little—can be a delicate balance.

. . . .

STEP 7. Break to Burp. Burping is especially important for a baby with a cleft palate because the cleft increases the possibility that she will take in too much air during feeding. Specialists offer a variety of ideas about how this practice should fit into your routine. Some recommend burping the baby once during the feeding, about halfway through, rather than many times throughout (as outlined here). Others recommend reading the baby's signals rather than looking at the clock. "The baby will give you a cue," advised one specialist. When the pause in the baby's suck-swallow-breathe reflex gets longer, she noted, it is usually time to stop and burp. Still others recommended stopping to burp after a newborn has consumed one ounce of liquid. However you decide to work this activity into your regimen, the goal is to make sure the baby feels comfortable and gas-free while eating, for the sake of efficiency and for her own happiness.

Feel free to explore a range of techniques for the burping itself as well—from gentle circles on the back to full-on patting. On the minimalist end of that spectrum, a few cleft-team nurses recommend simply straightening the baby's spine "while lifting and supporting the chest and head to elicit a burp." According to the What to Expect site, on the other hand, "some need a slightly firmer hand." Again, every case is different. If the baby burps, you've done it right.

. . . .

STEP 8. *Feed for Fifteen More Minutes, Making Adjustments if Necessary.* According to cleft-team feeding specialists, a baby's most energetic moments usually occur at the *beginning* of a feeding session. It is common, therefore, for a baby to take in less milk and lose focus as time goes on. One nurse recommended adjusting the bottle to increase the flow of liquid during the second half of the session as the baby's energy wanes. Another recommended doing as much as possible to keep the baby engaged during this lull, even if that means removing her swaddle and stripping her clothes to keep her from falling asleep. Still another offered a cool trick: use an extra finger to tickle the baby's cheek while she eats. "I hold the end of the bottle or nipple with my forefinger and my thumb," she explained, "then I push on the cheek with my remaining finger to encourage the baby to suck or remind her to stay on task and not fall asleep." In other words, the more you do to keep the baby awake and eating, the better.

Now, if *your* attention starts to peter out toward the end of the feeding session or if you feel tempted at this point to sort your mail or call your mother—or make goo-goo faces with the baby—you might want to hold off. Nurses advise caretakers to focus on the task at hand. "This time is all about feeding," commented one nurse, "not hugging, kissing, cuddling, and loving. When you are done with thirty minutes of feeding, you can do all that other stuff."

Other specialists *do* recommend having skin-to-skin contact with your baby during the feeding session to mimic the physical bonding of breast-feeding. This is a wonderful idea that *may or may not work for you* during the session itself. If your baby benefits from swaddling (as other specialists have advised), you may or may not wish to remove the swaddle and contend with her flailing arms. Also, some babies will require more attention in general than others during feeding. If your baby is getting enough nutrition in thirty minutes (more on the thirty-minute idea below) and staying focused throughout—enabling you to also keep her close to your skin—great. Otherwise, you may need to hold off on extra cuddling until afterward.

In sum, feeding usually requires concentration. "When you are breast-feeding a baby born without clefts," commented one nurse, "you can do two things at once. When you are holding a baby with a Haberman in your hand, it is very difficult to watch that other child." The second half of a feeding session may require special attention.

. . . .

STEP 9. Stop! After *Thirty Minutes, It's All Celery.* A common rule among feeding specialists on cleft teams is that caretakers should aim for a thirty-minute feeding session—not longer. If a baby doesn't get enough milk within that time frame, commented one nurse specialist, the best thing to do is stop feeding her. "At that point, the baby is starting to use up the calories," she said, "working to get the food." In other words, she is burning more calories than she is taking in. Perhaps you've heard the old adage about eating celery, which posits that the vegetable is so low in calories and, at the same time, so fibrous that people use up more calories chewing it than they gain. The same concept applies here.

According to the ACPA, if you are feeding your baby within a thirty-minute time frame and she seems sated after taking the bottle, then all is well. If your baby seems hungry after thirty minutes, however, or simply wants to keep eating, fear not. At the *next* feeding session, you will need to make some small adjustments, either to squeeze the bottle harder or adjust the bottle mechanism to increase the amount of milk she gets each time she swallows (depending on your setup). Fortunately, the array of new bottles on the market allows for these micro-adjustments. The feeding specialist on the team can offer tips, as well.

. . . .

STEP 10. We're Done! There's More. The feeding session may be over, but now you need to make sure that the milk or formula stays inside the baby's body as she digests. "They regurgitate if they're lying down," commented one nurse, referring to a common occurrence for babies born with CP. So, the best thing to do after a feeding session, she continued, is to keep the baby upright for a bit, whether you are holding her in your arms or putting her into some sort of seat. "I'm okay with the car seat or the bouncy seat for the first few weeks," she added. If the food is staying down, you're all set.

Related Issue: Napping after Eating. As often as caregivers may hear advice from cleft-team pros to keep the baby elevated after eating, the question of keeping her elevated after eating and then while sleeping can be somewhat controversial. Another cleft-team feeding specialist advised raising the baby's head while sleeping— even in the bassinet. "You need to elevate the head of the baby's mattress," she said. Now, it is important to note that the American Academy of Pediatrics has issued recommendations *against* elevating the baby's mattress. "Elevating the head of the infant's crib is ineffective in reducing gastroesophageal reflux," the report said, "and is not recommended." The group goes on to state that elevating the head of the crib can cause the baby to slide toward the foot of the bed, possibly compromising breathing. What gives?

In this case, the answer itself goes beyond the scope of this book. The process of finding the answer, however, does not. If you hear mixed messages from your baby's practitioners—on this or any other issue—be sure to press for an explanation from your child's pediatrician and consult with members of the cleft team. In so doing, it can never hurt to ask each party about the *other's* advice. If you're still unsure about an issue, tell them so—as clearly and honestly as possible—even if you feel silly for asking again and again. Medical research and recommendations can be confusing to interpret; it is the practitioner's job to help parents navigate these murky waters.

Feeding Session, in Brief

BOTTLE-FEEDING A BABY WITH A CLEFT PALATE

- Signs of hunger? Prepare a bottle.
- Briefly relax the baby and yourself: swaddle the baby and get into a comfortable seat. Do a little burp. Let her suck on your knuckle for a moment.
- Position the baby to minimize milk coming out of the nose. Upright is usually best.
- Prime the nipple of the bottle.
- Feed with the bottle for ten-to-fifteen minutes, with the baby in an upright position and the nipple positioned away from the cleft palate. Read her cues!
- Break to burp.
- Feed with the bottle for another ten-to-fifteen minutes. Stay focused! Keep the baby alert. Increase the flow from the bottle, if necessary, as the baby tires.
- At thirty minutes, stop.
- After the baby is done eating: cuddle, kiss, and have skin-to-skin contact. Keep her in an upright position.

POSITIONING
Ways to Hold the Baby during Bottle-Feeding

Now, what about sitting? Cleft pros and parents have offered several ideas for holding a baby during feeding, all of which involve keeping her in an upright position. The goal, as you experiment with these options, might be to find an arrangement that is comfortable for you and the baby while minimizing regurgitation (for the baby!). But none of these suggestions are hard-and-fast. Have fun with it.

The Upright Rock-a-Bye. For this position, you should start by holding the baby in a classic rock-a-bye-baby position; the baby should be lying in your arms, facing up. Next, slowly slide her body up one arm into a sitting position, so that her head is leaning against your upper arm. You can hold her in place by grabbing the front side of her leg with your active hand—so that you are essentially holding her entirely with one arm. "When you start in the lying down position and move to sitting," explained one nurse, "it helps to orient the baby. Then, after you get that down, you can put your hands anywhere." The goal, she continued, is for the baby to be sitting up while she eats. Another feeding specialist emphasized grabbing the thigh. "If you hold the baby by the thigh," she said, "it gives the caregiver control and tucks the baby in. This way, they are sitting in the crook of your arm and are positioned upright."

Facing You, with Your Legs Crossed. One feeding specialist described the way many men sit with their legs crossed openly. "When guys do a feeding," she said, "they tend to put them up on their knee, facing them. This is a good way to do it." Start by sitting in a chair and crossing your leg widely, with the calf or ankle of your bent leg resting on the knee of your upright leg. Then place the baby into the crook of your bent knee, facing you. "The baby should always be positioned so the chest is higher than the stomach and the head higher than the chest," this nurse continued. "It doesn't have to be bolt upright but definitely on an angle." You may need to use one of your arms to cradle the baby's head and shoulders.

Another specialist suggested several advantages of having the baby in a facing-you position. "When you are face-to-face with a baby, you are interacting with the baby," she said. "You can watch him, and he can watch you. You can see his cues. Babies respond well to that."

Facing You, Using a Footstool. While several feeding specialists have enthusiastically recommended the idea of holding the baby in such a way that she is both positioned upright and facing you, one added a suggestion to do so with the help of a small footstool, which elevates the caregiver's legs and relieves pressure on their arms. "Your seat must be comfortable," she emphasized. "That's important. The little footstool really helps." Whether you use a footstool or an openly crossed leg—or some other position—many parents and professionals recommend finding a comfortable, upright position that allows for face-to-face interactions.

The Chin-Lift. This *Chin Lift* relates to the position of a baby's head. A few cleft nurses recommend using a spare finger or thumb to actually lift the chin of the baby while she eats, in coordination with her sucking motions. "This is subtle," commented speech pathologist Allyson Goodwyn-Craine, about this feeding position. "The head should not be extended," she advised, but the chin should be lifted from the neck by about the distance of one finger for a newborn and two fingers for an older infant.

One mother tried this technique while using the Haberman bottle. "I used one finger to lift her chin while two other fingers squeezed the nipple," she said. "Talk about hand cramps!" She admitted that the position did not feel even the slightest bit comfortable—but it did the trick. "I'm not sure why this worked so well for Eva," she continued, "but she ate great this way." If your baby seems to eat more efficiently and happily with her chin lifted, wonderful. And if you can figure out a way to accomplish that position without injuring your hands, all the better.

Do Whatever Works for You. The positions listed above are yours to pick and choose among—or vary or reject—as you see fit. "I don't try to lock people into one method or the other when it comes to positioning the baby," commented one cleft-team nurse. "All of this is so stressful, anyway." We all have different bodies and preferences. When my daughter was a baby, I tended to feed her while seated on the floor in a crisscross-applesauce position (I was younger and less creaky then). The arrangement might have resembled the Seated-with-Legs-Crossed position combined with the Rock-a-Bye...but maybe not. The details aren't as important as the fact that the position felt comfortable. My daughter ate more or less contentedly and didn't spit up too much. I didn't get injured from the repetitive sessions or otherwise end up in physical therapy. Whatever method works best for you and your baby is the best one.

Traffic Detour: Wrong Way!
The Lowdown on Regurgitation, Spit-Up, Burps, and Reflux

Is your baby spitting up formula? Is milk coming out of her nose? Are liquids and air colliding and emerging from her body in ways, locations, and times that surprise you? It is important for parents of babies with CLP to know that fluids may frequently come *out* of our babies even as we think they are supposed to be going (or staying) *in*. Liquidy, drippy, and otherwise wet noses and mouths are not only common, but sometimes dramatic, and accompanied by burps or cough-sneezes. If you were to consider investing in a year-long supply of burp cloths or traditional cloth diapers to drape over your shoulder to protect your clothing, I would not stand in your way. But these wrong-way types of events, while common for babies with CP, can vary widely. It may be helpful to know about two common occurrences, so that you will be able to know how—

and whether—to react (other than by washing your shirts). Let's take a look at *esophageal reflux* and *nasal regurgitation*.

WRONG-WAY EVENT No. 1: Reflux. The first liquid-related, wrong-way event that can happen for a cleft-affected baby occurs when food that has already entered the stomach comes back up. It's called *esophageal reflux, gastroesophageal reflux*, or sometimes simply *reflux*. According to the Mayo Clinic, it is common for the *lower esophageal sphincter*, the ring of muscles that separates the esophagus from the stomach, to be underdeveloped in infants. When those muscles are weak, the food can turn around relatively easily. Basically, this sphincter is supposed to act as a traffic officer of the GI system, directing the food along as it flows through the intersection, as if to say, "Keep going, keep going, straight ahead, that's right." When that muscle doesn't function as it should, the traffic—i.e., the food—backs up. According to an article by cleft-team nurses in the Losee-Kirschner medical textbook, esophageal reflux can occur especially often in babies with clefts because their sphincter muscles may be weak, *and* they often swallow a lot of air while eating.

Everyday Reflux or Painful Reflux? Now that we've established that *reflux* refers to liquids that have traveled to the stomach and back, it is important to distinguish between the two ways reflux can play out. First, it can occur in a typical, everyday way, coming out of the mouth or nose as garden-variety spit-up. Spit-up happens all the time with babies—clefts or no clefts, but probably more often for babies with clefts—and can cause a lot of liquid mess but usually no pain. According to the Mayo Clinic and other sources, this type of reflux is normal and not a sign that a parent has overfed a child. And as we'll explore below, the liquid associated with spit-up can come out of a baby's mouth *or* out of a cleft-affected baby's nose. Caregivers should try to minimize it, nurses advise. But generally speaking, the occurrence is usually not bothersome to the baby.

Sometimes, however, reflux can be painful for a baby, usually because the partially digested food that comes back up the digestive tract can be highly acidic. According to the National Institute of Health, parents should look for signs such as vomiting, irritability, arching of the back (during or following feeding), coughing, refusal to feed, or poor weight gain. If you suspect your baby is experiencing painful reflux, which may be a sign of GERD (*gastroesophageal reflux disease*), be sure to talk with your child's pediatrician or with a pro on the cleft team. According to a study published in the *Cleft Palate and Craniofacial Journal*, GERD can be common in cleft babies—as many as 9 percent of infants born with CLP experience GERD as compared to less than 1 percent of the general population, the study says. Fortunately, a doctor can help address this issue, sometimes by prescribing medications.

WRONG-WAY EVENT No. 2: Quick Escapes. Now, let's talk about *nasal regurgitation*. Nasal regurgitation occurs when something comes out of a baby's nose, usually a liquid such as breast milk or formula. In some cases, the liquid that comes out of the nose has already been to the stomach—i.e., reflux. In other cases, nasal regurgitation occurs because of the hole(s) in the baby's palate or gumline. A substance enters the mouth, takes a quick turn, and emerges from the nose shortly thereafter, *without* having traveled to the stomach. Put another way, the path of the liquid can vary.

According to one feeding specialist on a cleft team, it is common for nasal regurgitation—of any variety—to occur during a feeding session if a baby takes in too much milk at once, or if she lies down right after a meal before she's had a chance to digest.

Nasal regurgitation is usually not dangerous, but it may be alarming. Some describe it as picturesque. But as one cleft team nurse commented, "You need to know that it can't hurt the baby. It is worse for you, but it is not harmful to the baby." Unless the baby is in pain, these occurrences are fine, even adorable. We can pack our diaper bags with endless burp cloths and then exhale.

Wrong-Way Digestive Events
IN BRIEF

What is coming out of the baby's MOUTH? Possibilities include:	What is coming out of the baby's NOSE? Possibilities include:
NORMAL SPIT-UP (everyday reflux that is not painful) or PAINFUL SPIT-UP (bothersome reflux that may indicate GERD)	NORMAL SPIT-UP (everyday reflux that is not painful) or PAINFUL SPIT-UP (bothersome reflux that may indicate GERD) or LIQUIDS or SOLIDS that escape through the nose immediately upon consumption, without traveling to the stomach

What to Do? If you are concerned about wrong-way digestive events, the best thing to do, as always, is to talk to a professional. In the meantime, cleft-team pros advise parents to try to avoid these events during feeding, particularly liquid that comes out of the nose. One nurse mentioned a slight risk that the baby could choke on (*aspirate*) some of that milk. She also explained that babies can become frustrated over the long term if milk comes out of the nose all the time instead of going down the throat. "They start getting more fussy about feeding," she said, "and don't want to work for it as much."

Fortunately, everyday reflux is usually readily solvable with methods you probably already know. First, you can follow the baby's cues while she eats so that she gets the right amount of food at the right time—not too little, not too much. "It's all about the suck-swallow-breathe," advised another nurse specialist on a cleft team. "You need to follow the baby's cues and behavior while you feed her." Also, you can keep the baby upright, she added. The more you can do to keep the baby's head and neck elevated, the better.

. . . .

It can be challenging to solve problems with feeding, whether we are investigating possible issues with reflux, air intake, bottle setup, positioning, or myriad other possible health or life circumstances. In some cases, we may need time, persistence, and professional help—even several times—to get to the bottom of an issue. Feeding a cleft-affected baby can be a doozy. Fortunately, resources abound. Professionals on the cleft team and other parents (and book authors!) are here to help.

Chapter 15

. . . .

But I Had Planned to Breast-Feed!

Nursing, Bonding, and the Flip Side

When we as parents learn the news of our baby's cleft lip and/or palate, we also find out that direct breast-feeding is probably not going to be possible. A cleft palate prevents a baby from forming a complete seal of the oral cavity, all but eliminating her chances of suckling at the breast. Medical people sometimes make the analogy of trying to draw liquid through a straw that has a hole in it: it doesn't work.

The loss of breast-feeding can mean a lot of different things to different people. Some mothers feel okay when they learn that they cannot nurse. Maybe they weren't planning on it anyway. The news may not be that big a deal. Thank goodness! Some adoptive parents and other parents, too, may have come to terms with feelings about nursing, even before they learned about their baby's CLP.

For others, particularly mothers, there is sadness, even grief. This news may mark the loss of a lifelong vision or at least a long-term assumption about our choices for our body and our baby. With cleft palate in the picture, mothers lose that choice. "Part of the relationship I'd dreamed of for nine months was over," writes Jessica Burfield, who, after six days of trying unsuccessfully to nurse her newborn, finally learned of her daughter's cleft-palate diagnosis. She realized she would never be able to nurse her baby.

"I couldn't believe how much it broke my heart" she said. "I cried and cried and cried over what I would never have."

What is this loss about? And what are some ways to move forward?

For the majority of parents I have spoken with, the act of breast-feeding offers two main opportunities: for a baby's nutrition and for mother-baby bonding. Decisions about a baby's nutrition—the choice between formula and breast milk—are personal, and in the case of cleft palate, unique. Many parents of babies with cleft palate choose to use formula. The few mothers who can pump milk and choose to do so—those heroic few—face all kinds of challenges (See more on this topic in the next chapter).

The loss of breast-feeding also means the loss of a fundamental way for mothers to bond with their babies—during the first year of life, no less, when a cleft-affected baby faces all kinds of special hurdles. If anything, parents and babies need *extra* opportunities for bonding during that time. "It is so heartbreaking," commented one cleft-team nurse. "Parents come to me and first, their world is kind of falling apart because they just learned about the clefts. Then you tell them about breast-feeding. It is just awful."

Sometimes, there is loneliness. One mother, Heather, recalled that her friends were having babies at around the same time. "All of them were nursing," she said. "It was hard to deal with accepting not being able to breast-feed. It was also hard not having anybody I could really talk with about not nursing, because all my friends were nursing." Just at a time when Heather needed someone to lean on to cope with these feelings, the people in her support network were engaging in the very activity that stoked her sense of loss.

Partners can feel it too. When I mentioned the question of nursing to one dad, he responded with immediate recognition, as if the topic were still fresh on his mind. "Our son is eight years old," he said, "and my wife and I still talk about this one." As a self-described hands-on parent, this father tried to do all he could to help his wife and baby during the early days after their son's birth. His wife, Cheryl, tried to nurse, he explained. But she seemed intensely frustrated by the failed attempts. "I felt helpless," he admitted. And her feelings—like those of so many other mothers—radiated to her intimate relationships.

Fortunately, researchers have studied the feeding and bonding activities of parents and their cleft-affected babies. A recent study shows that feeding a cleft-affected baby can cause great concern and frustration for parents, particularly during the first few days after birth. These difficulties can cause mothers to feel incompetent and can disrupt bonding with their babies during those first few days. Other studies show that mothers with cleft-affected infants feel less secure about their relationship with their babies and are more likely to show symptoms of post-traumatic stress and depression (see Chapter 11 for a broader discussion of bonding.)

When I first read these conclusions, I almost laughed out loud. If those researchers had been at our house during the first week after my daughter's birth, studying our feelings and behaviors with clipboards in hand, they would have had an easy time detecting those very emotions. We were totally stressed out! Did we have difficulties with feeding? Unfortunately, yes. Did I feel incompetent as a result? Absolutely, I did. Check! Check! All of the above.

Fortunately, there is a flip side to this coin. Research shows that the presence of a cleft and/or feeding difficulties do not affect the mother-infant bond at all over the long term—meaning months rather than weeks or days—as compared to the bonds of mothers with unaffected babies. In fact, scholars state that mothers of babies with clefts may even bond *more* with their infants than mothers of unaffected babies. And this bonding occurs without the mothers having nursed their babies! Caregivers may perceive their cleft-affected infants as especially needy, one study suggests, "leading to heightened activation of the 'attachment system' and caregiving behaviors that foster early secure attachment." We realize our baby needs extra help, in other words, and we develop a soft spot for her. This, too, is good news.

So, in the end, the loss of breast-feeding does not mean that we mothers lose a chance to bond with our babies; it's that we lose a chance to bond with our babies *this way.* And by extension, we lose an experience within our own bodies that facilitates that bonding. As much as I hate to say it, this loss is unique and cannot be taken back. But as any adoptive parent will tell you—or any partner or spouse, for that matter, who cares for a baby but does not nurse—there are many routes up the mountain. Skin-to-skin contact is an oft-discussed way to facilitate bonding, as is the simple but meaningful act of gazing into a baby's eyes. We can wear our babies on our chests. We can play with their feet or let them squeeze our fingers. And just wait until they smile! The opportunities are there, everywhere.

Also, there are ways to cope with this loss in the short term. The first is to honor the sad feelings. The American Cleft Palate-Craniofacial Association (ACPA) recommends: "Give yourself time and space to grieve this loss." Cleft specialists suggest seeking help from the professionals on a cleft team, particularly with feeding, but also with coping. One nurse recommended accepting help (even if we resist that idea) from friends and family with meals, cleaning, and other things, during the early days and weeks. While those forms of assistance do not necessarily relate to nursing or feeding the baby, they give us valuable time and space to clear our minds and work through our feelings. Last, we can cope by leaning on sympathetic friends and supportive people, particularly the ones who are good listeners (even if they happen to be nursing, themselves).

The feelings of sadness and grief may not go away for a while. And the stress of learning to feed the baby is real. At the same time, it might be comforting to know that despite all of the difficult feelings and stressful moments, bonding need not be diminished over the long term. Not by one tiny bit.

Chapter 16

. . . .

What's for Dinner?

Formula or Breast Milk:
Choices and Challenges

O f all the hotly debated topics related to parenting, few are so ripe for argument or so notoriously touchy as what to feed a baby. If the subject were to come up over Thanksgiving dinner (where some of the juiciest conversations take place within families), I'm sure I would break into a cold sweat, realizing that a friend or family member—let's name her Aunt Margo—has just caught a glimpse of the powdered formula peeking out from our diaper bag, that one of *those* conversations is about to take place. And I would hope, just as she frowns and remarks, "Oh, so you decided not to breast-feed?" that a tornado would suddenly hit the house or even a small kitchen fire might erupt, burning the potatoes but thankfully preventing her from going on to boast about how she breast-fed each of her three children thirty years ago and wouldn't you know that cousin Jimmy just won a promotion to senior vice president.

These conversations can be lively. And they can arise, in one form or another, at the doctor's office, where at the outset of a postnatal visit, a medical person asks parents a seemingly routine but obviously weighty question regarding the method they use to feed their baby: "Bottle or breast?" The moment illustrates why this topic deserves a spot on a top-twenty list of touchy parenting subjects, because not only is the question itself difficult to answer for some parents from a technical standpoint (more on this later)

188

but interwoven in our explanations can be feelings related to our personal identity. In considering what to feed a baby, we tap tender topics related to gender roles, the capacity and value of our bodies, our choices regarding time and resources, our obligations to nurture a child, our engagement with current scientific research, our response to opinions of all kinds—and in the case of CLP, our own baby's ability to feed from the breast.

Fortunately, not all parents feel sensitive about this topic. Not everyone wants to retort, "But the baby CAN'T breast-feed! She has a cleft palate! And can't you see it's complicated?" to metaphorical Aunt Margo—and in so doing, maybe choke up. But many do. And to make matters worse, we confront this issue when we feel exhausted and sort of loopy, either from childbirth or from the period of parenting that follows.

When a baby is born with CLP, parents face the immediate need to feed her. In this chapter, we will examine the question of what to put in a baby bottle, including a review of the options, a primer on exclusive pumping, some information from scientific research, and some stories of what other parents have done (and how they felt about it). Hopefully, this information will help with decision-making and just as important, peace of mind—first, in working through the options privately, and then going out into the world with our powdered formula and/or breast pumps to interact with the Aunt Margos (and others) in our lives. To be sure, there is no single, best answer to the question, *What's for dinner?* The ideal solution is the one that feels comfortable, desirable, and healthy for everyone involved.

What Are the Options?

When a baby is born with a cleft palate, professionals on cleft teams usually inform parents of the unlikeliness that she will be able to feed directly from the breast. A hole in the roof of the mouth, the pros say, prevents a baby from forming enough suction to draw milk from the breast (or for that matter, from a regular baby bottle).

I can imagine that if you are processing this news—even if you have heard it before—you might be wondering exactly *how* unlikely they mean. I sure did. After experiencing years of infertility, adopting our first child, and building up my hopes for breast-feeding our second (biological, cleft-affected) child, I wondered whether there might be some wiggle room or even a flicker of hope behind that "unlikely." The pros rarely say, "impossible," after all. And occasionally, someone cries out, "Yeah, but!" in an online discussion group, exclaiming, "I breast-fed my baby with a cleft palate!"

Those individuals may appear to speak LOUDLY in those comment boxes. Their excitement can be palpable, even infectious. But they have also won the breast-feeding lottery. One clinical nurse specialist on a high-volume cleft team commented that during her decades-long career, she has met only two mothers who were able to breast-feed a baby with a cleft palate. "They were both tandem nursing," she explained, "which means that they were also feeding another baby at the same time, a baby without a cleft." This situation can be the case with twins, she said, where if you feed one baby from one breast, the other breast leaks. "These were extremely unusual cases," she said. This news isn't always easy to handle. Some parents, mothers especially, feel deep disappointment and loss (as discussed elsewhere in this book).

Knowing it is highly unlikely an infant with a cleft palate will feed directly from the breast, parents are left with one or two options for feeding the baby, both of which involve using a bottle—infant formula or, if possible, expressed (pumped) breast milk.

Option 1: Formula. Infant formula, the powder sold in a can (or sometimes premixed in individually portioned, disposable bottles found in some birthing hospitals), can be purchased at almost any place that sells food, both in person and online. With formula, you measure the powder, dump it into the empty bottle, add the appropriate amount of water, and mix. Voila. Anyone can do it—

and by anyone, I mean partners, grandparents, babysitters, and other caregivers.

It is important to note that not everyone can *feed* a cleft-affected baby since, in many cases, this activity requires special preparation and concentration. But almost anyone can mix formula. In that regard, formula is a great equalizer. I mention these logistical details because while a discussion of "what's for dinner" often involves examining many different feelings, it also revolves around the most pragmatic of issues, such as whose body needs to be doing what activity at which time(s), for how long, and with what costs and benefits.

Option 2: Breast Milk. Another option may be to feed the baby pumped breast milk, which is referred to these days by the pros as *expressed human milk*. It is true that some women are not physically able to pump milk (or enough milk) to feed a baby, that some babies struggle to gain adequate weight from expressed breast milk alone, and that some women suffer from the after-effects of sexual trauma or other emotional or physical issues that limit their options. And of course, breast milk may be out of the question for adoptive parents and any number of other parents. So, this option may be on the table for some families but certainly not for all. *Exclusive pumping* refers to the act of using a pump, usually electric, to pull milk from a woman's breasts and then to feed the baby with a bottle in a separate sitting.

Exclusive pumping differs distinctly from direct breast-feeding or its popular cousin *supplemental pumping*. In this case, the two activities of expressing and feeding occur independently, similar to train tracks that run parallel but never cross. "If you pump, it is twice the work," commented one nurse specialist on a cleft team. So, when the intake nurse asks a new family whether they use "bottle or breast," he or she leaves out this incredibly challenging, often overlooked, or underplayed third option: both.

EXCLUSIVE PUMPING 101

Basics, Tips, and Resources

If you are considering pumping milk for your baby, here is a brief primer to give you a sense of what's involved.

Who Pumps? A biological mother pumps milk. As obvious as this answer may seem, it is critical, when examining our options, to point out exactly who will be doing what task at which time. While some parents purchase or receive donated breast milk via prescription from a milk bank, this option can be prohibitively expensive (one source estimates $3–5 per ounce). So, in most circumstances, only one person will be doing this job.

Equipment and Cost? Pumping milk requires equipment, some of it essential, some of it simply helpful, depending on physical considerations, individual needs, and personal preferences. As such, it can be difficult to calculate average costs because needs and preferences vary widely. Here is a list of tools, with brief explanations about their uses, compiled from recommendations from cleft team pros and experienced parents.

- **A Breast Pump.** Professionals and experienced mothers overwhelmingly recommend investing in a high-quality, double-electric *breast pump*, a machine that draws milk from the breasts. A *hand pump*, according to the pros, is not efficient enough for the volume and time required. Many hospitals offer rental services of high-quality breast pumps; some insurance companies will even cover this expense for cases of CLP.

- **Pump Accessories and Backup Accessories.** Every breast pump requires accessories in order to function, such as breast shields, valves, tubing, collection containers, and other extras to draw milk from the breasts and deposit it into containers (specific parts usually depend on the type of pump you use). Parents recommend buying at least two sets. "You might think this [backup] is unnecessary," writes Sylvia Noyes on the Global Big Latch On site, "but it's not. Having back-ups will keep you from frantically washing bottles and pump parts, using your precious pumping time," she explains. "Additionally, you never know when a part could give out, slip down the drain, or otherwise need to be replaced."

- **A Hands-Free Bra.** A hands-free bra allows a mother to pump milk without needing to use her hands to hold the equipment in place. Several mothers have referred to this item as a lifesaver since it allows a mother to multitask. Others find that even with a hands-free bra, the act of feeding the baby while pumping is still too awkward or inefficient to undertake regularly.

- **Lubricant.** The contact area between breast shields and the surface of the breast can become irritated or pained during pumping. A simple, baby-safe lubricant, such as olive or coconut oil, can decrease this discomfort.

- **Freezer Bags.** Milk storage is a topic unto itself since breast milk must be stored properly in order to be consumed safely later on (whether refrigerated or frozen). Many mothers freeze their milk in special plastic freezer bags designed for this purpose. Be sure to ask the cleft team for more information.

- **Nursing Cover.** A nursing cover is a smock-like covering that offers privacy while pumping but also allows a woman to see her chest. "Exclusive pumping can be isolating," commented one mother. "The more tools you have for comfortably pumping around others, the better."

- **Breast Pads.** Breast pads are disposable cotton inserts that fit into a bra in order to catch leaks in between pumping sessions; they prevent a bra and shirt from becoming soaked in milk.

- **Car Adapter for Breast Pump.** An electrical adapter that enables pumping on the go.

- **Manual (Spare) Breast Pump.** Many women recommend having a low-tech, alternate pumping method on hand for use during power outages or equipment breakdowns.

- **Coolers/Insulated Containers.** If you plan to feed your baby breast milk outside the home, you will need to store it properly to ensure it is safe to consume at mealtime. Insulated containers are a must.

- **Infant Formula.** Some families need or want to supplement their expressed breast milk with formula, depending on how much food the baby demands, how much breast milk a mother is producing, and other factors. For the sake of comparing (monetary) costs, the US surgeon general estimates the cost of exclusive formula-feeding at $1200–$1500 for the baby's first year.

- **Time.** While the cost of a person's time can be difficult to calculate monetarily, its value cannot be denied. "Breast-feeding is only cheaper [than formula-feeding]," writes Adriene Stortz on the Medium site, "if you believe that a woman's time has no value." While this mother writes about direct breast-feeding (as opposed to exclusive pumping), the idea may be even more applicable in this case. Expressing milk, by definition, requires time spent *not* doing other activities.

How Much Time Is Required? According to professionals in the field, a newborn usually eats eight-to-twelve times in a twenty-four-hour period or about every two-to-three hours. Some professionals advise pumping as many times as the baby eats or around every three hours. A typical session can last twenty-to-forty minutes, including setup and takedown. But this number depends, in part, on how long it takes to empty your breasts (an important consideration for maximizing milk production and for preventing *mastitis,* a painful swelling of the breasts often caused by infection). In other words, time requirements can vary. But one mother, who pumped for a typical duration of thirty minutes per session, estimated that she devoted about six hours per day to pumping and pumping-related tasks.

While pumping schedules can vary according to physical considerations and, to some extent, personal preference, here are two sample schedules, to provide a sense of the possibilities:

For eight pumping sessions in twenty-four hours:
7 a.m., 10 a.m., 12 p.m., 3 p.m., 6 p.m., 9 p.m., 12 a.m., 4 a.m.

For ten sessions in twenty-four hours:
7 a.m., 9 a.m., 11 a.m., 1 p.m., 3 p.m., 5 p.m., 7 p.m., 12 a.m., 3 a.m., 5 a.m.

It is important, even critical, according to pros in the field (and also experienced mothers), to pump regularly during the first three months of a baby's life—even through the night—in order to establish a milk supply. "Consistency is really important," commented one group of cleft-team experts in the *Cleft Palate-Craniofacial Journal*. As time goes on, however, a typical baby eats less frequently than before and consumes more milk per meal. A two-month-old, for instance, usually eats once every three-to-four hours. By age six months, feeding sessions may occur every four-to-five hours. Likewise, many women pare down their daily pumping schedule at various points during the baby's first year, depending on their supply and other factors. But situations vary.

Where Can I Find Support? Given the tremendous time and energy involved in exclusive pumping, many mothers rely on logistical and emotional support, both inside and outside the home. The feeding specialist on the cleft team should be an essential point of contact for learning the ins and outs of exclusive pumping (as always, the cleft team should be a family's first stop for information and advice). Lactation consultants, usually found at the birthing hospital, are also indispensable. But online groups devoted specifically to exclusive pumping can be enormously helpful as well, if not for medical advice, then for tips and emotional support. The two groups recommended most often by exclusive pumpers are "Exclusively Pumping Moms" and "Exclusively Pumping for Cleft Cuties," both private groups on Facebook (at the time of publication).

Other popular resources abound, both in terms of informational websites and hindsight from other mothers. Amanda Glenn's site, exclusivepumping.com, offers in-depth information, sample schedules, specific equipment recommendations, storage tips, books, and more. KellyMom.com is another popular site. (Remember, again, to use personal blogs and Facebook groups for tips and emotional support but not for medical information.)

Nutrition
What Does the Research Say?

Sometimes I wonder whether it is more confusing and overwhelming to learn about what to feed a baby than it is to actually feed a baby. Whether we hear from medical people that breast milk is the "gold standard" for babies or read about recent research that calls that recommendation into question, information and discussions on this topic seem to go in all directions, especially since the outcomes of recent studies seem to conflict with or debunk other work. One science journalist likened the experience of researching breast-feeding literature to watching a game of ping-pong. "One study will show a connection," she writes, "another study will tear it down."

Still, it is reasonable for expectant parents to seek basic information on the costs and benefits of the available feeding options—and in our case, to learn specifically what expressed milk and infant formula have to offer. First, let's explore and, hopefully, untangle some recent research on the merits of breast milk and formula, both for all parents and babies (clefts aside) and for babies born with cleft palate.

Immunity? One of the common arguments for feeding a baby breast milk is to help her fight infections—in other words, to boost her immunity. A large body of academic research performed in the late 1990s and into the 2000s concludes that breast milk offers long-term benefits for metabolism and immunity that formula does not (note that these studies refer to direct breast-feeding). So, it makes sense that the US surgeon general, the American Academy of Pediatrics, the American College of Obstetrics and Gynecologists, and other large national and international organizations have referred to these findings as they recommend breast-feeding. Doctors and medical establishments seem to agree, as stated in the *Journal of Perinatal Education* in 2015, that scientific data supports "unparalleled immunologic and anti-inflammatory properties of breast milk" and that breast milk promotes health and prevents disease.

Direct or Indirect Feeding? While the immune benefits of breast-feeding have been established in medical literature with regard to direct breast-feeding, a 2019 study published in the journal *Cell Host Microbe* distinguishes between human milk that is fed from the breast and that which is fed through a bottle. This research says that some so-called good bacteria—the bacteria that contribute to a baby's healthy "microbiome"—are transmitted through the skin of the breast but not through pumped milk. The study supports a theory about a dynamic back-and-forth between the baby's oral cavity and the woman's breast, saying that the microbiome provided by the mother is responsive to the composition of the baby's saliva. It also shows that factors—such as the cleanliness of bottles and nipples, storage methods, and even the acts of freezing, thawing, and reheating—can affect the quality of the expressed milk. In other words, while this study states that milk "microbiotia" are still poorly understood, the experience of direct breast-feeding offers benefits beyond pumped milk alone.

Cognition? While decades-old scientific research showed that breast-feeding benefited a baby's brain (in addition to her immunity), researchers now have evidence to suggest that those earlier studies were biased. We now know that the subjects (mothers and babies) who participated in some early research came to the table with certain, preexisting advantages or disadvantages. Nancy M. Hurst, PhD, RN, IBCLC, summarized the situation this way in an article for *CNN Health*: "The easy question—do kids who are breastfed have better outcomes? The answer is yes. The difficult question is: is it breast milk that improves their brain or is it that growing up with parents who are better educated and have better incomes makes a difference?" The issue of bias has moved to the forefront of the discussion on cognition—as our ping-pong ball flies across the net.

Pumped Breast Milk and Ear Health. Now let's look at research related specifically to cleft palate. Fortunately, researchers have studied the relationship between breast milk and ear health for babies with CP. Over the last thirty years, studies have shown a connection between breast milk and improved health of the middle ear, an especially pertinent concern for babies with CP given the high likelihood that these babies will experience recurrent fluid in the ears (see more on this topic in Chapter 21). One 2017 study published in the *Cleft Palate-Craniofacial Journal* shows that while feeding breast milk to a baby with CP for three months did not affect the need for ear tubes—the average age for ear tubes hovered at six or seven months for all babies with CP regardless of whether they consumed breast milk or formula—it did show that the babies who consumed breast milk were less likely to need further sets of tubes as time went on. More recent work published by some of the same researchers, however, has debunked those findings, showing no connection between breast milk and middle-ear problems for babies with CP, including the presence of fluid in the ear, problems with hearing, and the age at which a child gets tubes.

Dizzy yet?

The Nutritional Value of Formula. Now, what about formula? More often than not, medical research on the nutritional value of infant formula shows that using it is not as beneficial to mother and child as direct breast-feeding (again, this research pertains solely to direct breast-feeding) but at the same time, is nutritionally adequate. A 2016 study published in the *Journal of Gastroenterology and Nutrition*, for instance, concludes that while formula is inferior to breast milk, there will always be a need for it. "Breast milk is a dynamic fluid: it changes with gestational age, stage of lactation, within the same feeding, and from one mother to another," the authors explain. While these characteristics will never be reproduced in infant formula, the authors continue, recent advancements in formula "have brought the performance of formula progressively closer to breast milk" and have improved its safety. A clinical nurse specialist on a cleft team relayed a similar message. "Formula doesn't have the antibodies," she said, but it is nutritionally complete. "Formulas are excellent in this day and age."

So, Now What? As we can see, learning about what to feed a baby can be confusing. Not only is it difficult to keep track of recent research on the value of breast milk versus formula, but it is all the more challenging for cleft parents—and others in the small subset of families with similar circumstances—to find and parse information on the nutritional merits of *pumped* breast milk versus formula. Many professional health organizations officially endorse breast-feeding over formula-feeding—their websites usually include a statement of position—but these groups do not seem to take a formal stance on situations where direct breast-feeding is not an option.

Fortunately (and unsurprisingly), the pros on the cleft team have a lot to offer on this topic. Unlike some of the nurses and old-school lactation consultants in a birthing hospital—who, as we have seen anecdotally, do not always understand the logistics of feeding a baby with CLP—members of the team will likely be up-to-date on current research, appreciate the challenges of caring for a cleft-affected baby during her first year, and maybe most importantly, offer a nonjudgmental stance on the decision itself (the publications of the ACPA can be helpful for the same reasons). "It is so personal," commented one cleft-team nurse about this topic. While some new parents arrive in her office already feeling content to use formula, she said, others care deeply about the immune protection of breast milk. Her solution is to offer straightforward information. "I remain totally neutral with everyone," she continued. As always, the cleft team is a critical stop for information and advice.

Also, some general practitioners have started to discuss feeding options more holistically, acknowledging the wide variety of circumstances families encounter when determining what to feed a baby. One Harvard pediatrician acknowledges that "breast is best," on the blog for Harvard Medical School, but goes on to describe the many ways the matter can be complicated. Not all mothers can nurse, she reasons (and of course, neither can all babies). "When we demonize formula," she writes, "we also run the risk of shaming women who, for any number of good reasons, choose not to breast-feed." This doctor points out what cleft parents know keenly and what others—even some medical professionals—tend to overlook or perhaps forget to acknowledge: that in special circumstances, feeding a baby is not only physically challenging, but emotionally, logistically, or financially fraught. And in all circumstances—clefts or no clefts—the element of personal experience (as we'll discuss next) can and should play a role in a family's decision.

Given the back-and-forth, ping-pong-game nature of this research—not to mention the range of personal circumstances, feelings, and experiences of parents—there is no wonder the professionals on cleft teams tend to support parents in whichever path they choose.

Parents' Perspectives

When I asked the parents of cleft-affected babies about their decisions on what to feed their babies, almost all of their initial responses included either a sigh or a sigh-like expression. Many replied with phrases to the effect of, "Oh boy, where do I start?" A few simply chortled. The topic is weighty, they seemed to acknowledge. But the stories that emerged thereafter painted a variety of pictures. Whether a mother expressed milk exclusively, pumped for a while, and then decided to stop, or used formula right from the start, these parents had strong and diverse reactions during the early weeks and months of feeding their babies. While the value of medical research cannot be denied when considering what to feed a baby, the three stories below illuminate the many other factors of our personal lives that can—and should—also play a role in our decisions.

FAMILY STORIES

Jen Pumps Exclusively
THE STARS ALIGN...AND YET

By the time Jen gave birth to a baby girl with unilateral CLP, she and her husband, Aaron, had already decided that they wanted to feed the baby breast milk. "We were terrified of playing the formula game," Jen said. Not only had Jen suffered an allergic response to infant formula when she was a baby, but as an adult, she lived with severe allergies to milk, eggs, and nuts. "The decision came from a health-allergy standpoint," she explained. Jen and Aaron assumed that their daughter would be allergic to formula. But while exclusive pumping turned out to be a productive and satisfying experience for their whole family—since as we'll explore, everyone in the family played a role—Jen was quick to describe its challenges. "If [our daughter] had not been our only child," Jen said in retrospect, and if several other factors hadn't been in place, "there would have been no way I'd be able to do it."

Jen and Aaron were fortunate, to start, that Aaron was able to take a five-week parental leave from his job. So, the couple used that time to work out a two-person, round-the-clock, collaborative effort: while Jen pumped milk, Aaron bottle-fed the baby. And since Jen was recovering from a C-section and felt physically unsteady—and afraid to walk with the baby—Aaron and his mother arranged to be at the ready whenever the baby showed signs of hunger or needed a diaper change. It was only five weeks later, on Aaron's first day back at work, that Jen realized how little time she had spent holding her daughter. "When my husband was home, I wasn't bonding with her at all," she said. When he went back to work, it was almost as if she held her for the first time. "It was then that I realized what everyone meant when they talked about the smell of a baby's head," Jen said. So, the very assistance that made pumping possible during the baby's early weeks was also the factor that stood in the way of basic mother-baby bonding.

Eventually, Jen and the baby did begin to bond. And Jen settled into a routine that involved pumping and feeding sequentially. The two activities, repeated throughout the day and night, required an enormous amount of time—probably twelve total hours per day, she estimated. But the routine worked. Jen was able to produce enough milk to get the job done. And fortunately, the baby didn't just sleep well; she actually slept through the night from the time she was three weeks old. What's more, the baby did not undergo any presurgical orthodontic treatment (like NAM, Latham, etc.) that often involves significant time and energy. And Jen had no trouble learning to use a cleft palate bottle. "Feeding was easy," she said, adding that her daughter's soft palate, which was intact when she was born, played a role. In sum, the stars were very well aligned for this family. "We were very, very lucky," Jen said.

Despite all of these advantages, Jen felt pushed and pulled with regard to pumping. She loved giving her daughter nutritious breast milk and felt fortunate to be able to do so. But loneliness was an issue. "I had a ton of friends who had babies the same age—three within the same week," she said. "It is no fun to go to a barbeque with all those people and be the one to ask to go inside to pump and say, "I'll see you in forty minutes." Not only was Jen not seeing other parents, but she also wasn't seeing her baby. "That's forty minutes when I'm not with her," she continued. "It was very, very isolating."

Jen was certain that her feelings of isolation related to the fact that she was expressing milk rather than breast-feeding directly. Even when she pumped in her own home, she felt compelled to do so privately when houseguests were around. It turns out that her houseguests felt the same way—starting with her mother-in-law, who at an early visit asked her husband, Aaron's dad, to leave the room while Jen pumped. "She made my father-in-law stand out on the front porch," Jen said. "She told him, 'You need to go outside.' So, then I was super pressured to hurry up so Richard could come inside. It was one hundred ten degrees in July." While Jen laughed as she described her father-in-law's forays on the front porch, she also observed a social norm related to privacy. "There is something different about pumping in front of people than breast-feeding in front of people," she commented. "There isn't a baby involved!" So, Jen felt compelled to walk away from barbeques, family get-togethers, and the like, forestalling social awkwardness but increasing her sense of isolation.

While Jen and Aaron's extended family helped a great deal with the baby (that is, when they were physically in the house), Jen described her strong marriage as the lynchpin to the whole experience. During evenings and weekends, the couple divided household and baby tasks equally. "My husband is very laid-back," Jen commented. "I told him a few times that I wanted to throw the pump out the window, and he'd reply, 'Whenever you decide you're done, we're done.'" So, she—and they—kept going as a team. While pumping exclusively was taxing for both of them, their ability to communicate (and cooperate) as a couple played an enormous role in their success.

Had Jen been able to turn back the clock and decide again what to feed the baby, she probably would have proceeded in the same way. "It was worth it," she said. Jen was especially grateful to provide milk for her daughter at surgery time and was certainly glad to avoid potentially serious issues with allergies. But then, she sighed and reiterated her feelings of isolation. And she went on to describe just how many life factors had lined up in her favor to make pumping possible—starting with a resilient marriage, the support of an extended family, and a certain amount of financial freedom. Even after the baby's birth, additional factors surfaced that helped make life easier, like her easy temperament, her relatively minor cleft palate, and her ability to sleep and eat well. Overall, Jen emphasized that the decision to pump exclusively required tremendous time and resources. The challenges were real. In the end—on balance—she felt pleased with the decision.

What's Your Viewpoint? Like other mothers I spoke with who expressed milk exclusively for their babies, Jen made tremendous sacrifices in order to do so—as did Aaron and other family members. But it is important to point out how those sacrifices can actually vary from one person (and family) to the next. It is true that expressing milk requires a lot of time; that's the case for everyone. But the constellation of life circumstances and feelings surrounding the commitment—that is, our individual perspectives—can vary widely.

One person's isolation, for instance, is another person's respite. While Jen felt burdened by loneliness each time she set up her pumping equipment to begin her routine, another mother recalled how much she enjoyed pulling out her tablet during those moments to chat online with friends and fellow exclusive pumpers. While Jen described her strong marriage and sense of teamwork with her husband as key factors in her satisfaction with her decision to pump, another mother characterized her relationship with her (now ex-) husband as stressful and, at times, even abusive, with the tensions only rising as they argued over who would feed the baby while she pumped at 2:00 a.m. Other mothers describe financial pressures or a lack of support from family and/or health professionals. The list goes on.

The key, if you are in the process of deciding how to feed your baby, may be to consider your own, personal circumstances and to know that your feelings and instincts about any of these circumstances are unique—and valid. While I heard the phrase, "I wanted to throw the pump out the window" several times from mothers who pumped exclusively, each woman and family seemed to want to do so for different reasons. The commitment to pump is tremendous—and the parents who do it successfully often feel pleased and proud for having provided the best milk possible for their baby. But the stressors can be individualized.

FAMILY STORIES

Whitney Pumps, Then Stops
"I Felt There Was Something Wrong with Me"

When Whitney learned of her son's cleft lip at a twenty-week ultrasound, she was not entirely surprised by the news. Her husband, Jeff, had been born with CLP, as had a distant relative on her father's side of the family. Whitney also felt ready to accept the news that her son couldn't nurse. "I know a lot of women feel very sad that they can't breast-feed," she commented, "but I didn't feel that grief." Whitney's surprise came when she planned to express milk for her son but found the task—and the entire first three months after his birth—more difficult than she had anticipated.

"It did not go well at all," Whitney said about her initial experiences pumping milk for her baby. Right from the start, a lactation consultant in her local birthing hospital implored her to express milk. Whitney remembered that she visited the room several times to repeat the mantra, "'Okay, okay, keep pumping!'" Yet Whitney's production seemed low. "I could never really make enough milk," she said. And while it helped to receive a jumpstart of donated human milk from the hospital to mix with formula, none of the professionals in the ward seemed willing or able to either teach her to express more milk or to reassure her that her current production was normal. "I felt like the lactation consultant didn't know anything about how to stimulate milk supply in an exclusively pumping mother," Whitney commented. "She gave me a book that she probably hadn't read. It was about herbal supplements to increase supply."

While Whitney said she supports other people's decisions to use herbal supplements, she felt uncomfortable knowing that the advice wasn't supported by mainstream scientific methods. With the book in hand—but sure she wouldn't use it—Whitney left the hospital feeling discouraged. Even after returning home and receiving in-person visits from another lactation consultant, Whitney was never able to produce enough milk to fully nourish her son. She averaged about one-third of his diet while topping it up with formula.

As time went by, the pressure mounted. Whitney kept careful track of the amount of milk she produced during each pumping session, hoping that the numbers would climb, but they never did. And while she found tips and support from other mothers on private Facebook groups—particularly a group for exclusively pumping mothers of cleft-affected babies—certain comments on the forum actually made her feel worse rather than better. "Some people were posting [pictures of] their freezer stashes," she said, describing the common practice of freezing an oversupply of milk. Unlike those mothers who produced too much milk, Whitney fed almost all of her output directly to her son, usually bypassing refrigeration, much less freezing. "I wasn't ever able to get up to speed," she said. Feeling like an outsider in an insider's group, Whitney eventually decided to leave that forum. "I felt completely inadequate," she said. "I felt that I wasn't able to provide for this baby and that there was something wrong with me." No matter how hard she tried, she felt like her efforts were never enough.

Feeling frustrated and stuck (literally "stuck to the pump," as she described later), Whitney finally decided enough was enough. After three months of this routine, she packed up her industrial-strength rental pump and brought it back to the hospital. The result? Relief. "I was so happy to return that thing," Whitney said. "I just wish I had quit earlier." In fact, reflecting on the experience three years later, she felt all the more secure in her decision to stop. While she theorized that breast milk might provide vital nutrition for a baby with a serious health issue, she wasn't sure that her healthy son needed it. "It didn't make that much of a difference for this baby," she said. And it certainly didn't make enough of a difference, she added, knowing that she had felt so upset trying to produce it. "I think it is more important to be happy with your baby and know your baby is safe," she said, "than to feel miserable and trapped all the time."

During the months and years that followed, Whitney has tried to support other mothers who face challenges with regard to nursing or pumping, not only by helping them learn about the physical realities of milk production—which can be overlooked or underplayed by medical people—but by letting them know how easily bonding can take place without having to nurse. "You can be a great mother if you don't breast-feed or pump," she said. While those lessons only sank in for Whitney herself after three difficult months of expressing milk, she ultimately felt strong and free in her decision.

What Is "Normal"? Although Whitney was physically unable to produce enough milk to feed her baby, leading to feelings of frustration, anguish, and even shame, her physical capacity to produce milk was far more common—and normal—than she might have known. Studies show that "suboptimal" milk production can occur in 22 percent of mothers during the first few days after birth, particularly if the birth occurred by C-section but also as a result of several other factors. The figure jumps to 44 percent for first-time mothers. With professional assistance (such as the help of a knowledgeable lactation consultant), some mothers are able to overcome this early obstacle, but some aren't. Other research shows that all kinds of factors relate to low milk supply more generally, such as body mass index, maternal age, fertility treatments, or how soon after birth a mother starts pumping, just to name a few. It turns out that milk production can be a lot more complicated and challenging, physically, than many mothers realize.

As normal as these physical realities may be, many families haven't received the memo. "Mothers are led to believe that it's rare not to produce enough milk for their baby. In fact, it's not rare," commented one board-certified lactation consultant. To make matters worse, the language associated with the topic can be loaded. Just at a moment when a mother's most fervent desire may be to provide milk for her baby, she learns that her body is "suboptimal" or that "Breast is Best" (discussed in the next section). No wonder so many women feel inadequate. It was not Whitney's fault that her body produced milk as it did, just as it was no one's fault that her child was born with CLP. And it is certainly not a reflection of her capacity to mother.

FAMILY STORIES

Michelle Uses Formula from the Start
"I Can't Even Think about It!"

By the time Michelle's daughter was born with bilateral-complete CLP, Michelle had already spent eighteen weeks of her pregnancy on bed rest. And since she and her husband lived in a small, remote town, they had decided before their daughter's birth that they would travel several hours to reach an ACPA-approved cleft team in a large city. Michelle was well aware of the controversies surrounding the decision of what to feed a baby. "Feeding is always the big, scary issue," she commented. But the activity seemed out of the question both logistically and emotionally. Michelle remembered how the hospital staff had pressed her to try to breast-feed during the hours after her daughter's birth, not fully understanding the feeding limitations of babies born with cleft palate. A little while, later, when they asked whether she would "at least pump milk," Michelle refused. "I said, 'Look at me! I can't deal with that right now. I can't even think about it. No way.'"

Michelle's decision to use formula stemmed from a desire to be realistic about which activities she could do successfully and which she couldn't. "I just knew that if I couldn't pump or didn't have enough [milk] or something else failed, it would be too much emotionally," she explained. "That was the one thing I could control." While Michelle said she respects women who have the ability and desire to pump milk exclusively—"If you can, you should!" she commented—she also knew that the activity would not suit her—that expressing milk would be more of a burden than a boon.

Whether you decide to express milk, use infant formula, or offer your baby some combination of the two, each parent comes to the table with distinctly different life circumstances, physical health, opinions, feelings, and values. That wide variety only underscores the individuality of the decision.

What about Thanksgiving?
Choices in Private, Choices in Public

It is hard enough to decide what to feed a baby, but perhaps just as challenging to discuss that decision with others. Whether we are talking with a coworker, a dental hygienist, or a fellow parent standing next to us at the library story hour (or a family member at Thanksgiving dinner), most of us have met someone who not only doesn't understand a special health condition but also feels comfortable tossing off a comment that strikes a nerve (or chokes us up), even if they mean well. Unlike other kinds of personal decisions, parenting decisions tend to play out publicly. One way to manage these situations is, first, to make the best decision possible personally—realizing that that choice is yours alone to make—and then to tackle and, perhaps, try to reframe your interactions with Aunt Margo. A little historical context might help.

Why Is This Topic So Loaded? As we consider the lively conversations that can take place on the topic of what to feed a baby, it may help to know that the social dynamics have been shaped by powerful messages and movements in this country over the years. Baby-feeding trends have fluctuated dramatically over the last century or so in the US. At the turn of the previous century, approximately two-thirds of women were nursing their babies. Over subsequent decades, nursing behaviors declined, reaching a low point of about 22 percent in the early 1970s. Seeing this trend and hoping to reverse it, Dr. Penny Stanway and Andrew Stanway wrote a 1978 breast-feeding guide called *Breast is Best* to explain and promote the benefits of breast-feeding and to help women learn how to do it. Institutions had started to promote breast-feeding at that point as well. By the late 1900s and early 2000s, organizations like the American Association of Pediatrics and the World Health Organization were strongly recommending breast-feeding to doctors and families. The efforts were effective, in part, because the simple slogan "Breast is Best" (taken from the title of the book) was promoted by governments, medical organizations, and individual practitioners nationally and internationally.

Research shows that under ideal conditions, breast *is* best. Under ideal conditions, direct breast-feeding offers numerous health benefits, not to mention opportunities for bonding. But as cleft parents and many others know, a one-size-fits-all message such as this cannot—and should not—apply to everyone. Not only does such a slogan overlook the range of physical and logistical capabilities of some mothers, babies, and families, but it focuses on a body part, assigning no value to the element of personal experience. As a result, "Breast is Best" can stigmatize mothers who cannot nurse (or pump), due to physical circumstances, or who look at factors in their own lives and make a perfectly reasonable decision not to do so. When we see the 2012 statement from the American Academy of Pediatrics, "Breast-feeding and human milk are the normative standards for infant feeding and nutrition," or a 2017 statement from the World Health Organization saying, "Breast-feeding for the first six months is crucial," the message is clear: breast-feeding is a moral imperative.

Here is where Aunt Margo comes in. The messages and moral underpinnings of *Breast is Best* have reached a wide audience. People have listened. One result is that since the 1970s, more women are breast-feeding than before. Another result is that the women who breast-feed or pump exclusively often feel proud for having done so. As they should! Breast milk is healthy for a baby. And the activities of breast-feeding and expressing milk can be incredibly difficult. Even under the best of conditions—as we saw with Jen and Aaron—these activities can feel isolating, boring, frustrating, physically painful, and depleting (just as they can be immensely rewarding, nurturing, healthy, and wonderful). Women who breast-feed or pump success-fully should indeed celebrate their hard work.

But here's the rub. Those of us who can and do engage in these activities should also keep in mind our good fortune for being able to climb that mountain in the first place. Public policies, life circumstances, physical considerations, and other elements beyond our immediate control play an enormous role in aligning the stars, making breast-feeding or pumping possible. And so, the problem, socially, occurs when a successful nurser or pumper forgets about the element of luck and, reinforced by blunt messages passed on by revered doctors and institutions, allows her well-deserved pride to bubble over into superiority or judginess.

A second and far sadder result occurs for the families on the receiving end of those judgments, who, like Whitney, feel ashamed or inadequate when they either aren't physically able to breast-feed (or pump milk), when their baby is unable to nurse, or when for all sorts of valid reasons, they decide that they don't want to engage in those activities. Even worse, the "Breast is Best" message pits women against women. The horrible term "mommy wars" paints a picture of women squabbling when, in fact, our feelings and behaviors were likely shaped by unreasonably blunt messages sent by institutions. What a mess! If medical professionals and health organizations could encourage us to throw out the baggage, maybe all of us would feel more comfortable celebrating with one another when we succeed and thrive within our own choices. It is brave and heroic to breast-feed or pump exclusively; that's for sure. But given the myriad pressures and circumstances families face when a baby is born, it can be just as brave and heroic to decide not to.

Moving Forward. Fortunately, medical institutions have begun to take a broader, more inclusive view in their recommendations for what to feed a baby. The recent campaign, "Fed is Best," acknowledges the diversity of circumstances among families. Cleft teams, too, generally support parents in whatever choices they make. One clinical nurse specialist on a cleft team mentioned the importance of striking a balance between the two elements of nutrition and personal experience when deciding what to feed the baby. She also sympathized with the pressures families face as they confront this sensitive issue. "I think, sometimes, mothers want so badly to be able to nurse," she stated, "and feel like it is THE way." At the same time, "they need to understand that getting the nutrition into [their] baby is the most important thing." In other words, each path is valid. Nurturing a baby can take many forms.

Whether you feel committed to providing breast milk, equally sure about formula, or content to play it by ear after the baby is born, the decision of what to feed your baby is yours to make. As cleft professionals have mentioned, most of us come to the table—or at least pick up this book—with an initial sense of where we lean. My hope is that the current research on this topic, as dynamic as it is, and the experiences of other parents, perhaps just as dynamic, will illuminate the individuality and validity of this decision. I hope, too, that you can then feel comfortable pulling out your breast pump or mixing powdered formula at Thanksgiving dinner, and in so doing show the Aunt Margos in your life that you feel confident loving and nurturing your baby in the ways you see fit.

Early Days

Chapter 17

. . . .

What to Say?

Ideas for Family, Friends, and New Parents
A Two-Way Street

When Jessa first shared the news of her infant son's cleft lip and palate with close family members, their reactions surprised her. Ordinarily, Jessa felt supported by her parents and other relatives when challenges arose. This time, unfortunately, some of their comments stung. "My mom doesn't understand why my baby can't breast-feed," Jessa said. "My grandfather refers to my baby's cleft as a 'harelip,' and a friend's mom has told me that I need to 'warn people' before they meet my baby, so they aren't caught off guard by her defect." If the remarks hadn't been so upsetting, she noted, the collection of statements would almost be laughable. "I have handled these situations both well and not so well," she added.

Interactions with friends and family can feel stressful for the parents of kids born with CLP, as they did for Jessa. Some parents have strong and fresh feelings about the news of their child's condition that they haven't fully digested themselves, especially if they learn the diagnosis in the delivery room (as opposed to via prenatal ultrasound, weeks earlier). Some feel nervous simply *anticipating* the reactions of loved ones, realizing that the situation (and the relationships) can feel complicated. Yet here are friends and family, standing in a hospital hallway, balloons in hand, waiting to meet the baby. While a new parent may easily wonder, *What should I say to them?* it is also true that 599 out of six hundred of these friends and family were not born with CLP. A loved one may easily enter the room considering the very same question: *What can I say?*

This chapter is intended for both parties. If you are among the family, friends, coworkers, neighbors, or even medical staff in the delivery room who are waiting to meet the new baby, you may be wondering how to support a parent of a child born with CLP. The first two sections of this chapter offer suggestions for sensitive communications and active listening. The third is intended for new parents—because thoughtful communication, after all, is a two-way street. These messages and techniques are intended to help everyone involved, especially (if not until later on) the affected child.

For Family and Friends
Misunderstandings and Hot Words

Given the untold complexities of family interactions and relation-ships, it is difficult to explain Jessa's anecdotes (and related feelings) in a way that applies to all families. But it is possible to untangle—and hopefully clarify—some of the common misunderstandings that can occur in families or friendships when a baby is born with CLP. First, we'll explore ways new parents might feel about their baby. We'll also look at what *not* to say—not for the sake of waving fingers or lingering on the negative, but in order to suggest *why not*—to prevent hurt feelings. Then we'll move on to the good stuff: ideas for creating positive and supportive interactions that lay the groundwork for love and acceptance—that is, the interactions that everyone is probably hoping for.

A Juggling Act. To start, it might be helpful for friends and family to know how common it is for new parents to balance several feelings at once, some of them seemingly incompatible. Many parents of cleft-affected babies love their baby just as she was born, clefts and all. And, paradoxically, parents may love their child's face even as they choose to move forward with treatment to change it. "Before Danny was born," said one mother, "my husband and I thought, *It will be good to have surgery. The earlier our son has the surgery, the better.* But then, it hit us. As soon as Danny was born, we realized that we didn't want him to change. We thought, *That's Danny. That's his smile.*" Another mother described juggling many emotional responses at once. "I was overjoyed when my son was born," she said. "And worried. I also got really depressed. I functioned, but I was depressed. Some of my friends understood my reaction, but others didn't." New parents' responses vary widely, of course—but some are feeling many things at once.

So as a starting point, it might be safe for loved ones to assume—until you find out otherwise or *even if* you find out otherwise—that new parents see their baby as beautiful, before and after surgery, inside and out. It is very likely, too, that this sentiment of love and acceptance is the very one parents want to hear from you (and eventually wish to relay to their child). When new parents hear certain hot words or phrases, they hear the message that you, as a friend or family member, do not love their baby as is. They may also hear that you think *they* feel the same way. Those messages can feel uncomfortable and painful, especially when coming from someone they care about deeply.

Hot Words. Some unwelcome phrases are more obvious than others. "Harelip," for instance, is outdated. Decades ago, this term may have been the norm, but now it can hurt. It may feel strange or uncomfortable to learn that a once-common, perfectly fine word is now so powerfully negative as to insult people. New information like this can be hard to process. But many people affected by cleft lip and palate find the comparison to a rabbit demeaning. So, if you have an urge to use the term, even in a humorous way, please fight that urge. Incidentally, it might be a good idea to tread lightly with "cleftie" too. While some people find this word endearing (I've seen it used on social media to mean, "cleft + cutie"), in certain contexts, it can feel insulting, as if the speaker is name-calling.

Less obvious hot words abound, as well. For instance, CLP is officially considered a birth defect. Medical people use this word all the time in a clinical way, and it is still used regularly in research. The Centers for Disease Control uses the term as a header on its website, referring to CLP as, "one of the most common types of birth defects in the United States." The context here is clinical and probably not commonly received as hurtful (though to be honest, I think the medical establishment should look thoughtfully at this term and others). In any case, families affected by CLP have said they feel sensitive about hearing the word *defect* in everyday conversation. Why? Because it indicates that a baby is flawed or inadequate. And perhaps more problematic, the noun *defect* is only three short letters away from the adjective *defective*. With a stroke of a pen, the word goes from clinically acceptable to heartbreaking.

We all respond uniquely to the use of different words. "Defect" may bother some and not others. But all things considered, it is usually better to play it safe and choose another word rather than risk hurting someone's feelings (we'll explore thoughtful wording in a bit).

More than a Face. Likewise, many parents of kids born with CLP chafe at the implication that their child is either 1) broken or 2) fascinating in a clinical way. One father felt uncomfortable about the comments he heard from the staff in the delivery room following his daughter's birth. "I sensed some nurses gawking a bit," he said. They asked probing questions about CLP, he said, that seemed impersonal and cold. "One of them asked when the doctors would fix it. They were trying to learn, no doubt," this dad said. "But for me, it wasn't an 'interesting case;' it was my daughter!" Again, new parents may feel several emotions at once. They may struggle with the news of their child's condition. Some new parents do not bond right away—as could happen for anyone. Some of *them* may wonder when the doctors are going to fix it. But generally, they want to hear others declare their love and acceptance for this child and to hear that she is beautiful, before and after.

So what words are left? What can a loved one say? Actually, there is a lot to say! First—oh, my goodness—you can ooh and aah over this baby, as we'll discuss in the next section. But when in doubt about hot words, you can replace words like "fix" or "repair," which imply that a child is broken, with a word that describes a specific activity, without judgment. For example, if you are curious about treatment, you could ask, "When are they going to close her lip?" You could also use the word "difference" or "facial difference" to replace "defect" or "disfigurement." Even better, you can apply some tools of active listening, as described below.

For Friends and Family
Active Listening

ACTIVE LISTENING, STEP 1: Follow Parents' Lead. When Susan first learned the news of her daughter's CLP, she and her husband spoke with another family whose child had been born with an isolated cleft lip. "They told us, 'Clefts are no big deal. It's easy!'" she said. Years later, after her daughter had undergone several operations and other forms of treatment—with more to come—Susan pointed out that "easy" was hardly the way her daughter would describe her experience. Situations vary. While one child may undergo a single operation during infancy and that's it, another may have a sequence of interventions that span her childhood (and beyond). Moreover, every child and family will have a different take on how these experiences fit into their lives and identities.

Given this wide variation of emotional responses to CLP diagnosis and treatment, a realistic way to support a family is to see if you can meet them where they are. And there is almost no better way to do that than with an open-ended question. You might ask something like, "What does this situation [diagnosis, treatment, upcoming operation, etc.] mean for the baby?" or simply, "How is this experience going for you?"

The key is to try not to guess how new parents feel about a surgery or event, even if you know something about clefts—or perhaps, *especially* if you know something about clefts. One mother, Meredith, remembered hearing advice from her husband's parents, who had ushered her husband (their son) through cleft treatment some thirty years prior. "'It'll be fine!'" they counseled the young parents. "My in-laws are very optimistic about it," Meredith said, "because treatment went so well for my husband when he was a kid." But as Meredith commented later, her in-laws' comments didn't help. "I'm grateful that they didn't have to deal with some of the stuff that we are dealing with," she continued, "but it is hard that they don't understand. Sometimes, it makes me mad and resentful when they say, 'It is going to be okay!'" According to psychologist Paul G. Quinnett, MD, a mishap like this is common. "This is the mother lode of all mistakes in active listening," he states. "Do not assume you understand. Active listening does not mean telling your loved one that you 'know' what he or she is going to say; just listen and demonstrate respect for their thoughts."

The same concept applies over time. The treatment for CLP—and the impact of the condition on a person more generally—can ebb and flow throughout childhood, sometimes without notice. It is not unusual for a child to go several months or even years without treatment and to feel just fine about appearance, speech, and social relationships—smooth sailing. But it is also true that the tides shift. A child might run into trouble with teasing. They might feel nervous about a big operation. The best thing you can do is to let the family fill you in on what is going on *right now*.

ACTIVE LISTENING, STEP 2: Repeat Back. Perhaps you've asked some open-ended questions. Wonderful! Now what? Occasionally, new parents respond to open-ended questions with a request for specific advice. They may ask something like, "What should I do?"—and welcome your words of direction. Perhaps this question-and-answer dynamic is a regular and fruitful aspect of your relationship. Great.

Other times—maybe even a majority of the time, actually—words of advice tend not to go very far. As psychologist Thomas G. Plante puts it, "Advice-giving usually doesn't work, and often completely backfires." This professional goes on to introduce a body of research called *reactance theory*. According to a group of international researchers, people who are confronted with interpersonal "threats to their freedom" tend to resist those threats. We get defensive, in other words, when presented with unwanted advice because we sense our independence is jeopardized. We want to be able to make our own decisions. Whether we are a small child in the sandbox who ignores a parent's shouts of direction across the playground or a new parent who balks at Aunt Edna's ideas about our child, experts say that unwanted instructions will usually *not* be met with open arms.

Fortunately, there are many routes up this conversational mountain. One safe path may involve remembering that a suffering person will benefit a great deal from simply feeling heard. Other research shows that when a person feels understood, their sense of "personal and social well-being" is heightened. One study even links this feeling with certain responses in our neurobiology. What good news! Empathetic listening—just listening!—can go a long way in helping a hurt person feel better.

But what is the best way to listen effectively? According to psychologist W. Huitt, a key way to acknowledge someone's feelings is to summarize and repeat back their words. This concept may feel a little obvious at first, even clunky or overly simple. But the practice validates a person's experience and shows that you are listening. If a new parent tells you, for instance, about their experience of feeling surprised when they learned the news of their child's diagnosis and challenged by the subsequent search for a cleft palate or craniofacial team, you might respond with, "Wow, it sounds like learning the news about this diagnosis was really surprising for you. And then there was so much to learn about finding a team. How's that going for you now?" Seasoned professional conversationalists—Oprah Winfrey is a perfect example—demonstrate these patterns all the time; they comfort people by repeating back their words simply and empathetically.

Sometimes, a well-meaning person will try to console another by comparing their misfortune with something that seems more serious. "At least it's not cancer!" for instance, or "Be grateful it's not worse!" While this instinct is usually based on good intention— and may seem like a reasonable comment in the case of CLP—the gesture can belly flop. One mother was surprised to hear such comments from the staff at her birthing hospital. "The nurses and the obstetricians see the whole gamut of issues that children have," she said. "So, clefts, to them, are fine. It is all relative, right? But for me, it was a very, very big deal. I wanted to say to them, 'Don't blow it off as if it is nothing. You see horrible situations. Right now, for this momma in this room, the situation is pretty traumatic.'"

It is generally not helpful or productive to compare one person's pain to another's. New parents of cleft-affected babies probably *are* grateful that the situation is not worse. But they may interpret such a comment as dismissive of their feelings. "I know clefts are 'fixable,'" commented another mother, "but that doesn't make the journey easy by any means." The best substitute is to simply repeat back a person's feelings and thereby acknowledge that those emotions are valid.

The same concept applies to accidental comparisons. "I think one of my hardest journeys was relating to other moms," commented one mother. "I would get so jealous when people would complain about their baby's colic or sleepless nights when I was struggling with surgeries or stares from strangers."

The problem in these kinds of situations (which parents mention often) may *not* be that a friend wants to discuss a problem that is less intense or severe in comparison—since healthy friendships routinely involve a range of light and heavy moments. The issue here, instead, may be that cleft parents do not feel heard in the first place. Again, active listening comes into play. As a loved one or friend, you might spend some time listening to and discussing a cleft parent's intense news, say, about an upcoming operation. Then, after the person has been heard—truly heard—you might move on to another subject, perhaps by acknowledging the shift. "It feels odd to bring up the subject of my search for a perfect birthday outfit for my baby when your child has just had surgery. But can you believe….?" The key is to engage in active listening before making the transition. Many parents would welcome the discussion *and* the diversion.

ACTIVE LISTENING, STEP 3: Use Supportive Words and Gestures. As a corollary to active listening, certain simple verbal and physical gestures can go a long way in showing that you care. Many cleft parents have said that they appreciated hearing any and all traditional congratulatory expressions and baby talk. And the expression "wide smile" has come up as a lovely way to describe a cleft lip. You could say, "She's beautiful! Just look at those eyes and all that hair! And look at that adorable, wide smile!" When we as parents notice friends and loved ones interacting with our child in a regular way, we feel reassured that she will be okay. These gestures support *us*.

Another thing to keep in mind is that many new parents see a baby's arrival as not just a positive event but a joyous one—even if they also feel concerned about her health or other issues (as mentioned above). One mother, who shared part of her story in the book, *I Wish I'd Known…How Much I'd Love You,* described a conversation she had with a nurse immediately following the birth of her son by C-section. In her foggy state after the operation and upon learning the news of his cleft lip, she asked the nurse several times whether he also had a cleft palate. The nurse gave the same response each time: "'No, just a cleft lip, and he's beautiful.'" This mother was overjoyed. It is one thing for a parent to think they have a beautiful baby, she said, "but when someone else confirms it, it means so much more."

Wordless acts can go just as far. "I remember it being really comforting when my mother took her in her arms," said one dad in a video for parents, "and they passed her around and made goo-goo faces. You quickly realize that this is the baby you've been waiting for, and that she will be loved, and that we will get through it." *Oohs* and *aahs*, in all varieties, comfort everyone involved.

ACTIVE LISTENING, STEP 4: Comfort In, Dump Out. The last idea to keep in mind is a general rule of thumb for determining where to direct thoughts and comments. The "Ring Theory" of kvetching, as pioneered by a breast cancer survivor and endorsed by a clinical psychologist in the *LA Times* in 2013, has become a popular new standard for supporting an injured, sick, or otherwise suffering person during a time of trauma. First, let's imagine a series of concentric circles. The name of the affected person—let's say, a cleft parent (and later on, perhaps the affected child)—goes in the center ring. Then, working outward from the center, let's put the name(s) of the parents' very close loved ones in the second ring. Less-close relations go in the third and subsequent rings. The idea, then, is for a support person to determine where they belong among those circles and then to freely express their own problems, responses, and issues about the trauma to someone *less* involved in the crisis—not the other way around. It goes like this: comfort *in*, dump *out*.

If you feel shocked, for instance, by the look of your grand-child's unrepaired clefts and wish that surgery would occur sooner rather than later, those are valid feelings. Just don't tell your adult child ("dump") these potentially hurtful thoughts. Instead, seek that support from a person who is less involved in the situation. Then, comfort *in*. You could ask open-ended questions and *ooh* and *aah* over the baby. "My sister was amazing," one mother, Tara, said. "I told her first." Tara's sister didn't deliver any particular magic words, Tara admitted, at least not that she could recall. But she listened, asked questions, and expressed love for the baby—which was exactly the response Tara craved. The key is to remember that active listening, especially directed inward in the series of circles, will go a long way in reassuring new parents that their child and their family will be okay.

For New Parents
A Two-Way Street

Sara and Sebastian had a lot of worries when they learned the news of their child's CLP at a prenatal ultrasound. But they grappled especially with how to share the news with loved ones, particularly with Sebastian's family. "I was worried about how my mother-in-law would react," Sara said. "She has a tendency to focus on the negative." The couple feared that Sebastian's mother would share their news with anyone and everyone and in a way that, to them, felt gossipy.

TIP for NEW PARENTS: If Possible, Be Honest. Fortunately, the ACPA offers advice on situations just like Sara and Sebastian's. In its fact sheet, "For Parents of Newborns," the group counsels parents to be forthright with loved ones, especially at first, but also over time. Indeed, many of the parents I spoke with found it helpful to be as direct as possible, both in terms of sharing medical information and telling people how they feel. When Jessa, the mother who listed a string of unfortunate comments from family members, discussed the ways she handled those early conflicts, she noted that the best interactions were the candid ones. "I'm very brave with my mother and mother-in-law," she commented. "When they say something I find off-putting, usually I'm honest with them. I'll say, 'That's not the way I see it,' or, 'That's not what we're doing.'" All familial relationships are different. But many parents have found that honesty can go a long way.

TIP for NEW PARENTS: Plan Ahead. As you consider your interactions with loved ones, it might also be helpful to prepare your words carefully before picking up the phone or sending an email. This extra planning may feel a little contrived or overly rehearsed (and may not always be possible logistically). But in retrospect, many parents say they've felt best about the conversations that they thought through beforehand. The subsequent interactions felt more productive, they said, and less likely to push the same old buttons or provoke tired arguments. And in the end, these constructive interactions helped them cultivate the most informed, attentive support system possible.

SHARING the NEWS
Sample Email

SARA and SEBASTIAN'S LETTER to FAMILY

When I spoke with Sara and Sebastian about their experiences sharing the news of their daughter's CLP with loved ones and acquaintances, they described taking some time to compose a careful, honest email before sending it to family members. They also shared the note itself, in case it might be useful for other parents. While each of us will invariably use our own words in communicating with loved ones, this example might be a springboard for those of us who wonder, "What did they say *exactly?*" It is lightly edited for clarity.

Hi All,

We'd like to preface this news by saying, in the big scheme of things, everything is fine and it's all going to be okay, so before you read on, rest assured!

It appears our second sweet baby girl will be born with a cleft lip and palate. She will need several surgeries to repair them, the first likely occurring somewhere between birth and three months. We are in the process of getting more information regarding exactly what her cleft is like (right now we know it is just on her left side) and information on the recommended surgeons, baby bottles, and resources that can be most helpful.

We are very thankful that we live in this area and have amazing doctors nearby and that we know to expect this, so we can do our research and get as prepared as possible for her. It was difficult to hear the news, at first, because it was unexpected, because we had a lot of questions, and didn't know the implications, and also because it will be hard to see our little girl go through this process. Cleft lip and palate does not run in either family, but the doctors believe it is an isolated situation, where in the early development, the lip/palate just didn't grow together completely.

We are mentioning this now, so you know what to expect when you see her for the first time and know that it can and will be repaired, and so you have an idea of what we'll be going through. It will be a different parenting experience for us for sure!

We ask that her cleft not be a topic of conversation at the office or with anyone outside the immediate family. It is nothing to be ashamed of, but we'd also like for her not to be a conversational talking point or gossip. As her parents, we're trying to be the best advocates for her, and being fiercely protective is part of the job.

We are looking forward to falling in love with not just her first smile but also her forever smile. Please ask us any questions you have. We will keep you posted.

Sara and Sebastian

TIP for NEW PARENTS: *You Go First!* As Sara and Sebastian's story demonstrates, not only can you be as honest as possible when communicating with loved ones, but you can actually take the lead. Many cleft parents have mentioned their disappointment when people react awkwardly to the news of their child's condition—or worse, don't react at all. "When I shared the news, some people kind of shied away," commented one parent about the period after her daughter's birth. "These were people I thought would be there for me. Coworkers, for example, kind of disappeared."

These kinds of situations often call for proactive communications, as uncomfortable as that idea may seem during a moment of weakness. One mother, Celine, deliberately brought up the topic of her son's CLP with friends and recommended that other parents do the same. "Showing them that I was okay with it opened them up to asking me questions," she explained, though the questions she received sometimes began clumsily. "Some people would say, 'This is just my ignorance; I'm sorry if you are offended....'" But Celine tried to give them the benefit of the doubt. She would reply, "'I am not offended,'" and then she would answer their questions.

With time, Celine's friends began initiating conversations. "People love to talk to me about Jaden's clefts," she continued. "I say, be open about it. It makes a world of difference." As new parents with a cleft-affected child, you can do your part to encourage healthy conversations, first by simply bringing up the topic (rather than staying mum), then by demonstrating your preferred words, and if possible, by giving loved ones some slack if their questions come out less than perfect.

TIP for NEW PARENTS: *Try on Their Shoes.* Finally, we can be mindful of generational differences, not to excuse old-fashioned biases, but to be aware of our loved ones' personal histories, perspectives, and even conversational styles. In my interviews with cleft parents and in some cases, *their* parents, I noticed that grandparents sometimes described strong emotional responses to a diagnosis of CLP, especially if they hadn't known of the significant medical advances that have occurred in cleft care in recent decades. "My family was super supportive," said one new mother, Rachael, about the early days after the birth of her son. "It was hard for them, but they didn't tell me that until later."

Rachael explained that her father, especially, had felt shocked and enormously sympathetic when he saw pictures of his newborn grandchild. But he didn't mention those feelings for several weeks. "He finally said to me, 'I don't know how you get out of bed in the morning. This is devastating.'" Rachael's father cared deeply about his daughter and her new family, but he held off on relaying his strong feelings. So did Barbara, below.

FAMILY STORIES
"I didn't want to hold the baby or feed him"

A GRANDMOTHER'S VIEW

Barbara was not the least bit surprised when her daughter invited her to stand by her side in the delivery room during the birth of her son. "You have to understand the culture of the South," she explained. Barbara's family, like others she knew, was a tight-knit bunch. Raising a child—even birthing a child—was considered a team effort. Barbara bubbled with delight as she recalled how it felt to anticipate the birth of her grandson. Her job was to take a video. Her daughter-in-law would send updates to other family members. Both women would be there to hold her daughter's hand. Barbara couldn't think of a place she'd rather be.

When the birth day came, the mood in the delivery room was upbeat. And for the most part, Barbara recalled, the process went well. Barbara's daughter labored for several hours, as expected, followed by a relatively smooth delivery. But then the mood changed. "At the end, when he came out, and the doctor held him up, I glanced over, and I knew immediately that something was wrong." The doctor, once almost jovial, appeared stunned. "His face was completely white," she said. "There was no color. I asked, 'What is wrong?' I don't know what I did with the video camera at that point."

A few minutes later, someone informed the family that baby had been born with cleft lip and palate. Barbara was furious. "I wanted to hit the doctor," she said. "I thought, 'How could you have missed it? After all those ultrasounds?'" During her pregnancy, Barbara's daughter had undergone almost a dozen prenatal ultrasounds to monitor the baby's health, since she had been taking medications that were necessary for her own health even as they increased certain health risks for the unborn baby. For whatever reasons, none of those scans revealed CLP—even though the condition would have been visible at the time. So, the family didn't learn the news of the diagnosis until the baby's birth.

"It was such a shock," Barbara said. "I didn't know what to do. Hit him? My daughter was sobbing. We had all of that on the recorder—all of the sound, all of the conversation. I was telling her, 'It will be all right. We will love him.' I didn't believe we would, though, to be honest. I didn't. I don't know what happened to me. I told that to her to try to console her. But I wanted to hit the doctor."

Her feelings did not improve from there. "For the next week or so, I didn't want to hold the baby or feed him," she said. "I can't explain it." Family members visited, each excited to hold the baby. Not Barbara. But one day, she was in the NICU nursery. "It was my turn to check on him," she said. "The nurse said to me, 'I am going to hand him to you while I change his bed.' I thought, 'No, I don't want to hold him,' but I couldn't say that to her because he was my grandchild."

She paused to take a deep breath. "I sat in the chair," she said, "and I looked at him. Then, I can't explain it, but the cleft disappeared. That minute was a complete turnaround. I saw his eyes, his cheeks. He had my whole heart. But for those first nine days, I couldn't wrap my head around it, the shock of it. Other family members? Everybody else—everyone was shocked, yeah. But there was no hesitation for them. This was something that happened just to me."

As new parents, we can be as direct and honest as possible with parents and loved ones, to start. But we can also keep their journeys in mind. We can be patient with their clumsy words if we know they mean well. And we can do our best to be active listeners—and remember the two-way street—even through our own troubles. "Your support system is critical," advised one mother, "even if it is a system of people who love you dearly but have no idea what is going on with you." As the old saying goes, a child's health and well-being sometimes takes a village, whether that village is made up of friends, coworkers, neighbors, or family.

Chapter 18

. . . .

Why Photos?

I once asked a nurse on a cleft team for general tips for parents during the baby's first year. I expected she might talk about choosing a team, dealing with feeding issues, or managing surgeries. "Take pictures of the baby," she advised. "I highly recommend it. You don't have to share them. But at least you will have some."

This nurse echoed a common refrain in the cleft community: that parents need to take baby pictures in order to help a child understand her identity. We need to send the message that our child was—and is—loved as is. But this nurse wouldn't have brought up the topic if she hadn't noticed something else throughout her long career: that the task is easier for some parents than for others, especially early on. Why is this topic so important? And how can we move forward?

Who Am I?
A Child's View

Shortly after Shelly's son, Jack, finished his first year of cleft treatment, she made a small photo album of his early babyhood. The book was kid-sized, she said, and durable. Jack used to laugh as he yanked it off the shelf, especially as he toddled around, learning to walk. Then one day a few years later, when Jack was about four years old, Shelly took out the book again, to reminisce. This time, he saw the images of his unrepaired clefts and didn't recognize himself. "He kind of freaked out," she said. "He didn't want to see the pictures. We said, 'That is you! Look at how handsome you are.' We are proud of who he is. He said, 'That is not me!' He was not having it."

Coming to terms with appearance can be a long and winding process. All of us, to some extent, compare powerful cultural beauty norms with what we see in a photo or in the mirror. But for a person with a facial difference, especially a child, that process can also involve keeping track of several different appearances. Shelly's son balked when he saw images of his original baby face, prior to his lip-repair surgery. But it is true that his face might change again later, too, both from growth and from other surgical procedures. That's a lot of change to process. Without photos, it would be very difficult to grasp the progression. The images are key artifacts, breadcrumbs on a path to self-discovery.

Child-development experts use the term *remembered self* to refer to the internal picture a child develops over time as she develops a sense of self and belonging. Each of us creates a personal life story, they say, based on the stories and memories we hear—and see—from family members about our early experiences. While this internal picture, sometimes called *autobiographical memory*, is just one of several factors that the experts believe contribute to our personal identity, its importance is not to be underestimated.

There's more. Baby pictures can be a sensitive topic, too, because of the element of parental involvement. The very existence of a child's pictures—what, when, and how many—reflects the attitudes of parents. Under ordinary circumstances, many new parents take loads of pictures; it's a practice that has only expanded with the rise of camera phones and social media. Also under ordinary circumstances, other parents hold back. Some would rather experience an event fully than interrupt it with a camera. Some are simply not into pictures. A friend of mine smiles and rolls his eyes as he recalls how his parents took only a handful of photos of his entire early childhood. He was the third child in the family, he explains. His parents were tired.

Yet for many families, CLP is no ordinary circumstance. In this case, a lack of pictures can carry special, even profound weight as a child considers a parent's motivations and wonders what happened. "There is a hole in my life that will never be filled," writes one cleft-affected woman on the Wide Smiles site. "My parents were too ashamed of my face to have it photographed when I was born. I had a cleft lip, and they could not accept that. Now I am twenty-three years old and writing to retired doctors and distant hospitals just hoping that someone somewhere thought to take a picture of me." This woman pleads with new and expectant parents not only to take pictures but also to consider a fundamental shift in ownership that occurs when a baby is born—that baby photos belong to the parent *and* child. "If your child has a cleft, PLEASE take her picture," she continues. "Don't take it for yourself. Take it for your child, because it's your child's face, not yours, and someday she may want to know what it looked like." Technically speaking, the image of a minor may belong to his or her guardian. But this woman reminds us that emotionally speaking (if not for other reasons), the ownership is shared.

As distraught as this woman felt about her situation, it may be important to note that some kids grow up and don't feel strongly about pictures. The first time I spoke with Lisa, it was clear that while her ten- and eleven-year-old children, both born with CLP, had struggled at times with the intensity of their operations and other treatments—most recently with dental work—neither worried very much about cleft-related issues. "They are more concerned about hair and clothes and junior-high things than about CLP," she said. Lisa laughed as she described one baby picture of her son, in which he wore a pair of overalls that had a large, animal-shaped, cloth patch sewn onto the butt of the pants. Also pictured was his unrepaired cleft lip. "When he looks at that picture, his response is about the outfit," she continued, "not about how he looks."

No one can predict how today's baby will feel about her baby pictures down the line. It is possible that as a person grows and changes, she will feel just fine about those images, as Lisa's son did, or won't care much about them at all (except for the overalls). Yet it is also clear that baby pictures play an important, even critical role in a person's self-awareness.

Early Challenges
A Parent's View

Given that we can't predict how our children will feel about their baby pictures as they grow, it might seem relatively easy for new parents to forestall any potential problems. We could simply snap some photos early on, to cover our bases. As my grandmother used to say about such questions as whether to walk under a ladder or open an umbrella in the house, "I am not superstitious. But why risk it?" Just as it costs us almost nothing to walk around the ladder, you'd think that a similar, simple workaround would be true for taking pictures. We could just take some.

And yet...just at a moment when parents might be taking pictures, many are in crisis. Learning about cleft lip and palate and all it entails can be overwhelming, especially for parents who receive the news in the delivery room (as opposed to during prenatal testing, months earlier). Many are stressed out and full of worry. Some have never heard of clefts, much less know how to find someone to treat them. "Learning the news at delivery was horrible," said one mother. Some feel shocked by their child's unusual appearance and wonder whether this condition was their fault. Many have strong fears about other, underlying health conditions. Taking photos (much less taking deep breaths) can be hard to fathom when medical people are running into the delivery room, sounding the alarms.

One parent felt most vulnerable at a moment when others were celebrating—you guessed it—with pictures. "The low point came," she said in a video for parents, "when they announced over the loudspeakers in the [hospital] rooms that the photographer was there." Parents were asked to bring their babies to a central meeting room in the hospital to line up for photos. "My husband and I just agonized," she continued, "and decided that we really couldn't deal with this. We couldn't deal with having all the parents line up and say, 'Let's see your baby, let's see your baby.'" It can feel overwhelming to engage in a public ritual with strangers at a moment of palpable distress.

Picture-taking tends to be a relatively happy custom. Even in an age of smartphones and selfies, as people take considerably more photos, in general, than they did in years past, most of us take pictures to record good times, celebrate milestones, or mark moments of transition. Maybe we document our dinners or the antics of our pets. But do we take photos when we learn difficult news? Maybe not. Most likely we pause and set down our cameras, if not all kinds of other things in our lives. Dr. Ronald P. Strauss spoke about that very moment. "That is the crisis time," he said, "...and there is this natural inclination to hide away." So, it is understandable that we would want to call off our rituals of celebration and pull our heads and legs into our shells, like turtles in distress. These feelings are normal.

Two Journeys

And yet...there is good reason to take pictures anyway. We need to take pictures, if not with the other babies in the hospital, then in some other place that feels right. Our children will need them. The nurse (mentioned at the beginning of the chapter) is wise.

At the same time, we don't need to pretend that the act feels easy; it may feel odd, counterintuitive, and uncomfortable. As mentioned earlier in this book, the news of a child's health condition can feel jarring and frightening. Yet as inconceivable as it may feel in the moment, feelings change. Crises do resolve. While the cleft-team psychologist acknowledged that our initial response to our child's CLP may feel overwhelming, he went on to say that it is "not what the rest of life is all about." Our own retreat, if indeed we have one, will ease.

Some parents need time to come to terms with their child's differences. "I didn't want to get pictures taken at first," admitted another mother, Brenda, about her discomfort with the news of her son's CLP shortly after he was born. But then her own mother stepped in. The new grandmother acknowledged Brenda's feelings but reminded her that her baby was healthy. "My mom really helped me get through it," she said. "Finally, I thought, *You know what? He is who he is.*" For Brenda, the journey to acceptance took weeks, as well as the thoughtful advice of a trusted family member. But it did happen.

How many pictures do we need? "My photo albums are over-flowing with pictures of my son before, during, and after surgery," writes another mother about her early days with her son. "He will ask about his scar, and I will have photos and videos to help him understand." It is wonderful to have a lot of pictures. But the album doesn't have to overflow. We just need enough, which means being consistent with previous patterns, especially if there are siblings involved. It means having photos to answer a child's questions later on. And imperative is sending a message of love, acceptance, and respect for a child's ownership of her own image—even if our own love and acceptance arrived later than expected.

One parent turned the celebratory ritual on its head—she actually took pictures to cope. "The very best thing I did," she wrote for the cleftsmile website, "was take photos…hundreds and hundreds of them. They are my favorite memories of such an uncertain time in our lives." Indeed, the early days can be shaky times for parents. It is important to take pictures for the sake of the child. But as parents, too, we may find ourselves flipping through a baby album one day, thinking back on those early times and seeing the footprints of our own journey.

Chapter 19

. . . .

Supermarket Stories

Baby in Public

Like many parents of kids born with cleft lip and palate, Brittany and her husband learned about their child's CLP during pregnancy via prenatal ultrasound. Also like other parents, Brittany spent some of the remainder of her pregnancy anticipating how it would feel to bring their baby out in public—and in particular, whether she and her husband would hear rude or unkind comments from strangers. "How would the world respond to him?" she wondered. "We were very worried about that." So, after signing on with a cleft team, Brittany sought advice on the subject from her child's surgeon. Did he have suggestions, she asked, about possible responses to hurtful comments about their baby? "He said to us, 'I don't think you are going to have to worry about that,'" Brittany said. "He said that ninety-nine percent of the time, people will say that they love babies or say that their cousin has that, too."

Brittany wasn't sure whether to believe him. But in the weeks and months after their child was born, she and her husband found that their surgeon's predictions came to pass. "People were never rude or condescending," she continued. "I was still nervous to go out in public, though—nervous and ready for that one jerk who was going to be rude."

To a certain extent, as Brittany and her husband discovered, expectant parents may be pleasantly surprised by how smoothly their trips to the supermarket (or pharmacy or cookout) play out.

238

Many other parents report a similar story to Brittany's. "We got zero negative feedback," commented another mother. Still others, however, report having interactions with strangers about the appearance of their baby, some more positive than others. And unfortunately, a few describe hearing flat-out hurtful comments— which, even though infrequent, can have lasting effects, sticking to minds and hearts for years to come.

Whether they've received many questions about their baby or none at all, the parents I spoke with seemed to agree that the anticipation of a negative conversation can feel just as intense as the event itself. As Brittany aptly pointed out, the fear of interacting with "that one jerk"—whether she's standing in line behind us in the grocery store or replying to our pictures on social media—can keep us awake at night, full of fear and worry, even anger or heart-ache, wondering how we'll respond. I certainly lost plenty of sleep over this question myself, ruminating about possible responses that were tactful and…not so tactful. Fortunately, there are ways to approach these situations that do not involve arguing in line at the post office, crying in the produce section, or offering a rude stranger a complimentary copy of the *Wonder* book to teach her a thing or two about empathy (as plausible and constructive as those responses may feel at 3:00 a.m.).

This chapter explores four broad ideas to consider, based on parents' stories and insights, as well as input from cleft team professionals. While grocery shopping will likely change dramatically with any baby in tow, ideally, the interactions we have out in the world (or on Facebook) should be as stress-free as possible.

· ·

Supermarket Tip No. 1
Expect Attention

When I asked Shannon, the mother of Henry, about public inter-actions with her son, she recalled receiving a lot of attention from strangers—much of it driven by Henry's bubbly temperament. "Our son was the smiliest kid you have ever seen," she said about her trips around town with Henry before his lip-repair surgery. "He loved getting attention. He spent a lot of time smiling at everyone and you couldn't help but smile back at him. We only got positive feedback." Shannon didn't mind the interest from others, perhaps because Henry exuded such warm vibes—and also perhaps because Shannon described herself as outgoing with strangers. But other new parents dislike the newfound attention, particularly if they are unaccustomed to it. It can feel disorienting to be approached by someone in a store when, just weeks or months ago, we happily minded our own business, picking out broccoli or bell peppers in easy anonymity.

One way to deal with this new situation is to consider that *any* baby draws initial interest. Based on casual observation, it seems that some people make a second job out of interacting with babies. Most of us have probably seen the happy stranger in the super-market who spots a stroller and drops everything to speed-walk halfway across the store, knocking over display cases and innocent bystanders in order to enjoy a few sweet moments making goo-goo faces. Shannon's baby happened to have CLP, but he also drew people in by simply being a baby—in his case, an especially smiley, cooing, people-magnet. This new level of public interest may take some adjustment all by itself, with any baby. With a cleft-affected baby, new parents can expect increased interactions in public *and* possible questions about her unusual lip and nose. But as Shannon's story shows, the attention doesn't necessarily stem from the clefts.

Supermarket Tip No. 2
Consider Motivations

When parents of kids born with CLP described the questions and comments they received from strangers or acquaintances about their baby's clefts, several common scenarios emerged—some of them, they said, more uncomfortable than others. Yet before you decide how to respond to these different situations (which we will explore in the next section), it may be helpful to gauge a speaker's motivations. According to Marina Ebert, a researcher in the field of social cognition and child development, a key step in deciding how to respond to a stranger's questions is to "identify what lies at the core of the comment the person made." While at that moment there may be many factors that contribute to our decision about how to act, the simple act of considering the speaker's underlying motivations—whether they are outwardly negative or grounded in "innocent ignorance," as Ebert says—can go a long way toward reacting with a calm, level head.

Awkward, Basically Kind Person. When Rachel, the mother of Zeke, went back to work at a social services agency a few weeks after his birth, she brought a framed picture of him to display in her cubicle. She was proud to share the image with her coworkers, she said—but she also knew that it might elicit some questions. "When people saw my son's picture on my desk, there was a split second," she said, when they paused at the sight of his unfamiliar features. "A couple of times, people said to me, 'That is not what I was expecting to see.'" Rachel didn't mind receiving those responses, however, especially from people she knew. "I was not offended at all," she said, "because cleft lip is not that common." Other parents describe similar scenarios; they hear awkwardly worded comments or questions from people who probably mean well. In many cases, as Rachel noted, people in our lives may be surprised by our child's appearance because they have never seen a cleft before—a sentiment that many of us felt ourselves when we first learned about our baby's condition.

School-age children have been known to ask questions in public, as well—often in a decidedly clumsier manner than an office mate or other curious adult. The term *outside voice* comes to mind. Also, *no filter.* Several parents have described the following scenario. They're shopping quietly with their baby in Target when a child approaches, looks into the baby carriage, raises his eyebrows, and then asks his nearby parent, "WHAT IS WRONG WITH THAT BABY'S NOSE?" in a too-loud voice that sends his parent into cold sweats. A child may not know any better, but in making such a comment he pulls his parent into an impromptu, two-person act that shines just as much light on the parent's behavior as his own. One mother, Donna, was disappointed when such a situation happened at her local Costco as she was shopping with her daughter—and the nearby (other) parent did not respond gracefully. "The mom looked over, stared, and looked back, and never said a word to her child or to me. I think she was embarrassed, but that was a teachable moment for that mom. She could have talked about differences."

In retrospect, most parents attribute the discomfort of these types of situations to unfamiliarity and social awkwardness rather than unkind intentions. Several parents observed that young children tend to wonder whether a baby is in pain because of the clefts. "It is not that people are being mean or rude," commented another mother. "In fact, I think most of the time they are trying not to be rude. They just don't know the way to handle it."

As unintentional as these comments or stares may be, they can hurt us just the same. And ultimately, it is up to us, in the moment, to decide whether a person's motivations feel kind. But a majority of people mean well, most parents believe, even if they don't know what to say, ask a too-loud question, or give us more attention than we would like.

Silent, Avoidant Person. Sometimes, it is easy to tell if a person feels awkward but tricky to tell if the person means well. Shortly before my daughter had her first operation, while she was still wearing her NAM device full-time, I took her with me to the Dairy Queen at our local mall. As my daughter sat in her stroller, a man standing behind us in line caught a glimpse of her, flinched noticeably, and then pretended not to see her, looking downward as if he had taken a sudden, intense—and unbelievable—interest in the pattern of the floor tiles. I can only guess that this person felt extremely uneasy (and also that he had not had any formal training in acting). At the time, I felt ready to give him a short, friendly explanation, assuming that he probably felt more uncomfortable than anything else, but soon realized that he was not open to conversation. When I think back on the interaction today, though, my chest aches. It is difficult not to feel hurt and saddened by his behavior.

This kind of avoidant, awkward silence from a stranger, perhaps like that of the mother Donna saw in Costco, can be especially difficult to interpret because we have very little basis for explaining a person's behavior. With no verbal input—whether rude or just curious—we cannot surmise the person's underlying motivations.

One solution may be to consider the interaction as rationally as possible. A study published in the journal, *Sociology of Health & Illness,* examines parents' descriptions of public encounters with their autistic children. It introduces the distinction between "felt" and "enacted" stigma, the notion of identifying whether a stranger has actually spoken or behaved in a negative way in a public encounter, or whether the parent in the situation simply projects or perceives a negative response. The study states, "Although they are analytically separate, the two types of stigmas often merge in the experiences of the parents." In other words, it can be easy to jump to conclusions. While the Dairy Queen man sent a negative message by social avoidance—and while it hurts me even today to think that he behaved as awkwardly as he did simply because of the appearance of my child—I can't presume, having heard nothing from him, that his underlying intentions were negative. The Texas-based advocacy group Parent Companion recommends that parents approach public interactions with a positive guess. "Assume the best," the group suggests about the strangers we encounter, "unless you have a definite reason to assume otherwise." As we'll explore later, we don't owe a person a response. But in the absence of convincing evidence, it may ease our minds to make a positive assumption about the other person—or at least check an initial urge to assume the worst.

Rude Person. Once in a while, a parent hears a comment that stings. Amber, the mother of June, described smooth sailing during the first few months after her daughter was born. "For the most part, no one made any comments," she said. "People would say, 'Oh, my gosh, she's so cute! How old is she?' The usual stuff." But one day, after attending an Easter service at her local church—where she also happened to work full-time—Amber was surprised when a woman from the congregation approached her as she stood in a common room holding her baby. "She said to me, 'You know, I was really taken aback when I saw your daughter's face. You really have to warn people!'" Amber was stunned. "I didn't know how to respond," she said. "I just walked away. It was so weird. This woman went out of her way." In this case, a stranger made a comment that a parent perceived as flat-out hurtful.

Words like these can feel painful and infuriating. Even the *thought* of words like these can send a concerned parent tossing and turning in the middle of the night. Truth to tell, I hesitated to share Amber's story at all. But given the unfortunate reality that these kinds of interactions do happen—even outside of the context of parenthood and CLP—it might be helpful, even especially important, to consider a speaker's motivations right now, during a (hopefully) quiet moment.

To start, we might note the difference between *rudeness* and *meanness*. According to social worker Signe Whitson, rudeness is a behavior that involves "inadvertently saying or doing something that hurts someone else," while meanness involves hurting someone intentionally. As upsetting as Amber's story may be, it is probably fair to say that the woman at church did not intend to cause pain. In fact, of all the stories I have heard from parents about their interactions in public—and while, of course, each story is open to interpretation—I don't think I heard a single one that involved purposeful unkindness.

That said, mental health professionals are quick to point out how harmful rudeness can be. Several scholars and psychologists have said that even minor incidences of incivility can have long-lasting, negative effects on our well-being. So, no matter how we decide to respond—and as important as it is to consider a speaker's underlying motivation—we should make sure to honor our shaken-up feelings. They are normal and okay.

Angelic Person (False Alarm). Every so often, a parent anticipates a negative or uncomfortable public interaction, then has an experience that restores faith in the kindness of others. Maude described taking her daughter, Sylvie, to a casual weekend event in her small town. "I took her to a community hike for babies," she said, noting that the event took place during the very early days of her maternity leave, before her daughter's first operation. As Sylvie sat in the stroller looking out at the world, a little boy approached. He seemed curious. Very curious. "The boy comes over and keeps looking and looking and looking," Maude said. At this point, Maude was starting to feel some flutters in her stomach. "I'm preparing in my head, getting ready to say that she was born that way and that it doesn't hurt." Finally, the boy blurted out a question—but it did not relate whatsoever to CLP. "He asked, 'Why is she wearing a hat?'" Maude paused to laugh. "I ended up saying 'Because it's cold outside!'"

As stressful as it may feel to anticipate awkward or negative reactions in public, sometimes a stranger, whether an adult or child, surprises us with compassion or even indifference. "For kids, it's nothing," Maude commented in retrospect. "The cleft doesn't mean anything to them."

Facebook Person. As daunting as it may feel to interact with strangers in public spaces, some parents feel just as vulnerable posting pictures on social media. "I was really worried about Facebook," commented one mother, Marla. She was quick to note that "private" groups were not the problem. "I had a lot of support from the Cleft Mom group," she said, adding that she was pleased to make contact with other parents through that carefully administered, private group. "That part was really cool." But the larger world of Facebook made her nervous. "I was really scared of putting my daughter's picture on Facebook itself," she acknowledged, "just on my own page."

Recent research into internet behavior confirms, perhaps unsurprisingly, that the relative anonymity of online communications can lead to interactions that are less civil than they would be in real life. A study from the University of Wisconsin refers to this behavior as "the Nasty Effect." Psychologist Maria Konnikova explains that physical factors (or the lack of them) play an important role. "Without the traditional trappings of personal communication like non-verbal cues, context, and tone," she writes, "[online] comments can become overly impersonal and cold." It's no wonder cleft parents feel nervous about Facebook. Who wants to encounter "the Nasty Effect" just at a moment when we feel particularly vulnerable?

The upside of this situation is that those of us who use social media have tools at our disposal that vary from the ones we might use in the grocery store or the pharmacy—including the popular option of being proactive with the material we post (as discussed in the next section) and depending on our comfort levels, even refraining from posting at all.

. . . .

Supermarket Tip No. 3
Prepare "WISE-ly"

So, now what? At this point, maybe you have considered the element of increased attention in public—for any baby, regardless of CLP. And maybe you have thought about the underlying motivations behind the comments you might hear in public. But then, there is the question of what to actually *do* when an interaction takes place (or doesn't take place) at the Costco or the church hall or the community hike for babies.

Start Early. When we think about interactions in advance, we are already helping them go as well as possible. So, to begin, you can continue reading this chapter. Professionals on cleft teams recommend going even one step further, by actually practicing what we might say in certain situations. Whether we're fielding a well-meaning question or an awkward—or rude—comment or stare, they advise practice and more practice. "Right from the beginning," said one clinical nurse specialist on a cleft team, "when people start asking about the cleft, families need to be working through the answer."

Then, perhaps, we can refer to the flight safety instructions we hear on an airplane before takeoff. "Take care of your pain first," advises sociologist Christine Carter, PhD, from the Greater Good Science Center, who writes about how to handle rude or mean comments. As a rule, when we are interacting with a person who asks a question or makes a comment, we might remember that we don't owe them anything. As one nurse on a cleft team put it, "People don't deserve an answer." It is okay to assert our own desire to feel comfortable.

What to Say? Then, we can prepare an actual statement to say to strangers. The idea here, as odd as it may sound, is to prepare a few sentences that you *may or may not* use at the moment—or may use with some variation—depending on your mood, the setting, the timing, and how you perceive a speaker's motivations. (In some cases, you may choose to simply walk away, using no words at all, as Amber did—and as explained in the framework below). But to start, as one cleft-team nurse specialist recommended, you might prepare a few short, honest sentences, followed by—and this part is key—a transition to another topic. I like to think of these sentences as a *truthful-statement-plus-diversion* strategy. It's a template that you can edit or adjust, in the moment, depending on the situation. "You can be matter of fact," the nurse explained. "Give them a brief, truthful answer and a transitional topic." Here is an example, which is a slight variation on an example given by this nurse:

> *I see you're curious about my baby. She was born with a cleft. She's doing really well! Her doctor is so pleased. I'm looking for clothes for her for a holiday party. I just love this outfit!*

When to Say It? Once you have come up with a statement that feels workable, you can decide how and when to use it. The Maryland-based Center for Adoption Support and Education developed a tool for children who receive uncomfortable questions from others about adoption. The method, called "W.I.S.E. Up!," offers a simple acronym for deciding how to respond. While this method is designed for children in adoptive families, it applies to anyone receiving questions about difference—in this case, parents of cleft-affected babies, and perhaps later on, their children themselves. The method can be empowering for individuals and families because, as noted in the academic journal *Pediatric Nursing*, it is "based on the premise that adoptive children are wiser about adoption than peers who are not adopted." The same truth applies to cleft-affected individuals and families. The method offers four options for behavior:

W Walk away or ignore what was said or heard.

I "It's private and I don't have to answer it." [Ignore]

S Share [what you are comfortable sharing].

E Educate others about adoption [or CLP] in general.

Walk Away, Ignore. The first two options in the framework, *Walk Away* and *Ignore*, involve offering no response at all or giving only a short statement, something like, "That's private information." Amber, the mother who heard a rude comment about her baby while at work at her local church, reported that she responded only very briefly to the speaker and then walked away. "The situation was tricky because I worked there and I couldn't be rude," she explained. "If I had had time to respond, I guess I would have been honest with her. Luckily, it happened so late after my daughter was born. I was already mentally prepared."

It is important to remember that these types of very uncomfortable situations may occur rarely. Still, according to the parent support organization Parent Companion, it is all right to feel angry—or to feel however you feel in the moment—and want to walk away. "The unfortunate reality is that some people stare and make rude comments," the group writes. "Sometimes we are in a calm state of mind and can help educate the person who has made the inappropriate remark." Other times, we aren't in the mood. "Both kinds of reactions are normal and to be expected," the group continues. Even if we try to give the rude or thoughtless person the benefit of the doubt or assume a positive motivation, their question, comment, or stare can hurt or anger us. It's okay to walk away.

Share/Educate. Some days, a question from a stranger may feel nonthreatening, even comfortable. If you feel ready to share and/ or educate, you might deliver a version of your *truthful-state- ment-plus-diversion* sentences. The idea is to tell the truth in a simple, sincere way that feels easy to you. If you are in the mood to teach or if you realize midstream that the interaction feels safe, you might delay your transitional sentence and even answer another question—or not! Fortunately, this idea works like a template. You can vary the words—and add and subtract content—based on the situation, your interpretation of the person's motivations, and your mood.

A slight variation on your *truthful statement*, as the W.I.S.E. framework suggests, is to educate people about CLP more generally instead of focusing on your child (and then to include a diversion, of course). You might say:

Yes, my child was born with a cleft. Maybe you've seen the ads for charities like Smile Train. Treatment in the US has improved a lot in the last few decades. Hmm, I just noticed that these eggs are on sale. Wow, look! Can you believe that all twelve of them are broken?

A second variation, assuming you feel comfortable, is to elicit a question, particularly in the case of awkward silence. One mother, Dasha, described being proactive when people stared at her child. "I learned to say, 'Do you have a question for me?'" she said. This approach can work particularly well with curious children. "I remember asking people, 'Do you want to ask a question—because it is okay if you do,'" Dasha said. "Then, a lot of times, they asked questions." By taking the initial, brave step of speaking about the topic—with kids and adults alike—you can go a long way in putting people (including yourself) at ease. After hearing the person's question, you might follow up with some variation on the truthful-statement-plus-diversion sentences.

Being proactive can help ease our interactions on social media too. Marla, the mother who felt nervous about posting pictures of her daughter on her personal Facebook page, eventually decided to take the bull by the horns. When she shared pictures of her daughter after she was born, she included a simple phrase alongside. Marla wrote, "'Eva was born with cleft lip, and she is the most beautiful thing we have ever seen.'" The key here was Marla's forthrightness, not just in bringing up the topic, but in sharing her emotions. "We signaled how we felt about it," she said. As a result, Marla received no negative responses at all. "The comments were all positive," she said. "People wrote, 'Look at those eyes, look at that smile.'" She described her approach in this case as similar to the process of choosing a baby's name. "If you tell people about a baby's name once you've made the decision," she said, "you'll only get positive comments. The same thing happened to us with those pictures." By posting loving comments under the photo, she actually provided a model for her friends and acquaintances.

Responding to public interactions can feel daunting, as it did for Marla and so many others. But whether you decide to walk away from a person, engage briefly, share, or educate—in real life or online—the key is to feel comfortable and prepared.

. . . .

Supermarket Tip No. 4
Forget about Home Runs

Public interactions can be taxing for new parents. Some days (perhaps all days), you may feel tired and not in the mood to be generous with a stranger who asks an awkward question. "It takes a lot of mental energy to be willing to teach," admitted one mother. She found it difficult just to leave the house with her daughter. "I did it," she continued, "but there were situations when I wanted to grab a kid's parents and say, 'Teach your kid that staring is rude!'" Teachable moments can be draining—as can public interactions in general. And sometimes, the last thing we want to do is educate someone who has just hurt our feelings.

Fortunately, when it comes to making decisions like whether to teach a person or just walk away, you don't have to hit a home run every time. The "W.I.S.E.-Up!" framework, along with the *truthful-statement-plus-diversion* sentences, can be useful tools to have in your toolbox, but you don't have to master them right away. It is okay to mess up—to reveal a little too much personal information, for instance, or to misread a person's awkward question. As cleft teams have advised, practice really does make a difference, whether you're assessing people's motivations, gauging your own moods, or deciding which kind of response feels best for a particular situation.

When considering how to react to public interactions, you might also consider the fact that your baby isn't listening. One mother mentioned feeling pressured to answer questions smoothly and gracefully in order to model positive messaging to her child. This impulse is spot-on—we *do* have an obligation to model body-positive messages to our child. As one nurse specialist noted, "Your answer [to a stranger] is what your child is going to grow up hearing. What you say is what they are going to say." But not yet! For now, the baby just sits there, gazing at her toes! So, the stakes are low, if nonexistent, for a baby at the start. Parents get a beautiful, built-in, months-long grace period in which to work out the kinks before their child understands.

One mother, Tiffany, described some initial slipups. "We live in a rural area," she explained. "I remember one time—more than one time—when someone asked, 'What is wrong with your baby?'" The people in her small town, she reasoned, had likely not seen CLP before, especially her son's bilateral type. "I would like to think that I was always patient," she said, starting to laugh, "but when you're at Walmart and trying to get something…I was not always that way!" To get it right is *not* to satisfy a stranger's desires, necessarily. To get it right is to consider various scenarios in advance, make a plan, practice your words, and then do your best job assessing and responding to a situation as it happens. To get it right is to do your best to honor your own feelings.

As the weeks, months, and trips to the grocery store go by, your interactions in public—and the anticipation of those interactions—may feel easier, whether you're responding to an awkward stare, a too-loud question from a child, a comment on Facebook, a false alarm, or an awkward but basically well-meaning inquiry. Maybe you'll goof up your lines at first (I know I did). But eventually, through interacting with others about your child's condition, you will have an opportunity to model strong, positive messages to your child, giving her tools to feel empowered—and hopefully, as time goes by, giving yourself the tools to feel empowered as well.

Chapter 20

. . . .

The Clinic Visit

Tips for "The Mother of All Doctors' Appointments"

The first time I called my daughter's cleft team to make an appointment for her, the coordinator recommended that I schedule the visit for a "clinic day." *Huh?* I thought. Until then, I had presumed that a "clinic" was a building. As in, *It's Sunday and Billy's got an earache; let's go to the walk-in clinic on North Main Street.* I wondered, *Isn't every day a clinic day?*

It turns out that, in the context of cleft lip and palate, a clinic day is a gathering of all or some of the specialists on a child's cleft team to visit with patients. The individual members on the team may work from separate physical locations for some of their time but convene in one place on a regular basis—say, once or twice a month—to consult with families. From a family's perspective, a clinic day is another name for a child's annual visit with the team. It may include three to five (or more) appointments wrapped into one. The visit can be surprisingly long. It can be tiring. Yet seeing all those experts convene to care for our child can also remind us why having a team is so amazing. And hopefully, the act of reconnecting with caring practitioners will feel productive and reassuring, even fun. One parent described the clinic day as "truly, the mother of all doctors' appointments." Here are six tips to help it go well—both now, during babyhood, and during subsequent annual visits as the years go by.

TIP No. 1. Bring Rations. The choreography of a clinic visit varies from team to team. In some cases, a child and family sit in a single exam room while professionals cycle through to conduct visits. A family might see the surgeon, for instance, as well as the speech-language pathologist, the clinical nurse specialist, the geneticist, and the audiologist or ENT—sometimes, with overlap. Other teams shuttle families back and forth to the waiting room in between visits with individual specialists. In any case, a 9:00 a.m. clinic appointment could reasonably last until noon, 1:00 p.m., or even 2:00 p.m., with no predictable break.

I get cranky if I go too long without a snack or a cup of coffee. I lose my ability to think clearly, listen well, and ask pertinent questions. My kids start to lose their marbles too (and so does my husband). I realize that this is a doctor's appointment, not a hike up Mount Kilimanjaro. But the visit will shape decisions about my daughter's health—and our family life—for an entire year. So, for good measure, I always throw a few bananas into my bag. Incidentally, one year the bananas served double-duty. As my toddler daughter snacked, the surgeon looked for evidence of a palatal fistula (a tiny hole in the palate). We all huddled around, mid-snack, watching to see if little bits of banana would come out of her nose as she ate. (TMI? Not for a cleft parent!)

TIP No. 2. Ask about Bagels (and Sneezes and....) As you plan for an upcoming visit with the team, you may anticipate conversations about significant treatment. *Does my child need surgery? Orthodontics? Speech therapy?* These are the big-ticket topics that can make our brains buzz beforehand, and certainly afterward if we learn about imminent action.

It is just as possible, however, to come to the visit with small questions too. Cleft lip and palate can affect daily life in countless ways, especially as a child grows. *Is it okay that my child can't really bite into substantial foods, like bagels? My child sneezes a lot (snores at night, and has a constant runny nose)—does this behavior relate to the clefts?* These questions may seem minor in comparison to the big ones—and they are! But they affect our lives in tangible ways. And you never know when a small question will unearth a bigger, underlying issue.

"No question is a stupid question, no matter what," commented one mother, Valerie, about her family's annual visits to the team with their three-year-old daughter. "If you feel it is stupid, it is not. You know your child best. Ask it!" Valerie described these questions—and the courage sometimes required to speak up about them—as important parts of a parent's role in advocating for their child. Cleft professionals agree. One surgeon described the ability to listen to families' concerns—all of them—as one of the most important characteristics of a good cleft team.

If you're not sure you'll remember all the issues that can come up on a day-to-day basis, it may help to jot them down as they arise rather than wait until the meeting approaches. "I write down my questions right away," Valerie continued, "because I know I am going to forget them."

Also, as the visit progresses from one professional to the next, don't be afraid to ask people to repeat their names. These kinds of inquiries may feel silly or embarrassing, but it is better to ask a question than to wonder who is talking. Some teams are not only large but also change in composition from year to year, if not among the team members themselves, then among the residents or fellows who accompany them into the exam room. You might say, "I'm sorry, I missed that. Do you mind repeating your name and your role?"

TIP No. 3. Make Plans for Your Young Child. One of the unfortunate aspects of having a team visit with a baby, toddler, or very young child is that the patient needs to be present in the room. As mentioned above, the appointment may last more than three hours. Even the calmest of one-year-olds will be tempted to grab the doctor's exam tools off the wall countless times during that visit. (I am referring to the instruments used for ear and eye exams, which are often fixed to the wall just above the exam bench, right within a kid's reach, like toys or candy in a checkout aisle. Who came up with this arrangement?) And what parent can sustain a serious, important conversation with doctors while redirecting a child? "Okay, yes doctor, I see. He needs major surg—put that back! Jimmy, I said, put that BACK!"

One solution is to bring distractions like toys, crayons, a tablet, etc. "I'm not going to lie," commented one mother about her preparation for the annual appointment. "In our family, it's bribery at its finest. My daughter likes little toys, so I bring a bag of them." Given the importance of the visit, this mother pulls out all the stops to make it comfortable. "It helps your child, it helps you, it helps everyone," she continued. Even better, bring a trusted person—if at all possible—to provide an extra set of ears and to take the child into the hallway or back to the waiting room if necessary.

TIP No. 4. *Make Plans with Your Child as She Grows.* An older child will likely restrain herself from playing with the exam tools on the wall (although if she's tempted, I don't blame her. Three hours!) Yet a parent may want to prepare, instead, for sensitive conversations with the surgeon and team.

Some parents of older children have expressed concern about how conversations about appearance can feel jarring to a child (even as one of the goals of cleft treatment is to improve self-confidence). Best intentions aside, some surgeons talk about people's faces in astonishingly frank terms. A surgeon might look at a child and say, "She's got a collapsed X, protrusion of the Y, and asymmetry of the Z. I could fix that." The *New York Times* journalist and cleft parent KJ Dell'Antonia described such an interaction during a team visit with her ten-year-old daughter. "The consultation took us both aback," she writes. "Hearing her face so bluntly discussed was upsetting for my daughter." Even if you agree with your surgeon's ideas, your child may find the conversation unsettling for being so direct.

What to do? If you sense that your child feels uncomfortable or bothered by these conversations, you should know that it is okay to take some control of the narrative. "It's fine for parents to tell doctors: 'Please do not use language that will echo in her head for years,'" Dell'Antonia advises. Another option is to ask up-front for an adults-only conversation following the initial exam. (A staff member may be willing to stay with your child in the waiting room if there is no one else available to do so.)

Another way to prepare for potentially sensitive conversations is to consider the element of teamwork between parent and child, especially as a child gets older. By the time a child is a preteen or teen, she may be conversing directly and successfully with members of the cleft team about treatment options and may participate actively in decisions about her care. Wonderful. But it may also be helpful to consider beforehand what you know about how your child feels about aspects of appearance Is your child curious about—or resistant to—changing parts of her face? If so, why?

One mother thought she knew how her daughter felt about the appearance of her nose until she pursued a conversation with her—several times. "As I pressed a little more," she said, "I was astonished to find out that my daughter felt disappointed that [her nose] was not symmetrical." Every child and parent communicate differently, of course. But it may be useful to have a conversation (maybe more than one) with your child before the visit. If you are both on the same page beforehand, you can help her get the information she needs. You can ask follow-up questions she may not have considered. These conversations are all about trust (on a child's part) and active listening (on our part).

TIP No. 5. *Sharpen Your Pencils.* When I asked Simone about her most recent annual visits with the cleft team with her teenage son, she let out a little laugh. "You go to seven appointments," she said. "You're there all day, you're exhausted, and you have no idea what anyone said when you're done." Conversations with team members on a clinic day can involve a surprising, even overwhelming amount of information exchange—such as learning diagnoses, hearing about options, asking questions, and more. And as much as a child's role in the annual visits will evolve as she grows, the goal of the visit remains largely the same as the years go by, usually to assess and discuss *now* and then to act *later*. Sometimes, team members recommend treatment and lay out a time line without asking for very much parental (or patient) input. Other times, decision-making happens later on, at home, especially for procedures that are considered optional or are not strictly time-sensitive.

Written notes can pay dividends in both situations. As important as it is to come to the meeting with questions, it is just as valuable to leave the meeting with your own record of the discussion. That way, when *later* comes, you won't find yourself asking, *What did the orthodontist say about that treatment? What happens, again, with recovery from surgery?* I take an old-school approach by purchasing a small, coil-bound notebook for every person in the family (and incidentally, every pet). Two kids plus one dog and one cat equal four cheap, grocery store notebooks that I use as a repository for day-to-day health questions, notes from doctors' appointments, questions for parent-teacher conferences, and the like. My notes are sloppy but located in one place (and the old-fashioned notepads could easily be replaced by a smartphone).

The clinic visit can tax our brains. In a few days or weeks, we may forget the details—and there may be many details! As simple as this idea may seem, the notes we take during a visit can be extremely helpful and reassuring when we need them most.

TIP No. 6. Expect More. After a child's annual visit with the team, there will almost always be a follow-up appointment to make, an item to buy, a decision to consider, or a resource to check out. This cycle never ends (with medical appointments and with practically any other kind of appointment). In a way, the myriad tasks that parents take on before, during, and after these visits are emblematic of our role on the cleft team. One nurse specialist from the Children's Craniofacial Association describes a parent's participation in team care as critically important to the success of the treatment. "Parents whose children have health or developmental issues," she writes, "have been thrust into the role of advocate, researcher, observer, educator, coordinator, and all-round mountain mover."

While an annual team visit often involves keeping track of a lot of moving parts—while also providing snacks, asking questions, keeping notes, and yes, moving mountains—hopefully, the "mother of all doctors' appointments" will also feel informative, clarifying, and reassuring that our child is in good hands.

Chapter 21

. . . .

Early Hearing and Speech

Midway through Courtney's pregnancy, she and her husband splurged on a $150 specialty 4-D ultrasound in order to enjoy some keepsake pictures of their unborn baby. The couple didn't anticipate a prenatal diagnosis of unilateral cleft lip and possible cleft palate. "I was devastated," Courtney said, as well as overwhelmed, especially by the constellation of issues related to CLP. The idea of surgical repair—to the lip, to the palate—seemed logical to her, even unsurprising, since she had seen shows and ads on TV about cleft-affected kids. Feeding challenges seemed understandable too. But Courtney and her husband hadn't realized that a person born with cleft palate could have hearing loss or problems with speech. This news immediately made sense when they learned about the anatomy of the mouth and ears. But the couple felt sideswiped—and scared—by the realization that their child might encounter even more challenges than they first realized.

As daunting as this situation felt to Courtney and her husband—and to other cleft parents, as well—the good news is that hearing and speech can be managed. The specialists on the cleft team are ready to help. And while management and treatment can require effort and diligence from parents (and later on, from the affected child), many parents feel relieved to see how treatable these conditions really can be. In this chapter, we'll hear more from Courtney and her family as we explore these two issues, starting with hearing and moving on to speech.

Hearing during Infancy

Hearing loss can feel stressful for us, as parents, not only because the issue sometimes comes as a surprise when we learn the news of our baby's cleft diagnosis, but because hearing, in general, can have profound effects on a child's growth and development. Experts suggest that even mild, untreated hearing loss can affect social and emotional growth, speech and language development, and later in childhood, academic achievement.

But did you notice a key word in that last sentence? *Untreated* hearing loss can be problematic. Fortunately, hearing loss can be addressed. And according to experts, when hearing issues are detected early on, the related challenges can be decreased and even eliminated. "Our daughter failed her hearing tests at birth and struggled with infections for years," said another parent in the book *I Wish I'd Known…*, "but with four sets of ear tubes and lots of checkups, she now has perfect hearing." Before we discuss treatment (more to come on ear tubes), let's look at some basics of the relationship between hearing and cleft palate.

Types of Hearing Loss. There are two types of hearing loss, one relatively unusual for babies with CP, and the other much more common.

Sensorineural hearing loss is a permanent hearing loss that cannot be cured through medicine or surgery; it is caused by damage to the acoustic nerve or other parts of the *inner ear* (the innermost part of the ear). While babies born with cleft palate are more likely to have this type of hearing loss than unaffected babies and while it is associated with genetic syndromes, its occurrence is reportedly quite low among babies with isolated clefts (cleft lip and/or palate not occurring alongside a genetic syndrome). The Craniofacial Center at Seattle Children's Hospital characterizes sensorineural hearing loss as occurring in a "very small number of babies" born with CP. And one recent study on hearing outcomes among 338 children born with CP showed that none of them were born with this type of loss. Sensorineural loss can be caused by certain illnesses, a lack of oxygen during birth, and genetic factors.

Conductive hearing loss, in contrast, occurs when sound is unable to move through the other two parts of the ear (the *outer ear* and *middle ear*) in order to reach the inner ear. This type of hearing loss occurs frequently among infants born with CP—one study states it occurs in 82 percent of cases—and usually happens when something obstructs the pathway such as wax or fluid. While conductive hearing loss causes short- and long-term problems, if left unattended (as mentioned above), it is relatively easy to correct and is usually temporary.

These two types of hearing loss can occur alone or in some cases, together (called *mixed hearing loss*).

A Common Culprit: Fluid. Given how often babies with cleft palate experience conductive hearing loss, it is important to know about a likely cause—fluid in the ear—and why it can be problematic. The space of the middle ear is supposed to stay dry. Under normal circumstances, fluid will show up from time to time, sometimes in the form of mucus from a common cold. But also, under normal circumstances, the *Eustachian tube* opens every so often, allowing any such fluids to drain away.

The Eustachian tube is a small tube that connects the middle ear to the throat. It opens when we yawn, swallow, change elevations, or suffer from a cold, in order to equalize pressure (thus, the occasional popping sounds in our ears). But can you guess which muscles control the opening and closing of that tube? Yes, indeed, the muscles of the soft palate—which, of course, may not function as they should in babies born with CP. To complicate matters, the Eustachian tube itself is typically underdeveloped in infants (all infants) and located in a horizontal position, making drainage less effective. So, while it is common for all babies to get fluid in the ears, it is even more common for those with CP. As speech-language pathologist Ann Kummer explains, the temporary hearing loss caused by fluid in the ears feels like you are trying to hear when you've put your hands over your ears or when someone has turned the volume on the TV way down. One cleft-team audiologist stated its effects more bluntly, that fluid "acts like an earplug."

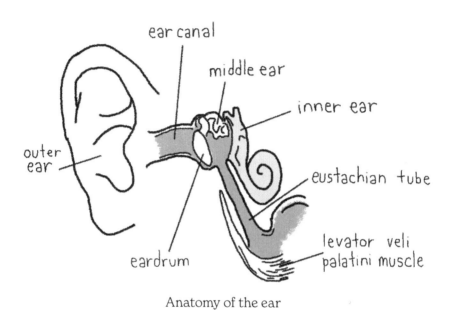

Anatomy of the ear

Let's go one step further. When fluid sits in the middle ear, it can get infected. Ear infections, which are sometimes treated with antibiotics, are common for all babies and especially for those with CP. As parents, you will usually be alerted to infections when your baby fusses and cries, tugs at the affected ear(s), has a fever, etc. (see below for a complete list of possible signs). But here's the thing! Hearing loss can occur when fluid sits in the middle ear *whether infected or not*. One recent study published in the journal *Clinical Medicine and Therapeutics* states that *otitis media with effusion* (fluid in the ear that is not infected, sometimes called *glue ear*) occurs in 97 percent of children born with CP during their first two years of life.

So, while it may be clear that you need to seek help from a doctor for an infection—because your baby will probably let you know—you may or may not notice signs when fluid is present but uninfected. One way to find out about fluid is to ask a doctor to examine the baby's ears. As Kummer emphasizes, it is important for you, as parents, to make sure those exams happen on a regular basis.

A Parent's To-Do List for Hearing: Three Tasks

The most important mantra to keep in mind with regard to protecting and helping your baby's hearing is *vigilance*. Why? Because the challenges associated with untreated hearing loss—of any type—are profound (as mentioned above). Ongoing attentiveness is necessary both in terms of finding out whether there is a problem and then, if necessary, treating it.

A parent's responsibilities with regard to hearing basically fall into three categories: making timely appointments with specialists whenever directed by the cleft team (usually for hearing tests and possible treatment), asking for frequent ear exams from the pediatrician during the baby's first year (and beyond), and paying attention to a child's hearing at home.

HEARING TASK No. 1. Pick Up the Phone! Make Appointments with Specialists. Formal hearing tests are critical for babies with cleft palate because hearing specialists can detect hearing loss that we, as parents, cannot identify on our own. Fortunately, a member of the cleft team will likely give you some direction with regard to hearing tests—and the appointments you'll need to make in order for your child to receive them—during very early infancy. But you will also receive information about your baby's hearing right from the start, at birth.

Every baby born in a US hospital receives a newborn hearing test (often called a hearing *screen*), the results of which are up or down: a baby passes, or she doesn't pass. If your baby passes the screen, wonderful! But remember that testing doesn't end there. It is important to follow up with the cleft team to learn their recommendations (see questions for the team, below). The *audiologist* (a specialist who tests hearing) or the *otolaryngologist* (usually referred to as an *ear, nose, and throat* surgeon or an ENT) on the team will be your point person for hearing. This specialist may recommend certain tests starting at least at age nine months and recurring once or twice a year until age five, as recommended by the ACPA for all babies born with cleft palate. But most hearing specialists recommend a *complete audiological evaluation* by the age of three months in order to take a baseline measurement of a baby's hearing. These hearing tests—and future tests—gauge a baby's responses to sounds. They are usually performed by an audiologist. None are invasive or painful.

If your baby does not pass the newborn hearing screen, a doctor at the hospital (and the ENT/audiologist on the team) will recommend the complete evaluation as soon as possible or by age three months. Whatever the outcome of the newborn screen, it is important to remember the value of timely hearing tests and treatment, to ask all your questions (no matter how small!) when you meet with the cleft team, and most of all, not to lollygag when you learn about something that needs to happen next.

HEARING TASK No. 2: Ask a Doc for Frequent Exams. Next up, it is important to make sure your child receives regular ear exams in order to stay on top of that pesky menace—fluid, which could show up in the middle ear at any moment (how's that for a recipe for parental stress?). Remember that fluid can be infected or uninfected. If you suspect your baby has an ear infection (see a list of common signs, below), you should contact her pediatrician. The pediatrician will examine your baby's ears with an *otoscope,* a handheld device with a pointed end that is usually mounted on the wall. The tool is necessary for ear exams (along with a doctor's expertise) because the eardrum—and any fluid behind it—are located too far into the ear to be detected with the naked eye. But as speech-language pathologist Ann Kummer suggests, you should ask for exams even if you *don't* suspect infection. "Every time you visit the doctor, ask her to look carefully in the ears," she says.

Heads Up! While your baby's pediatrician will check her ears several times during his first year (the American Academy of Pediatrics recommends a schedule of seven well-child appointments during year one) and while it is advisable, as Ann Kummer indicates, to ask the pediatrician to examine her ears during other visits whenever possible (at a sick visit, for example), it is important to consult the pros on the cleft team on a regular basis *as well.*

Hearing specialists have mentioned a gentle warning to parents about the seemingly simple act of examining a child's ears: not all pediatricians possess the specialized training or skills of an audiologist or ENT. Some pediatricians may detect fluid in a child's ears and understand its significance, but others may not. There is no fault in this difference; this is why generalists are generalists and specialists are specialists. But it is important to stay on top of ear-related visits with the cleft team no matter what (and to speak about this issue with the team if you have questions).

HEARING TASK No. 3. Pay Attention at Home. There are two things to keep an eye on at home with regard to hearing: the possibility of ear infection(s) (as mentioned above), and a baby's behavior and general developmental milestones. The ACPA offers some common signs of infection. If you notice any of the following behaviors in your baby or otherwise suspect a problem, you should call your child's pediatrician. Signs of ear infection include:

* fussing and crying more than usual,
* tugging at the affected ear(s), indicating discomfort,
* eating and sleeping poorly,
* having a fever,
* showing poor balance, and/or

* appearing to be tuning out when spoken to.

As parents, you can also pay attention to a child's hearing during day-to-day life. One doctor suggested, in the *Journal of Clinical Medicine and Therapeutics,* that parents should observe their baby's reactions to sound and watch their interactions with other children. "Any abnormalities warrant expert evaluation," he said. In a curious twist, however, professionals also acknowledge that parents are not always able to judge. Recent research shows that parents sometimes err on the side of missing a hearing problem when one is actually present.

So, what to do? You can keep an eye out for certain behaviors and then (perhaps unsurprisingly) consult with the pros on the cleft team. The developmental milestones below, published by the Harvard Medical School, reflect typical behaviors in babies who hear normally. If your baby does not demonstrate these behaviors—or if you can't tell (since as the research shows, it's difficult!), or if you feel at all concerned about your baby's hearing—be sure to pick up the phone and call the team. The key is to observe your baby at home, of course, but also to lean on the experts and ask as many questions as necessary in order to feel comfortable.

Typical Developmental Milestones in Babies with Normal Hearing

Harvard Health Publishing, Harvard Medical School

0 to 3 months. The child blinks, startles, moves with loud noises, and quiets down at the sound of the parent's voice.

4 to 6 months. The child turns his or her head to the side toward voices or other noises. The child appears to listen and then responds as if having a conversation.

7 to 12 months. The child turns his or her head in any direction toward sounds.

Publishing HH. Hearing Loss in Children. Harvard Health. Accessed March 11, 2021. shorturl.at/PRZ35

Treatments for Hearing Loss: Hearing Aids, Antibiotics, and Tubes. As always, it is important to ask the audiologist or ENT on the cleft team about treatment for hearing loss, since recommendations will vary depending on several factors that are beyond the scope of this book. But it may be helpful to know about a few typical paths and to have questions at the ready. Hearing aids are a common treatment for babies born with sensorineural hearing loss and in some cases, conductive loss. These devices have come a long way in recent years technologically speaking; they are smaller than they used to be and are available in many styles. Hearing aids can be invaluable for understanding the spoken word. The ability to hear consonants, in particular, is critical for a baby's comprehension and ultimately, for the development of speech and language.

Treatment for conductive hearing loss often involves addressing the problem of fluid in the middle ear. When fluid is infected, a child's pediatrician or ENT/audiologist may recommend antibiotics. Antibiotics are common medicines for ear infections in all infants, clefts aside. But if infections start to recur over time—as they do for many cleft babies—or if uninfected fluid sits in the middle ear over time, the specialist on the team may recommend pressure-equalization tubes (sometimes called *grommets, myringotomy tubes, tympanostomy tubes, ventilation tubes, PE tubes,* or just *tubes*).

You might think of a PE tube as the world's smallest air vent. This plastic or metal tube is inserted directly into the eardrum by an ENT through a very short surgical procedure. The procedure typically involves three surgical steps: making a tiny incision in the eardrum, draining any existing fluid that might have built up, and inserting the tube into the hole.

An ear tube usually stays in place for six-to-nine months, during which time it allows air to flow between the middle ear and the outside world (the atmosphere), thus preventing the buildup of pressure in the ear. A PE tube also allows new fluid to drain out of the middle ear as necessary, thus reducing the likelihood of further ear infections, subsequent exposure to antibiotics, and of course, conductive hearing loss. As a child grows, the tube usually falls out and the hole usually heals on its own. In many cases, the professionals on the cleft team will schedule the insertion of ear tubes during another surgical session such as a baby's palate-repair surgery. Some babies get ear tubes once and that's it; others receive several tubes (or pairs of tubes) during their infancy and early years.

FAMILY STORIES
Courtney and Violet, Part 2

Fussing and More Fussing! A Bumpy Start

As daunted as Courtney felt when she learned the news of her daughter's cleft lip and palate at a 4-D prenatal ultrasound, the shock of the diagnosis—and the subsequent torrent of related information—softened as she learned about clefts. By the time Violet was born with unilateral-complete CLP, this second-time mother not only knew about the risks of frequent ear infections but also almost assumed her daughter would need ear tubes at some point. "Infections are extremely common in cleft babies during the first year," she informed family and friends on her private blog.

Courtney was surprised, however, when Violet came down with her first ear infection only eleven days after birth and experienced a tangle of low- to medium-grade health issues during the weeks and months that followed. Thankfully, a round of antibiotics did the trick for the early infection. But Violet developed a rash on her face that didn't go away, even after she stopped taking the medicine. Could Violet be allergic to the antibiotic? The baby also resisted eating from the Haberman bottle; she fussed and cried during almost all feeding sessions. Could she have reflux? Or a food aversion? Courtney was pumping milk, an endeavor that not only required tremendous time but also brought her own diet into the equation. She also wondered whether her technique with the Haberman was somehow inadequate. Should she ask for more training from the cleft team nurse? Or change bottles entirely? There were so many balls in the air! And the baby didn't seem to stop crying. Violet's very energetic three-year-old sister added even another variable: a succession of illnesses that likely originated from her preschool. Courtney joked that their family practically lived with their pediatrician.

As other parents of cleft-affected babies have seen, the early months of Violet's life involved a lot of fussing on Violet's part and a lot of problem-solving for her parents, in a near-constant rotation of issues involving fluid in the ears, problems with feeding, and reflux. These issues can be challenging to sort out. But one by one—and with a lot of help from professionals—Courtney and her husband found solutions. Courtney was relieved to see immediate improvements in Violet's mood once she began taking medication for reflux; her crying ended during feeding sessions, and her milk consumption improved. What's more, the family began receiving free, in-home help with feeding from their local Early Intervention program, a huge boon given their one-hundred-mile distance from the cleft team (during a pre-Zoom era). "I can use all the help I can get," Courtney said at the time.

Violet's fussing did not end there, however: it abated during mealtimes, thank goodness, but persisted at almost all other times of the day and night. At around age three months, Violet's pediatrician discovered a second ear infection and prescribed antibiotics. But he had also discovered uninfected fluid several other times during that period and suggested to the family that fluid itself can cause discomfort whether infected or not. At this point, Courtney and her husband felt frustrated and exhausted (and sick themselves).

Enter ear tubes. Fortunately, Courtney had developed a trusting relationship with the ENT on the cleft team—and their discussions had included the prospect of ear tubes almost from day one. While the ENT acknowledged that most cleft babies receive ear tubes during palate-repair surgery at around age ten months, Violet might benefit from early insertion, perhaps at around age four months via a separate surgical procedure. Courtney immediately agreed. "I couldn't take the constant screaming," she said.

The procedure would be short, about fifteen minutes of operating time. Courtney felt good about this decision. The sooner she could stave off discomfort and possible hearing loss, she reasoned, the better.

About five weeks after the ear tube procedure, Courtney took her daughter to a postoperative appointment with the ENT and audiologist to look at the tubes and check the baby's hearing. As Violet underwent various attention-grabbing hearing tests, she sat on her mother's lap, facing away from her. "I started to get nervous when she didn't seem to turn her head at the low noises," Courtney said. But the audiologist, who could see the baby's face, had no such worries: Violet had responded to the sounds with her eyes.

As circuitous as the journey felt to Courtney and her husband during Violet's early weeks and months, the outcome felt straightforward. Violet aced her hearing test and all but stopped fussing. The ear tubes were a success. Eventually, she would receive a second set. And the anticipation of upcoming lip- and palate-repair operations weighed on the whole family. But at this moment, Courtney felt enormously relieved.

To Tube or Not to Tube? And When? According to the Children's Hospital of Philadelphia, ear-tube insertion is the most common surgical procedure performed on children in the United States. Yet it is important to know that specialists vary in their philosophies on the use of PE tubes and, in particular, the optimal time to insert them. Some ENTs/audiologists on cleft teams recommend tubes for babies who have recurring infections, as indicated above. Others recommend it preventatively for those with no fluid in the ears (whether infected or not) since fluid occurs so commonly among babies with CP. Still others recommend "watchful waiting" of about three months before insertion, because an initial problem could go away on its own. Opinions vary.

One way to navigate these murky (and sometimes stressful) waters is to know about the risks and benefits of ear tubes—and then to ask as many questions as necessary to feel comfortable with your baby's treatment. The risks associated with PE tubes include scarring of the eardrum and *persistent eardrum perforation*, meaning a hole or tear in the eardrum that does not heal. Several sources characterize these complications as low; one study published in the *Cochrane Database of Systemic Reviews* places the risk of scarring at one-third of one percent. It is possible, too, that a tube will fall out early. So, some doctors prefer to wait up to three months to make sure the fluid is persistent, and tubes are necessary.

In contrast, cleft professionals suggest that proactive insertion of ear tubes can have particular benefits for babies born with CP. A longitudinal study published in 2020 in the *Ear, Nose & Throat Journal* examines a range of "current best evidence" to suggest that while typical babies may benefit from a wait-and-see approach, "high-risk" babies, like those born with cleft palate, have a more urgent need. In these cases, the chances are low, the author says, that fluid will go away on its own, leading to the conclusion that a waiting period can adversely impact speech and development. In other words, when cleft palate is involved, many professionals believe the benefits of tubes—and their early insertion—may outweigh the risks. "Tympanostomy tubes are a safe, effective, and time-tested intervention that can improve quality of life," the author states.

As always, we must trust the professionals who treat our children. "A good working relationship is essential," advises Dr. Diane L. Sabo about the interactions between parents and hearing specialists. It is important to ask all your questions, hear a doctor's reasoning, and feel comfortable with subsequent discussions and treatments. Sabo also reminds parents of the impact of hearing on other aspects of a baby's development. The goal of the team approach, she suggests, is to "maximize a child's ability to learn."

Here are some questions to ask the audiologist/ENT:

- My baby passed/did not pass her newborn hearing screen. What do you recommend for further testing? Do I need to make those appointments myself? What number should I call?
- What is your approach to the use of PE tubes? When is the best time to insert them and why? For our baby in particular? What are the risks and benefits?
- Is there anything I need to do to coordinate medical records between my baby's pediatrician and the professionals on the cleft team?
- How can I best monitor my baby's ear health at home? Under what circumstances should I contact you and/or the baby's pediatrician with concerns?

Speech and Language during Infancy

A couple of weeks after Violet's palate-repair surgery at age nine months, Courtney wrote a jubilant blog post. "We've joined the No More Surgery (For Now) Club," she told family and friends (for a description of Violet's early experiences, see the first part of this chapter). Yet as ready as Courtney felt to take a break from all things CLP, she also felt eager to enroll Violet in a local Early Intervention (EI) program for some early help with speech. Courtney liked the idea of getting a head start on speech shortly after the palate operation. While the speech-language pathologist on the cleft team had not recommended EI specifically for Violet, Courtney saw the free, state-run program as a sort of bonus. She knew that the period after palate repair was an important time for speech and hoped that the one-on-one speech therapy sessions with a community-based speech-language pathologist would give Violet a leg up. And Violet seemed to have already made some exciting strides: she was starting to push her tongue against her new palate and was saying "mamamama." "Music to my ears!" Courtney exclaimed at the time.

Courtney didn't anticipate that her daughter's early start would begin with anything other than flying colors. "The EI [intake assessment] really hit me hard," she said. "I thought I would be so overjoyed to get her in the program, but when I heard the words 'delayed,' it made me very depressed." The pathologist informed the family that Violet had demonstrated a 25-percent delay in language, meaning that, at age ten months, she was using language at a five-to-seven-month level. Her motor/cognitive skills were also delayed by about 20 percent. While this professional suggested that Violet's cleft palate and early reflux might have caused the delays, Courtney wondered whether she was to blame. "It just bothered me with all we have had going on this last year I haven't had as much time to play with Violet as I did with my first child," she said.

As upsetting as this situation felt to Courtney (and may feel for other families as well), it is important to know that speech-and-language delays are normal—and usually solvable—for a baby born with CP. It is equally important to know about the critical role of the speech-language pathologist (SLP) on the cleft team, the myth that every baby born with CP needs speech therapy, and how Early Intervention programs, which exist in every state in the US, *can* be valuable, even essential, for a child born with this condition—given some behind-the-scenes legwork from her parents. We will discuss these ideas below, then explore important tasks for speech and language during the baby's first year.

Late Arrival? It's Okay. The word *delay* can be hard to hear, as it was for Courtney when she learned the news about Violet. But it may be reassuring to consider the context of cleft palate and the bigger picture of short- and long-term growth. When a baby spends the first nine (or so) months of life with an opening in her palate—a period that typically involves experimentation with the speech sounds that involve the roof of the mouth—there's no wonder speech is affected. Research shows that cleft-affected babies may start speaking later than babies born without clefts and that when they do begin to speak, the sounds they make may be delayed to some extent too.

But in a way, we don't need the research to tell us these things. If you close your eyes, say the word *papa*, and consider the buildup of pressure required inside the mouth to produce that initial P sound, the news makes sense. In order to pronounce P, you need an intact palate to close off the mouth from the nose. So, in the context of cleft palate—not to mention the context of hearing problems during infancy—understandably a baby might be delayed.

Also—and this is a big *also*—let's not forget that a delay means that something arrives late but does indeed arrive, sometimes after surgery alone and other times after surgery *and* some additional help and hard work. According to the ACPA, about 80 percent of children born with CP show normal speech development once the palate is repaired. And the treatment of speech has come a long way over the last several decades. While it used to be common for children born with a cleft palate to enter school with speech problems, the ACPA also suggests that recent improvements in both cleft surgery and the early management of speech issues have erased most of those differences. "We now believe that the speech expectations for children with repaired cleft palate should be much the same as those for children without clefts," the organization states in its booklet, *The School-Aged Child*. The long-term goal for a child born with cleft palate, according to the cleft team at Seattle Children's Hospital, is "to have speech that is easy to understand by the time they reach kindergarten."

So, while a child's speech journey may require more time, intervention, and diligence than we may have expected (we'll explore important tasks and milestones for the first year, below), it is important to know that a longer path is normal and okay.

A Family's Key Ally: the SLP on the Team. If it feels daunting to learn about the importance of increased vigilance with regard to a child's speech, rest assured that the cleft team provides a built-in leader. The speech-language pathologist on the team is an expert on the issues associated with cleft palate (as mentioned above) and should be a family's go-to person for speech and language during a child's entire cleft journey. But what does this person actually do?

During a baby's first year, the SLP will assess her early speech development (called *prelinguistic speech*) by age six months and then continue to monitor speech, language, and palatal functioning on a regular basis through formal speech evaluations in the years to come. Some SLPs also work with babies (and parents) on feeding and swallowing during the first year, often in coordination with a cleft-team nurse.

You might think of the speech-language pathologist on the team as a sort of Sherlock Holmes. As mentioned above, the SLP does a lot of sleuthing in order to evaluate a child's speech and language on an ongoing basis, come up with solutions, and then either treat issues that arise or, in the case of speech therapy for example, possibly refer a child to other professionals to do so. The SLP will then act as a point of contact with those other professionals to make sure treatment is on the right track and if necessary, offer assistance.

The SLP will also communicate with other members of the cleft team on the many issues that relate to speech. He or she will work with the audiologist or ENT on issues related to hearing (since as we know, hearing and speech are intimately related), the dental/orthodontic specialists on the position of the teeth (as they relate to speech), and the surgeon with regard to the condition of the palate (since again, the palate has an enormous impact on speech). Such communications both inside and outside the team are excellent examples of why team care is so important and so effective.

Community Speech Programs? Yes! But… As we saw with Courtney and her daughter, Violet, some families pursue early speech services outside the cleft team through free, state-run programs in their area. It is important to know about these programs since they are usually available to all children born with cleft palate (regardless of family income) and since some health insurance policies do not cover services (or offer limited coverage) with other providers. Plus, their assistance can be invaluable. Early Intervention programs, sometimes called Early Intervention Birth to Three (or something similar), offer one-on-one speech therapy with a speech-language pathologist inside a family's home. These programs also offer help with feeding during early infancy.

But time and again, professionals have mentioned a caveat to keep in mind—and speak up about if necessary. In most circumstances, a speech-language pathologist on a cleft team has undergone more training on cleft-related speech issues than the speech-language pathologists practicing in the community, say at an Early Intervention program or a local school. "The problem is that graduate schools do not require cleft and craniofacial courses in order to become a speech-language pathologist," explained one cleft-team speech pathologist. So, it is common to find SLPs in the community who have undergone no course work at all on this condition. And while the SLPs in the community *can* be enormously helpful to families—as Courtney recalled later, their speech therapist not only helped their daughter but felt like family—it is very important for the SLP on the team to act as the leader, or hub, on all things speech-related, especially as a child grows. "If a child is getting speech therapy with a community pathologist," the SLP said, "we [on the cleft team] try to make up any gaps by having close contact with the therapist, to talk about what we are seeing and make suggestions for things to work on in therapy."

Communication among the pros, in other words, is critical. As with other areas of cleft care, if you're uncertain about how to handle this issue, be sure to check in with the SLP on the team (see some sample questions, at chapter's end).

Speech Therapy after Year One? Surgery? Maybe, Maybe Not. The speech diagnoses that sometimes emerge at the end of year one and beyond can seem confusing and esoteric to families. Whether a speech-language pathologist is telling us about our child's *articulation* and *resonance* or explaining her *compensatory misarticulations,* the concepts and lingo can feel more complicated than baseball. Also, the interventions for speech disorders are not one-size-fits-all. "Everyone comes in thinking that their child needs speech therapy," commented one SLP on a cleft team. "That is not always the case."

As different as each case can be, speech experts generally describe a few types of common situations and interventions for children ages one to five(ish) who were born with cleft palate. We will explore them very briefly here.

Speech-language pathologist Marty Grames suggests in the book, *Comprehensive Cleft Care: Family Edition*, that 70-to-80 percent of children born with cleft palate will need speech therapy at some point during childhood, usually starting at around age three. Grames also explains that a child born with CP should *not* receive speech therapy simply because she was born with CP. Rather, the service should be offered by a qualified pathologist when a child shows evidence of a speech disorder.

Now, you may remember that Violet saw a speech therapist in her community *without* first being diagnosed with a disorder and also without having received an initial referral from the SLP in her cleft team. This path turned out to be productive for Violet because the two SLPs—from the EI program and the cleft team—communicated about the case and because Violet's problems were solvable with speech exercises. (And it is possible that Violet would have received a diagnosis from the SLP on the team at a later date anyway.) Communication between the pros, as always, is key.

Some children born with CP need special speech-related surgery, usually between ages four and seven, to lengthen or otherwise correct the back of the palate to prevent air from escaping between the mouth and nose during speech. This lack of closure in the back of the mouth, called *velopharyngeal dysfunction,* or *VPD,* occurs in 15-to-25 percent of children born with cleft palate (even after palate-repair surgery) and can cause a nasal tone of voice and lead to difficulties making certain sounds.

A few children have problems making precise sounds (called *articulation*) due to issues with their teeth and jaws. As mentioned, some children struggle with speech because they also have uncorrected problems with hearing. And as one speech pathologist noted, some children experience delays in speech development that are unrelated to CLP. So, not only do situations vary, but we must rely on the expert advice of the speech-language pathologist on the cleft team to help us navigate them.

A Parents' To-Do List for Speech and Language

Here are five tasks to do during infancy to help your baby with speech and language. These tasks are doable! In fact, you may be doing some of these activities already.

SPEECH & LANGUAGE TASK No. 1. Lean on the Team and Stay on Top of Hearing. I know, I know! I've used the phrases "lean on the team" and "be sure to stay on top of hearing" enough times to drive someone crazy. But the impact of hearing on speech cannot be understated. Cleft-team pros are always reminding parents of the importance of getting (at least) annual hearing tests and keeping an eye out for ear fluid and infections—as recommended by the audiologist or ENT on the team. Likewise, the speech-language pathologist (SLP) should become a family's trusted ally and frequent contact in order to stay on top of speech and language.

SPEECH & LANGUAGE TASK No. 2. Encourage Certain Syllables and Words. It is important to keep in mind that a baby's speech and language typically grow by leaps and bounds during her first

year. According to the ACPA, a baby's first two years of life are the
most important years for development in these areas.

Now, if you are thinking, "Hold up! Really? *Now?*" I see your
point. A baby doesn't say many words during his first year, it's true.
But the lead-up to "Mama" or "Papa" actually starts as early as age
two-to-three months, when a baby starts to make *cooing* sounds
and continues when she makes *babbling* sounds at around age six
months. The all-familiar "goo-goo, gaa-gaa" sounds are actually
(and amazingly) part of the process of learning to speak—a process
that we can observe and encourage. This is true for all children,
born with clefts or not.

There is a lot you can do to help this process along, any delays
aside. Speech-language professionals often encourage parents to
incorporate certain speech activities into daily routines during
the baby's first year. Your involvement makes a huge difference.
Bath time, snack time, and diaper changes are convenient times
to practice speech, since your physical positioning during these
activities—specifically, that you and your baby are facing each other
and holding your heads more or less at the same level—will work
to your advantage. But any time of the day will work.

The following exercises represent a compilation of written recommendations from cleft-team speech-language pathologists (cited
at bottom), as well as input from six additional cleft-team SLPs
(interviewed for this book). While it is always best to follow the
advice of the SLP on your cleft team about activities to undertake
with your baby during her first year, this information may give you
a sense of what to expect and give you a springboard for questions.

**WAYS TO ENCOURAGE EARLY SPEECH
DURING YEAR ONE**

**A Compilation of Recommendations
MAMA Sound Group**

A baby with a cleft palate may be able to make certain sounds
easily before her palate is repaired. These include "L, M, N, W,

Y" sounds and all vowels (SLPs call these sounds *low-pressure consonants*, *nasal consonants,* and *vowel sounds).* Speech professionals recommend encouraging a baby to make these sounds since she will likely be able to perform them successfully.

Words in the "Mama" Group: "more, mom, me, mine, meow. no-no, nana, nose, night-night. hi, happy, hot, hug, hat, head. water/wawa, wow, whoops, whee, yeah, yes, yummy, you."

Task: Model Correct Speech. Professionals encourage parents to model different sounds while talking to a baby. For example, you could use simple "la-la-la," or "ma-ma-ma" sounds or say any of the words above. You can also attach speech sounds to actions. You could say "aaah," for example, while watching bubbles float or "oooh" while pushing a toy train. Or you could say, "mmmm" or "yum, yum" during mealtime.

Task: Encourage Imitation. AGE TWO-TO-THREE MONTHS. You can imitate the sounds your baby makes at two-to-three months of age and encourage her to mimic sounds back to you. If she says "aaah" or "maa-maa," for example, you should say those words too. You could even turn her sounds into simple words. If she says "ma," you could repeat "ma" and then say, "Mama. I am your Mama." These teaching tasks also promote bonding as you "talk" back and forth with your baby, touch her hands, smile at her, and look at one another in the eyes.

You can also practice taking turns, with activities like "Peek-a-Boo," blowing kisses, and waving hello and good-bye. Standing in front of a mirror is a fun way to encourage imitation. The cleft team at Seattle Children's Hospital recommends taking turns clapping your hands, opening and closing your mouth, and making silly sounds that emphasize use of the lips and tongue (for example, "no-no-no" and "wee-wee-wee"). Believe it or not, taking turns will teach your child about the back-and-forth that happens with conversations.

Age Six Months. By the age of six months, a child born with cleft lip may be able to say "Mama," even though it requires the use of the lips. You can imitate that! It is good to continue imitations at this age.

Task: Speak Correctly. According to cleft-team profession-als, it is very important to use correct pronunciations when you speak with your baby. Mimicking an incorrect sound can reinforce that sound. You don't want to reinforce bad habits, even if they sound cute! One cleft team suggests that as you practice saying words by modeling them correctly, you should praise your child for *any* attempt she makes to produce sounds.

PUPPY Sound Group

A child with an unrepaired cleft palate may *not* be able to say certain sounds, such as "ba," "ga," or "da." These syllables are part of a group of sounds called *pressure consonants* and include "B, D, F, G, K, P, S, T, Z, SH, CH, DG, and TH." If you make a "buh" sound to yourself very slowly, you will notice that the "B" requires a buildup of pressure in your mouth before you produce the sound, followed by a burst of energy as the "B" comes out. To achieve this kind of pressure, you need to have—you guessed it—an intact palate. Your baby may not be able to make these sounds until after her palate is repaired. This is fine! And remem-ber that the SLP on the team is ready to help.

Words in the "Puppy" Group: "bye, ball, baby, bottle, book, bath. pop, poppa, peek-a-boo, puppy, dada, diaper, duck. two, toy, teeth."

Task: Model Correct Speech. AGE TWO-TO-THREE MONTHS. Remember that a child with an unrepaired cleft palate may not be able to repeat these words back to you. That is fine! The key is to expose her to the sounds even if she does not respond. Simple words that may be age-appropriate include "baby," "ball," "puppy" and "daddy."

If, by some chance, your baby is starting to produce some of these consonants—wonderful! Speech-language pathol-ogists recommend praising the baby and reinforcing those good sounds. But also note: if you hear extra air coming out of her mouth or nose as she makes these sounds (called nasal emission), SLPs recommend you simply ignore it.

Task: Encourage Imitation. AGE: AFTER PALATE REPAIR. After your child's palate-repair surgery, you can use the same imitation games (above) to encourage the use of age-appropriate pressure sounds. One cleft team recommends using farm animal sounds, which draw from a combination of "mama" sounds and "puppy sounds." These include words like *baa, moo, neigh, meow,* and *woof.*

Early Speech Development in Children with a Cleft Palate. Seattle Children's Hospital Patient and Family Education. Aug2019.pdf. Accessed March 31, 2021. shorturl.at/ikF18

Kummer, PhD, CCC-SLP AW. Cleft Lip and Palate: Effects on Communication Development. Presented at the: Cincinnati, OH. shorturl.at/afhzG

Hardin-Jones M, Chapman K, Scherer NJ. Early Intervention in Children with Cleft Palate. The ASHA Leader. shorturl.at/qvyV1

Lucille Packard Children's Hospital. Handout: Tips for Early Speech Stimulation. 2014.

SPEECH & LANGUAGE TASK No. 3. Discourage Certain Syllables and Words. There are certain speech behaviors that cleft team SLPs recommend *discouraging.* These are bad habits in the making. The throat is a common culprit. If you notice that your child is using her throat to make certain sounds, such as grunting, growling, or other throaty-sounding syllables, the best thing you can do is ignore the behavior and model correct speech (remember, you never want to mimic incorrect speech). You could respond with a sound you know your baby can make, like "ma-ma-ma" or "oooh." One cleft team suggests that if your child says, "uh" for "truck," you can respond with, "Yes, truck! Beep-Beep!"

It is normal for kids to experiment with throat sounds to some extent, such as when they imitate truck or animal sounds. The key with cleft-affected children, though, is to know that this behavior can become a bad habit down the line. Speech-language pathologists use several terms for specific errors such as *glottal stops* and *compensatory misarticulation*. You don't want your child to practice these sounds too much.

SPEECH & LANGUAGE TASK No. 4. Don't Bother with Bubbles. In the mid-to-late decades of the previous century, speech-language professionals recommended that babies practice certain non-speech activities in order to strengthen the speech muscles of the mouth. Professionals thought that teaching a cleft-affected child to blow bubbles, whistle, and suck through a straw would help treat problems with *velopharyngeal function*. This line of thinking has since been widely disproved, but unfortunately, some clinicians—particularly community pathologists not trained in CLP issues—continue to recommend these exercises to families, as well-intentioned as they may be. "SLPs have known for years that these tasks offer little resistance to the velopharyngeal mechanism," suggested three speech professionals in the *ASHA Leader*.

If the SLP on your cleft team has recommended you pursue services in the community (such as Early Intervention), be sure to keep this information in mind and, as always, ask for recommendations on how to proceed.

SPEECH & LANGUAGE TASK No. 5. Feed Your Baby Lots of Language. Now let's talk about language. So far in this chapter, we've used the terms *speech* and *language* in broad ways—but it may be helpful to know that professionals do not use these words interchangeably. SLPs use the word *speech* to mean how we say words. The word *language,* in contrast, is all about meaning.

Language refers to the things we understand and how we express ourselves with words. It is important to know that even though a baby with a cleft palate may experience delays of both types, she still needs to learn as much language during infancy as any other baby—and for that matter, as much language as possible. The SLP Ann Kummer emphasizes the importance of teaching a baby a lot of different words, even sentences, during infancy. "You want to stimulate language development," she suggests.

When it comes to language, you might think of your baby's brain as both a sponge and a time capsule. As cleft-team professionals suggest, the two elements of language—*receptive language* (the ability to understand language) and *expressive language* (the ability to use it)—may not necessarily develop on the same time line. So, even though a baby may not *use* words and language, you can assume that she is listening and learning. The language you pour into your baby's brain, in other words, has great value even if she waits until later to express herself. It is also important to note that there is a wide range for the onset of speaking for *all* children. "Children develop at their own rate," state experts from the ASHA. So, as parents, you can expect to wait for speech and language to emerge outwardly—and, meanwhile, help her as much as possible as that process plays out.

As you speak to your baby during infancy, you can keep a few things in mind. According to an array of professionals, the primary way infants learn language is through interactions with you, a parent, or caregiver. Stanford psychologist Anne Fernald describes this early learning as "linguistic nutrition and exercise." When we talk with a baby in "an engaging and supportive way," she explains, we can "nurture brain development and build a strong foundation for language learning." In order to feed and exercise our baby's brain, in other words, we need to talk with her. We need to do so directly by looking in her eyes and really engaging with her—rather than allowing her to overhear conversations in passing. And we need to do so often.

As you speak to your baby during infancy, cleft team pros recommend three activities: *imitating, expanding,* and *modeling.* If your baby speaks a single word, for example, "Mama," you can *imitate* that word (as you would with speech development, mentioned above). You could also acknowledge her effort in a positive way and then *expand* the single word into a string of words, such as, "Yes, mama! That's right! I am your mama." Finally, you can *model* speech and language by adding brand new information, such as, "My name is Amy. I am your mama. I love you!"

A more straightforward interpretation of these directions, according to the pros, is to simply use language with your baby as much as possible. Basically, you want to talk and talk and talk with your baby. You could look her in the eye and narrate your life, whether you are giving her a bath, feeding her a bottle, or changing her diaper. What are you doing as you mix up her formula? What are the different parts of the bottle? How much water do you use? All these events can be described. Professionals also recommend cuddling and reading books together. You could also sing to your baby (even if you can't sing!). As your baby grows, the talking can become more interactive, with plenty of give-and-take (which improves parent-baby bonding, to boot). But the key, no matter how you do it, is to feed a baby plenty of language, directly, early, and often.

QUESTIONS FOR THE CLEFT TEAM

Here are some questions to ask the speech-language pathologist:

- What activities do you recommend doing at home with regard to speech and language during the baby's first year?
- How often will you evaluate speech and language? What can I/we expect during those evaluations? Afterward?
- Do you recommend contacting Early Intervention to help with feeding and/or speech? If so, do you recommend any provider in particular? I am/we are aware that some speech-language pathologists in the community lack training in cleft palate-related issues. How do you recommend proceeding?

Violet Takes Off

One August day, about three months after palate-repair surgery, Violet wandered across the living room, picked up a stray copy of *Goodnight Moon*, waved it in the air, and with all the ease and simplicity in the world, uttered a sound that had so far been unattainable. "Book," she said, smiling. "The B sound almost made me cry," Courtney said. "I [had] thought she wouldn't be able to say B for a long time because it requires so much pressure in the mouth."

Courtney went on to explain that Violet was still substituting G sounds for Ds, saying *gog* instead of *dog*, for example. But the speech pathologist from the Early Intervention program had introduced some new exercises, the SLP on her cleft team had been in touch with this person to oversee the whole affair, and the mother-daughter pair had been consistent about practicing at home. So, Courtney felt optimistic.

Fast-forward to age two and Violet was thriving. Her ear tubes defied the odds by staying in place for an extraordinarily long eighteen months, at which point she received a second, larger set. Her speech, too, had improved so dramatically that the speech-language pathologist in her EI program determined that she was ready to "graduate." Meanwhile, even as Violet received annual speech evaluations from the SLP on the cleft team (and would continue to do so for the near future), this person, too, determined that additional treatment was not necessary. "I'm just shocked that my sweet baby is almost seven," Courtney remarked years later, "and [is] happy, healthy, confident, has the healthiest teeth in our family, and [is] just beautiful inside and out. We've been very lucky."

Situations vary widely with hearing and speech. Some children face more challenges with these issues than others. The early months can feel tricky to navigate, especially when the baby is fussing and crying at 2:00 a.m. with no indication as to exactly why. And getting help with speech, in particular, can feel confusing when we hear about options for outside providers such as Early Intervention. But fortunately—and above all—the cleft team is ready to help. And when we are vigilant as parents, these conditions can be managed, if not immediately, then with time.

Presurgical
Treatment

Chapter 22

. . . .

My Story, Part 3

Marry Me, NAM Treatment.
Now, Please Go Away.

The idea sounded exciting, at least at first. Our cleft team recommended that my daughter wear a *nasoalveolar molding* (NAM) device for her first few months of life to prepare her mouth and nose for her first operation. I appreciated this treatment right away, even revered it. I never anticipated that the experience would feel at all bumpy. Heck, I never anticipated much of an *experience* at all. Why would I feel conflicted about a tiny, pink orthodontic appliance?

NAM treatment readies a cleft baby's mouth for lip-repair surgery in the way a house painter preps a room before painting. If you've ever painted a room, you may have discovered that the *before* work often requires a surprising amount of time. Just at a moment when you've gotten your clean, silky, beautiful brushes ready to go and you're anticipating how satisfying it will feel to dip one of them into a puddle of Burnt Umber or Snowfall White, an imaginary voice, perhaps sounding a lot like my father's twenty-five years ago when I decided, on a whim, to repaint my childhood bedroom, gently advises you to *stop right there*. First up, you must sand and clean and tape. Likewise, the NAM prepares a baby's mouth over a few months—and incidentally, also involves sanding, cleaning, and taping. The appliance looks similar to an orthodontic retainer for a baby but functions more like braces. Aided by an astonishing amount of caregiver involvement, the treatment actually reduces the spaces of a baby's clefts—in her lip, in her gums—before surgery, so that the surgeon can have an easier time operating. It even reshapes parts of her nose. No drop cloths are required (though burp cloths come in handy).

When my husband and I first learned about NAM at a prenatal consultation with the cleft team, the surgeon admitted that this relatively new treatment would require a lot of time and effort from us, between the weekly appointments and frequent daily maintenance tasks. But it would enable him to get optimal results come the surgery. The orthodontists on the team presented a slide show of clinical before-and-after photos of babies who had used the treatment. In ten minutes, my husband and I looked at more cleft lips and gumlines, in all their shiny, fleshy, somewhat disorienting glory, than we had ever seen or imagined seeing. But we were able to envision how the treatment manipulates the parts of a baby's mouth. *Amazing*, I thought. We had already felt excited about the idea of working with this particular surgeon and team, but with NAM in the picture, the prospect seemed all the more appealing. It felt like an opportunity we didn't want to pass up—another reassurance that our baby would receive excellent care, that she would be all right.

Then our daughter was born, and I realized that I wanted to gobble her up—not tape her up. While the NAM appliance resembles an orthodontic retainer or braces, it differs from those treatments in that it is held in place by a web of accessories that affix directly to the baby's face. The arrangement had seemed perfectly acceptable prenatally, when I had considered it in the abstract, on other people's babies. Back then, I assumed that, upon meeting our daughter, my husband and I would want to hurry up and repair her clefts. I had worried in my most private, choked-up moments whether I would bond with her at all, or think she was cute. But now, when I saw that her lips and cheeks would be pulled and strained by medical tapes and rubber bands and that her nostrils would be forced open and upward by wire stents—and realized that I *did* think she was cute and *did* want to be able to see those cheeks and lips and sweet, little nostrils—my emotional winds shifted.

All at once, I couldn't decide which aspect of this treatment was the worst part. During the early weeks after my daughter's birth, I was already lamenting that I could not nurse her. With the NAM in place, I could barely kiss her. "It looks barbaric," my husband stated blankly a few weeks in, as we sat in our living room staring at our rigged-up baby. *What did we agree to?* I thought. Sure, our surgeon had told us about infants' remarkable resilience. But what about my resilience? After all the early discussions and enthusiasm, I now felt a queasy, sinking lump in my stomach. *Should we forget it? Make an early, clean break?*

Well, we didn't forget it, as tempting as that prospect seemed. We kept going, not as a long-term decision but as an in-the-moment choice to simply not stop *then*. We thought of the long view: that we wanted to do all we could to help our baby. And it turned out that NAM really did come with a hefty to-do list for us, as caregivers.

For NAM treatment to work, the device needs to be worn nearly 24/7, with proper tension—exerted by rubber bands and tapes applied to the face—to keep everything engaged and humming along. The face tapes need to be replaced each time they loosen, usually as a result of getting wet. And since the device is worn by a crying, drooling, sloppy, human baby, they need to be changed several times a day (or at least they did in my daughter's case). So, my husband and I did a lot of taping. We prepped tapes, we taped tapes, and we retaped the tapes. When we weren't taping, we were monitoring the state of the tapes—while also eating, sleeping, working, and tending to our older child (who thankfully, didn't need to be taped). Errant tapes began showing up on household objects and clinging to our pant legs.

My husband will be the first to admit that he didn't enjoy the daily NAM tasks because of his general intolerance for fumbling with small objects at all hours. But I didn't mind them. The duties appealed to my overly developed appreciation for order. I remember fiddling with the strips of tape and struggling, at first, to affix them properly but then happily tweaking my technique to get the angles and the tensions just right. Not for nothing, either. When the face tapes were fresh and clean and perfectly positioned, rays of sunlight streamed through the bedroom window. Choirs sang, temporarily easing my ill feelings toward a device that insulted my daughter's sweet face. The at-home tasks for NAM might be a perfect match for any parent who self-describes as a "Bert" rather than an "Ernie" in the classic *Sesame Street* trope (oh, how I envy the carefree Ernies). These duties seem to offer caregivers a sense of control when, in the larger sense, we might feel very little control. Nervous about surgery? Here is something to do, a way to contribute.

But, unfortunately in my case, there was how my daughter felt about it. By my unscientific assessment of cause-and-effect, my daughter cried and fussed with the NAM in place and did *not* cry and fuss when the NAM was not in place. Given that she wore the device nearly 24/7, you can guess how often she cried and fussed. My husband and I purchased sound-dampening materials for her bedroom—rug pads, soft pillows, quilts to hang on the walls—in order to preserve our sanity and prevent our neighbors from hearing any late-night commotion. Now, it is true that this constant fussing could have occurred for any number of reasons, such as troubles with reflux or pressure in her ears, both of which my daughter experienced during infancy. And she never seemed to experience outright pain from the NAM, just low-to-medium-grade annoyance. But during the occasional twenty-four-hour periods when the skin on her cheeks became too irritated to withstand the tapes, we gave her a NAM vacation and watched her transform into a smiling, cooing, different baby. Perhaps unsurprisingly, in these moments, I became a smiling, cooing, different parent. *There's your face!* I'd exclaim. It was as if we had been driving on a highway in a rainstorm and then passed under a bridge or overpass, producing a few blissful moments of respite.

And so, the weeks passed. We continued to tape. My daughter continued to fuss. But then, at a moment when we almost weren't looking, she started to make progress. *We* started to make progress. It seemed that the more time we all spent sanding and cleaning and taping (the pros did the sanding; we did the cleaning and taping), sure enough, millimeter by millimeter, the smaller the spaces of her clefts became. Each time we visited the team, I felt creeping bubbles of excitement when I saw how well the treatment was working. It didn't hurt that the orthodontic people on our team were remarkably supportive, whether they were staying late at a weekly appointment to get the adjustment of the appliance just right, replying to our texts during off-hours to troubleshoot, or generally cheerleading our efforts. I never told them about my hot-and-cold feelings for the device because I felt so overwhelmed by their generosity and genuine desire to help our baby. It felt satisfying to know that my actions were making a difference. Sure, I disliked the device. But by overseeing its use, I was actually helping my daughter.

An infant's first connection to the world is arguably through her lips. Upon leaving the womb, a newborn's earliest physical actions begin with an unprompted journey to her mother's breast. Medical people call this trip the "breast crawl." At arrival, still physically unable to see much more than a fuzzy blur, she makes initial human contact with her lips, facilitating feeding but also bonding. Now, of course, babies aren't born wearing a NAM device; the treatment usually begins a couple weeks after birth. But the point of connection continues into a baby's early months when she self-soothes with a pacifier in her mouth or rests, soft and mushy-faced on someone's warm chest.

It pained me that my baby's face was covered up, depriving her—and me—of these elemental interactions. And the fact that her lips happened to be shaped in a special way, fleetingly so, made my heart ache all the more. But on the morning of our daughter's lip-repair surgery, when we greeted the orthodontist and surgeon and they examined her NAM device for the last time, they smiled at us warmly, as if to say, "Here we are! Job well done. She's ready!" And I realized that we had prepped the room. The walls were as smooth as can be. The prep-work didn't feel very glamorous, sure. And there were times when I came *this* close to calling the whole thing off. But for a moment that morning, my chest swelled. I realized I had made a difference. I felt like a full-fledged member of the team.

There is another perspective I am seeing eight years later when I look at my daughter now. She loves horses. And third grade. She is a passionate kid, belting out Beatles songs from the backseat. "I want YOU!" she sings with an abandon that almost makes me blush. "I want you so ba-a-a-d, it's driving me mad, it's driving me MAD." She doesn't understand the lusty lyrics, of course. But even more, she doesn't understand or even remember some of her early experiences during infancy. I would like to think that, in some small way, she is living out the *love* part of the love-hate relationship every day, having forgotten or never realized those moments that drove *me* mad. I can also see that some of the challenges of parenthood relate not just to difficult tasks, like late-night wakeups and constant schlepping (though, of course, those challenges are real), but to the persistent requirement that we make thorny decisions. *Do we trust this babysitter? Should one of us cut back to part-time? Which school is best?* These choices can be messy, with trade-offs and imperfect solutions, even in the best, most fortunate of circumstances, even when we do our most thorough and thoughtful homework.

Our cleft team gave us an opportunity to make our daughter's life better and easier, in part by allowing us, as her parents, to shoulder some of her burden. Her cleft treatment is far from over, as are its related decisions. But I hope that NAM helped make her journey a little more carefree than it otherwise might have been. I'm sure it made me a more resilient parent.

Chapter 23

. . . .

YIPPEE-I-O

Presurgical Infant Orthopedics
Basics and Decision-Making

When Joelle and Kurt first learned that their son would be born with CLP, they knew nothing at all about clefts. One week later, they'd learned more than they'd ever imagined. "It was like a whirlwind," Joelle said. Not only did the couple discover that they needed to sign on with a cleft team, but they found out that choosing a team would involve considering a type of treatment called *infant orthopedics* (IO), sometimes called *presurgical infant orthopedics* (PSIO), that would prepare their baby's mouth for lip-repair surgery. The information seemed overwhelming, at first, especially when Joelle and Kurt realized that there were different types of IO, that there is some debate among professionals as to which one is best, and that any given cleft team might offer one form but not another—or none at all. But before they knew it, the terms "nasoalveolar molding" and "Latham treatment" were rolling off their tongues as easily as any other common household phrase.

It is natural to feel overwhelmed by this kind of situation—and to want to learn more. This chapter offers basics on three methods of infant orthopedics (IO) that are currently available and shares insights from professionals and parents (we'll hear again from Joelle and Kurt) on the sometimes-tricky task of considering IO as you choose a cleft or craniofacial team for your child.

297

Three Methods
Braces for a Baby

Of the three methods of infant orthopedics currently offered by cleft teams in the US, Nasoalveolar Molding (NAM) treatment is probably the most popular, followed by Latham treatment and lip taping. We'll address all three methods here.

In the preceding chapter, we explored the idea that NAM treatment works much like braces for a baby. In fact, all three types of infant orthopedics function this way. An infant doesn't have teeth, of course, so she can't wear braces, literally. But the broad goal of these types of interventions, like the popular regimen for teenagers, is to move parts of the mouth to better locations—in this case, before a baby's lip-repair operation. When the spaces between the clefts are made smaller, the surgeon on the team can close the gaps more easily, achieving a better result upfront and also reducing pressure on the surgical stitches over time. Depending on the size of the gap(s) of a baby's clefts—and the type of IO and the consistency and accuracy of its use before surgery—the treatment will slowly push the segments of the lip and gumline closer together over weeks or months until, eventually, under ideal conditions, the segments touch. Certain types of IO can also be used to manipulate and reshape parts of the baby's nose. (IO usually does not reduce the gap of a cleft palate.)

The idea of presurgical orthopedics may sound strange or overly involved, at first, especially if you are new to cleft lip and palate. But the treatments can do a lot to help a baby and, in many cases, play a prominent role in a family's experience during their first year.

Nasoalveolar Molding (NAM) Treatment

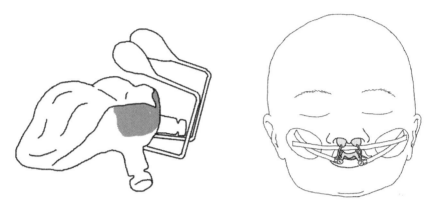

NAM treatment, bilateral: appliance (at left)
and as worn by a person (at right)

How It Works. Nasoalveolar molding (NAM) treatment, which has been used by cleft teams since the mid-1990s, involves three basic physical components: a custom-made, removable mouth plate; an array of special medical tapes; and depending on the situation, a nasal *stent* (or two). NAM treatment usually begins a few weeks into a baby's life and continues until lip-repair surgery, for a total of a few months. Many professionals advise that a baby wear the device 24/7 (with a daily break for cleaning) during that time.

The Plate. While face tapes are probably the most visible parts of NAM treatment, the removable acrylic plate is where a lot of the action takes place. Let's use a brief analogy. Have you ever seen a pair of custom orthotics made for someone's feet? These special shoe inserts match the shape of a person's foot; they're made with special molds. But let's imagine what would happen if someone were to change the shape of the surface of the orthotics by adding a bulge in one spot or taking away a bulge in another spot. The new bumps would feel painful and annoying, right? Also, the alteration would accomplish nothing since an adult's foot is not malleable.

Now, let's turn back to the NAM. The custom-made acrylic plate of the NAM can be sanded and manipulated to create little hills and valleys, which, in a baby's case, can actually change the shape of her gumline—since during a small window of time in early infancy, these body parts *are* malleable, like clay. As a dental person on the team (usually an orthodontist or a pediatric dentist) adjusts the plate each week, this "molding" process pushes the segments of the mouth closer together—and is entirely individualized.

THE CLEFT GUMLINE 101

The St. Louis Gateway Arch

Infant orthopedics can be useful before a baby's lip-repair operation because they reduce the gaps in her lip and gumline (let's set aside the nose, for now). But cleft professionals also consider the *shape* of these features as well.

Let's picture, for a moment, that the area of the baby's gumline—where the teeth will eventually emerge—is supposed to be shaped like the St. Louis Gateway Arch. This arch shape is the ideal contour of a person's gumline. If you look at the gumline of a person born without clefts—or even at one of those funny, old-fashioned, wind-up toys shaped like human teeth that go CLACK-CLACK-CLACK on a tabletop—you will observe that perfect arch. When a person is born with CLP, the sides of the dental arch are sometimes situated too close together, like a doorway instead of an arch. One of the goals of NAM and Latham treatment is to push the sides of the doorway outward.

There's more. When a baby is born with CLP, the segment of the gumline in the very front of the mouth—located at the top of the doorway—is usually sticking out too far. In other words, her doorway-arch is too tall. Infant orthopedics use various methods to pull that segment, called the *premaxilla*, inward (NAM and lip taping use medical tape; the Latham uses an elastic chain). So, these two actions—expansion on the sides and retraction in the front of the mouth—will turn the baby's doorway into an ideal St. Louis arch.

Why the Tapes? Given how much time and energy caregivers will devote to the taping duties of NAM treatment, it is important to know what these thin strips of medical tape actually do. When applied properly—and it is important to note that proper application is key—the tapes serve several functions. First, they ensure the mouth plate is held in place and thus able to do its job. Also, when applied to the outside of the cheeks and across the upper lip, the tapes move the segments of a cleft lip closer together. Last, the tapes pull the premaxilla, the front-most segment of the lip/gums (mentioned above), to a more advantageous location (usually inward) before surgery. The exact number of tapes and their arrangement depend on cleft anatomy and other factors. Some tapes are linked with tiny rubber bands (see Chapter 24 for details).

The Nasal Stents. A few weeks into NAM treatment, the orthodontic/dental specialists on the cleft team may add one or two nasal stents to the appliance to manipulate the shape of the nose: one stent for unilateral clefts, two stents for bilateral. A nasal stent looks like a bent Q-Tip®; it is made with thin, durable, L-shaped wire and a soft acrylic knob. Over weeks or months, the action of the stent(s) will push a baby's nostrils forward and upward, making the nose appear less flat, molding the nostril(s) to appear rounder, and reducing the width of the nose overall. And amazingly, the nasal stents of the NAM device will actually stretch and lengthen the central strip of skin between the nostrils (called the *columella*), which, as discussed elsewhere in this book, can be short or non-existent for cleft-affected babies.

Time and Energy Required. While the NAM plate and its tapes and stents are the tools of NAM treatment, caregivers are the lynchpins for the whole affair. Without weekly visits with the pros and daily attention from parents to maintain the device and ensure it is placed correctly on the baby's face—and worn 24/7—NAM treatment will not be effective. Simply put, NAM treatment relies on constant use by a baby and, therefore, tireless work from her parents.

Weekly visits with the orthodontist/dentist on the team can last anywhere from thirty minutes to an hour or longer. So, depending on distance and logistics—not to mention other considerations like the scheduling of meals, naps, etc.—caregivers can count on devoting significant time to these trips. "It took us an hour each way to get to the office," said one mother, "plus traffic, plus lunch, plus the visit itself. Also, I was pumping [breast milk]. It took all day!"

The time required for daily tasks can be difficult to estimate because these duties vary from one child and situation to another. Some cleft-team dentists require that caregivers remove and clean the device daily, a task that can take about fifteen minutes. But probably more important, the NAM requires constant, low-grade monitoring by a caregiver to make sure the tapes are affixed properly to the baby's face. If a tape comes loose after a meal, bath, or drooling episode, a caregiver needs to change it. After the baby has grown accustomed to the NAM device (usually around two weeks after treatment begins but sometimes sooner), a parent might devote several minutes to cleaning and taping several times a day—and that's it. But the monitoring never ends. And a parent may also be required to troubleshoot, at times, if a baby develops a sore in the mouth or seems bothered by the newly reshaped mouth plate or nasal stent following a weekly adjustment with the team. For more information and lots of tips, see Chapter 24.

Day Care and the Issue of Caregiver Training. As variable as the time commitment may be for NAM care, the question of training can become an important factor for parents who are considering how to arrange their work and family lives after the baby is born. Even on the lightest, easiest days of NAM treatment (let's set aside the weekly visits for now), the person who cares for the baby will need to know how to maintain the device. And while these daily tasks for NAM treatment are not difficult to learn or execute once a caregiver gets up to speed, they are specialized and require time.

Some parents find that this situation makes their baby ineligible for traditional child-care programs, where providers may or may not be able to accommodate these special needs. "There was no day care that would take him," said one mother about her early search. "I don't know what I would have done if we hadn't had my sister-in-law [to take care of the baby]" she said, describing her own obligation to go back to her teaching job. "I would have had to leave my job." Another parent, in contrast, found a day care that not only accommodated her son's NAM treatment but rose to the challenge with adeptness and even excitement. Situations vary.

Availability. A national survey published in 2019 in the *Cleft Palate Craniofacial Journal* indicates that fewer than half of all cleft teams in the US offer some method of presurgical orthopedics—and of that half, about 88 percent, offer NAM. Given that the ACPA currently lists somewhere around one hundred seventy approved teams in the US and six in Canada, a back-of-the-envelope calculation yields seventy-to-seventy-five teams in the US that offer NAM. Some families have a hard time finding an approved team in their area, much less a team that offers NAM. Availability can be a deciding factor.

Eligibility: A Matter of Timing. While access to NAM can be an issue for families, as can their ability to comply with its demands, cleft professionals indicate that most babies born with isolated cleft lip and palate are physically able to receive the treatment and benefit from it—provided it occurs during the window of time after birth when a baby's mouth is still malleable. "We recommend the NAM to almost all of our parents," said one clinical nurse specialist on a cleft team. But the timing must be right.

According to cleft-team orthodontists writing in the book *Comprehensive Cleft Care: Family Edition*, the tissues and cartilages of a baby's mouth and nose are malleable during the first three or four months after birth because, during that time, *maternal estrogen* is flowing through her body. Estrogen is a hormone that most of us have probably heard of. But we may not know that a mother passes on a burst of it to a baby at birth. The hormone actually makes the baby's body parts flexible, allowing her to fit through the birth canal at delivery. Fortunately, for advocates of IO, this hormone sticks around in the body afterward. Every baby's cleft (and/or other) diagnosis is different, of course, so it is important to ask someone on the cleft team for advice about your own child's case. But a baby's eligibility for NAM (and other forms of IO) often has a lot to do with timing.

Outcomes: Now and Later? NAM, like other forms of IO, can be somewhat controversial. As mentioned already, the treatment may be difficult to obtain and requires loads of work from caregivers. But there is also some debate among medical researchers about its benefits. On one hand, there is evidence to suggest that this treatment brings about positive outcomes. On the other hand, those claims have not been proven definitively over the long term.

Let's look first at some evidence in favor of the treatment. A collection of studies discussed in the journal, *Pediatric Dentistry*, shows that NAM can reduce the extent of a person's clefts prior to lip-repair surgery and improve symmetry, structure, and the lining of the nose. Other studies indicate that NAM is linked with the results just mentioned plus reduced chances that a child will need surgery on the nose later in childhood. NAM demands a lot of work for caregivers, admitted one cleft surgeon. But he thinks it is worth the effort. "If we don't invest in it," he said, "a child will have a compromised result." So, there are a lot of medical professionals on cleft teams who advocate strongly for this treatment, saying that it makes an enormous difference for a child in terms of possible surgical outcomes, both functionally and aesthetically, especially in the short term.

On the other hand, research about NAM leaves some important stones unturned, particularly questions about aspects of long-term facial growth. One orthodontist explained that the treatment is exceedingly difficult to study, technically speaking. "There are a lot of variables," she said. It can be challenging to create a study that isolates these factors, thus allowing researchers to compare apples to apples.

A Match? Opinions from Pros. If you are considering your options for infant orthopedics and wondering whether NAM is worth the effort, you are not alone. While cleft-team pros have mentioned that nearly every baby with CLP is eligible for NAM, they also point out that certain babies are more likely to benefit from it than others. Three main factors tend to affect outcomes, they say, for a baby at lip-repair surgery: 1) the severity of a child's diagnosis, 2) how well caregivers adhere to the NAM protocol, and 3) how well a surgeon operates. "There is a lot of controversy over which of these methods is best," commented one cleft surgeon about the different types of IO. But this surgeon went on to emphasize the value of either NAM or Latham for the more severe forms of CLP. "For the bilateral and the unilateral-complete, it is important to use one or the other," he continued, in order to lay the groundwork for the best possible surgical outcomes. Other surgeons and orthodontists have made similar comments.

Also, as sensitive as this subject may be among professionals, some cleft team pros have pointed out that surgical skill plays a role in the outcomes of lip-repair surgery as well, whether it relates to the methods a surgeon uses to solve certain problems or to outright ability. One cleft-team orthodontist described working with four different surgeons who each achieved different outcomes.

What Do Parents Say? When I asked Gina about her experience with NAM, she admitted that her early months with her baby felt like a blur. "I was in autopilot mode," she said. "I had the appointments scheduled, and I didn't stop. It was really hard." At the same time, she felt proud, even elated, by the wonderful results. "My daughter has an impeccable repair," she continued, "and the surgeon said it was due to me being so diligent [with the

NAM]." Another mother recalled feeling troubled by the NAM, at first, because she couldn't hug her son and bond with him the way she wanted when he was wearing the device. As he grew more comfortable with it, however, she did too. And this mother, like the first, was thrilled to see her son's progress. "[NAM treatment] starts out as a scary thing," she continued, "but then it becomes more positive." Still another parent looked back at the experience years later and described NAM treatment as one of the most challenging yet rewarding tasks she had undertaken as a parent. Opinions (like mine, as described in the preceding chapter) tend to be mixed and strong.

Bottom Line. Professionals and parents praise the NAM for its ability to relocate the segments of the lip and gumline and improve the shape and symmetry of the nose, especially in severe cases. And while research on NAM is incomplete, the treatment is shown to reduce the chances of further operations for a child as she grows. But fewer than half of the ACPA-approved cleft teams in the US offer NAM, so availability can be a major issue. And even when families do have access, some, through no fault of their own, are unable to comply with its demands.

Latham Treatment

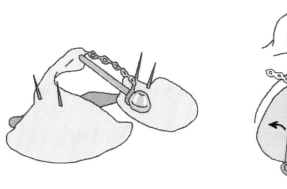 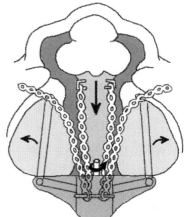

Latham treatment: unilateral appliance (at left) and bilateral appliance, as viewed from inside the mouth (at right)

How It Works. Latham treatment, developed in the 1970s, is another method used by cleft teams to manipulate parts of a baby's mouth before lip-repair surgery. The Latham appliance roughly resembles a palate expander; it is made of two narrow, acrylic plates that fit over a baby's gums on the upper right and left sides of the mouth and connect in the center with a hinged metal bar. In the center of the metal bar is a tiny screw.

Unlike a palate expander, which attaches to an older child's teeth, the Latham device is *pin-retained*, meaning that the acrylic plates are held in place by small, metal pins that extend directly into the baby's gums (gums are officially called *gingiva,* but you may also hear the terms *gum pads, gum ridges,* or *alveolar ridges*). Once the device has been inserted by way of a short surgical procedure during early infancy, it stays in place until the orthodontist on the team removes it (usually at the outset of lip-repair surgery, in a single round of general anesthesia, just before the surgeon operates).

The exact setup and mechanics of the Latham appliance vary for unilateral and bilateral clefts. The unilateral appliance moves the segments of the baby's gumline closer together through the turning of the tiny screw. This action requires help from a caregiver, who must tighten the screw on a regular basis, usually nightly for about six weeks, per instructions from the orthodontist (who will guide you every step of the way). The bilateral appliance, in contrast, includes an additional wire-and-pulley setup at the front of the mouth that pulls the premaxilla inward. (The *premaxilla* is the segment of a bilateral cleft located at the front-most area of the mouth, as mentioned above.) After the bilateral appliance is inserted, the orthodontist on the team tightens the bands of the pulley every one-to-two weeks to rein in that segment. In the case of bilateral clefts, caregivers may or may not be instructed to tighten the tiny screw.

These two actions of the Latham—realignment of the gum-line with the screw and/or retraction of the premaxilla with the pulley—will maneuver the baby's gumline to form a desired arch shape, enabling a surgeon to perform lip-repair surgery more easily.

Latham treatment does not manipulate a baby's nose. But some cleft centers use other methods to reshape the nasal tissue. The DynaCleft® Nasal Elevator System, for example, is a small hook that pulls and reshapes the nostril (see image, below). The hook is held in place with medical tape which, believe it or not, attaches to the baby's forehead.

Time and Energy Required. There are both challenges and benefits associated with the Latham device in terms of time and energy. On one hand, the Latham requires a short operation to place the device inside an infant's mouth. As professionals point out in the book *Comprehensive Cleft Care: Family Edition,* this early surgical pro-cedure—and its related use of general anesthesia—comes with risk, as would any operation. But once the device is in place, caregivers will usually only need to turn the screw once each day, a relatively quick task. There are no tapes to deal with. The entire treatment period lasts for weeks rather than months. And the weekly office/team visits are usually short.

Availability. According to a 2019 national survey, about half of approved cleft teams in the US offer some form of PSIO (as mentioned above). Of that half, around 15 percent of teams offer Latham treatment. Given that there are about one hundred seventy ACPA-approved teams in the US, we can probably conclude that twelve or so offer Latham. So, families' access to this treatment can be even more difficult than for NAM.

What Do Parents Say? Parents of babies who undergo Latham treatment tend to mention both its ease—once the device is inserted—and its shock factor. "The Latham was no big deal," commented one mother about her son's experience with the treatment. While she recalled that the appliance became clogged with formula and gunk, the messiness never caused any harm or inconvenience (cleft team pros generally clean the appliance at weekly visits). The experience was relatively stress-free overall for everyone involved. And this mother felt pleased that she did not need to teach caregivers how to use it. "It was nothing for the babysitter," she continued.

Another mother, whose two children both underwent Latham treatment, described the pin-retained device as primitive and extreme. "The Latham looked like a torture device," she said. And the surgical procedure used to place it, she continued, was emotionally trying. But once inserted, the device did not cause any problems for either of her children. While this mother recalled giving her son infants' Tylenol at night when she and her husband turned the screw, the appliance didn't seem to cause her kids much pain or bother. She also described how odd it felt to use a common household tool to care for a tiny baby. "The Latham is sort of like a palate expander," she explained with a chuckle, "except that instead of using a key, you use a screwdriver." She recalled joking with her husband each time they turned the screw. "We would say [to each other], 'Okay, you get the baby, I'll get the Phillips-head.'"

Outcomes: Opinions from Pros. Professionals on cleft teams have pointed out both advantages and drawbacks of Latham treatment. "We have had great success with the Latham device," commented one nurse specialist at a large cleft center, "especially for bilateral clefts." She acknowledged that the treatment can be challenging for infants and parents, particularly during the first week following insertion as a baby recovers from the procedure and reacclimates to feeding. But this nurse also pointed out that the treatment ends in around six weeks. A cleft surgeon echoed those words as he compared Latham treatment to NAM. "The Latham is faster and easier for parents," he said. "It has all kinds of advantages."

But professionals also describe some drawbacks to Latham treatment. One cleft team orthodontist commented that while Latham treatment can prime a child for wonderful outcomes in the hands of a skilled surgeon, the treatment (alone) does not target the nose area at all, oftentimes leading to so-called "revision" operations on the nose later on.

Bottom Line. Parents and pros praise the Latham for being relatively effective, easy on a baby (once the device is inserted), and not labor-intensive for caregivers. The appliance must be inserted surgically, however. And without the use of additional methods (such as DynaCleft®), the treatment does not manipulate parts of a baby's nose, which according to some professionals, can lead to additional operations for a child in the future. Some parents chafe at the idea of inserting metal pins directly into their baby's gums to keep the appliance in place, though others find it no big deal. Availability can be a prohibitive factor for this treatment since it is offered by only around 10 percent of cleft teams in the US.

Taping the Face
a.k.a. Face Taping or Nasolabial Molding

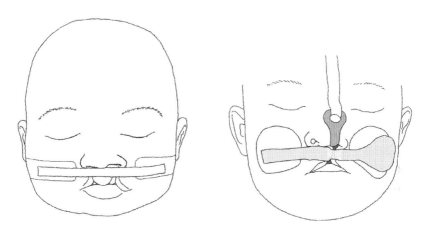

Taping: bilateral (at left) and unilateral, with DynaCleft®
Nasal Elevator System (at right)

How It Works. Face taping is a low-tech, low-cost method of pre-surgical infant orthopedics that is far simpler in structure and execution than the NAM and Latham treatments described above. Lip taping has not been studied at length in medical literature, but it is often recommended and overseen by cleft teams across the US, especially those who do not offer other forms of PSIO.

Lip taping functions exactly as it sounds. Caregivers place strips of medical tape on the baby's cheeks and/or upper lip in order to move those parts of the face closer together prior to lip repair. In most cases of lip taping, there is no internal appliance involved. One of the goals of this treatment is to pull a baby's premaxilla (the segment of the lip/gumline located directly under the nose) toward the space of the cleft, thus reducing the gaps in the lip and gum and easing the way for a surgeon during lip-repair surgery. Remember our discussion, above, of the St. Louis Gateway Arch? If the baby's gumline is supposed to be shaped like that famous monument but starts out shaped more rectangularly, like a doorway, lip taping can lower the top of the doorway, thus approximating—but usually not perfecting—the shape of the arch.

Exact methods of lip taping vary widely from team to team, ranging from the very simplest of regimens overseen in an ad hoc fashion by a surgeon or nurse to a much more formalized treatment involving regular office visits and possible nasal stents, all directed by an orthodontist or pediatric dentist. But generally speaking, a taping routine resembles the regimen used for NAM treatment, minus the acrylic plate. To start, a caregiver may be instructed to apply *base tapes* to the baby's cheeks in order to provide a foundational layer of support. Then, the caregiver applies narrow medical tapes called *Steri-Strips*™, which, when attached to tiny rubber bands, do the work of moving the segments of the lip together. Some teams use a taping system called DynaCleft® to manipulate parts of the baby's face (and/or nose). With lip taping, the arrangement and tension of these tapes are important, since in most cases the tapes are a solo act, doing all the heavy lifting of this treatment with no mouth plates or other devices to act as anchors or otherwise help the process along. So, technique does matter.

Taping may feel awkward, at first, for caregivers, but it often becomes second nature—since as parents have mentioned, a caregiver can expect to change the tapes with astonishing frequency as a baby drools, spits up, takes a bottle, smiles, cries, and basically acts like a baby.

Time and Energy Required. Lip taping requires time and energy from caregivers, both for daily tasks and regular visits with the team. Day-to-day tasks usually involve prepping the tapes—which sometimes need to be cut to size and affixed to rubber bands before they can be used on the baby—applying the tapes to the baby's face, and then monitoring and replacing the tapes when they become wet or loose (see the next chapter for tips on taping). It is hard to predict how often a parent will need to change the tapes. One mother shares on the Cleftopedia site that she performed the task up to twelve times per day (to her frustration), but others have been able to do it far less frequently. While the monitoring never ends, the job of replacing the tapes usually requires only a few minutes each time.

Lip taping may also require weekly visits with the cleft team, though the frequency of these visits varies from team to team and baby to baby. One orthodontist I spoke with asks families to check in virtually—and often—during the first week of treatment by sending daily pictures of the baby. This way, parents can perfect their taping technique and gain confidence. During this early stage, families may visit the office weekly, but soon thereafter, once every two weeks and then later, once a month. The frequency typically goes down, she said, after the tape has done its work and the treatment is "stabilizing" the positions of the mouth—and in the case of this professional's team, the nose.

Outcomes: Opinions from Pros. As often as cleft teams in the US use lip taping for their patients, the method has been largely overlooked in medical literature. So, we must rely on the opinions of professionals. Unfortunately (and confusingly), their ideas seem to vary widely, from outright negative views, on one hand—which can be hard to hear for parents who do not have access to NAM or Latham—to much-better-than-nothing and positive opinions on the other. "Lip taping would be my last choice" for presurgical methods, commented an orthodontist on a cleft team who specializes in NAM. Without a mouth plate, he explained, the movement of the mouth can be exceedingly difficult to control. "With a unilateral case," he said, "the tape cannot move the segments [of the mouth] proportionally. The segments collapse." And unlike NAM treatment, he continued, the nose is left untouched (remember that while some teams use nasal stents or the DynaCleft® Nasal Elevator System along with the tapes, others do not). A nurse on another cleft team explained that patients who do lip taping with her team tend to undergo what she characterized as "a hard repair followed by one or two revisions." meaning that after initial lip-repair surgery, a child may need to undergo follow-up operations later in childhood to adjust the shape or function of the lips, gums, and nose.

Yet professionals also say that taping a cleft lip is far better than doing nothing. "Our team offers NAM," commented one nurse on a cleft team, "but some families live far away, and it is not an option for several reasons. So, we also do taping, which has obvious benefits." The surgeons on her team, she continued, can get good results without NAM or Latham. Another cleft team nurse had a similar opinion. "I am a big believer in taping," she said. "There is nothing in the literature that has shown how well this works one way or the other, but I will tell you anecdotally, that in my years of experience, everyone says, yes, this works."

It is important to consider that lip taping can vary dramatically from situation to situation. While one team may offer taping as a very simple "it can't hurt" option when other options are not available, others go about the treatment more elaborately, with refined techniques for positioning the tapes and manipulating parts of the nose. One orthodontist at a large cleft center, who calls her lip-taping regimen "nasolabial molding," described positive out-comes for the babies she treats with taping, especially with regard to the shape of the nose. When nasal stents are used properly with taping, she commented, the devices can lengthen the baby's col-umella and "add curvature to the nasal form." She also disputed the common claim among professionals that a baby's dental arch needs to be perfectly aligned during infancy, since the arch tends to change shape anyway during a child's first seven or eight years of life, requiring reshaping prior to bone-graft surgery.

These opinions, in all their variety, indicate that while some professionals have a decidedly negative opinion on taping, others not only offer sophisticated versions of the treatment but describe outcomes far more optimistically.

What Do Parents Say? Parents who have used face taping with their babies generally offer positive reviews. "I was glad to have used this process," writes one mother on the Cleftopedia site, who described a reduction in the size of her daughter's unilateral cleft from 18mm at the time of her birth to 8mm at the time of surgery. While this mother expressed frustration with the at-home tasks associated with taping—which were very time-consuming with her especially drooly baby—she was grateful overall to have had the opportunity to do it. "I am amazed with her results," she added.

Another mother described the process as overwhelming at first, especially since at the time she was still coping with the news of her son's clefts. Still another expressed dismay at dealing with ongoing problems with skin irritation. But all three parents said that this method helped their babies. "[Taping] brought the rosebud even with the sides of [my son's] mouth," the second mother continued, referring to the baby's premaxilla. "I never imagined it would do that."

Bottom Line. Some cleft professionals take issue with lip taping because it does not move the segments of the mouth in a predictable fashion before lip-repair surgery, leading to possible follow-up operations as a child gets older. Also, in contrast to one of its IO cousins, NAM treatment, this low-tech method may not manipulate parts of the nose. It is also not reviewed in medical literature. But many parents and professionals describe lip taping as a viable, doable option when NAM and Latham are not available. Not only is this method far better than doing nothing, they say, but it helps parents feel empowered as we help our child's surgeon obtain better results through surgery.

Decisions, Decisions

A few weeks after Joelle and Kurt learned of their son's CLP—and after their initial round of whirlwind research—they went to prenatal consultations with two cleft teams. The first team, located about twenty minutes from their home, proposed a very simple taping regimen. "The surgeon said that he offers what is best for his clients," Joelle said. "He doesn't do the Latham or the NAM because a lot of families travel from neighboring states. They cannot come up once a week for a visit. It is not a good fit."

Members of the second team, in contrast, offered Joelle and Kurt information on both NAM and Latham, showed them before-and-after pictures for each treatment and predicted that their baby would be eligible for either one. The couple had a good feeling. The logistics, however, gave them pause: this second team was located over two hours away. Given their current work obligations and plans for the baby, this decision felt awkward. So, Joelle and Kurt took a few weeks to mull over their options. With time, Joelle realized that while she felt comfortable with the first surgeon and team, the skills, manner, and communication of the second team gave her a confident feeling. Also, the idea of doing NAM in particular seemed exciting. "The Latham is drilled directly into the mouth," she commented. "It was a definite turnoff for me. It is an old-school way of handling the issue, at this point." While the couple acknowledged how labor-intensive NAM would be—and all the more challenging with a commute— they mapped out some ways to rearrange their work and child-care plans to accommodate it. After a lot of discussion, Joelle and Kurt decided to sign on with the second team.

Looking back on the decision a few years later, Joelle realized how fortunate she was to be able to pursue NAM for her son, not only because of its availability but also her own ability to comply with its demands. "If I had had another child or a different work situation, we would never be able to pull that off," Joelle continued. "It was a full-time gig."

Considering the Circumstances. While Joelle and Kurt were able to choose between the NAM and the Latham—and between two ACPA-approved cleft teams located within a two-hour driving radius—not all families have these options. As mentioned above, some families do not live near an approved team, much less near one that offers more than one type of IO. So, availability can be a major issue, even a prohibitive one. In some cases, effectively, there is no decision to make.

It is also true that situations vary, availability aside. "We tried to do NAM," explained one father about his early efforts to obtain the treatment for his daughter. But during the first few weeks of his daughter's life, he and his wife had also decided to switch surgeons within their cleft team, a process that involved some unfortunate administrative delays. So, by the time the family could even make an appointment to have an initial NAM consultation, their daughter was already a few months old—too old for the treatment to be effective. Another parent described starting NAM treatment with her son but stopping when, without exaggeration, he threw up every single time the device was placed in his mouth. Still another parent, like others, described the physical distance to the cleft team as just too far and inconvenient for her family.

One nurse specialist on a cleft team commented that she sees these kinds of situations all the time. "We have an orthodontist [on the team] who has started offering NAM treatment," she explained. But while some families in the area opt to take advantage of this treatment, she said, others don't or can't. As a result, her team sees many children who end up using no IO at all or do rudimentary taping. "For some patients, NAM is completely unrealistic," she said.

Weighing the Options. As challenging as it can feel to learn about IO and make decisions about a plan of action—including the larger decision of choosing a cleft surgeon and team—it may be helpful to keep three steps in mind: 1) ask the team lots of questions, 2) have candid conversations at home, and 3) make a decision that feels comfortable and workable for your family—with no pressure or guilt. "I would say for parents to be really honest with themselves," advised one cleft team orthodontist, "and not hard on themselves, about what their resources are."

Learning about presurgical treatments can be overwhelming. In all their variety, infant orthopedics have obvious benefits and drawbacks, whether they relate to time, energy, finances, caregiver investment, surgical intervention, short- and long-term outcomes, or other factors. Also, the decision to pursue a presurgical treatment is almost always linked with the large and important decision of choosing a cleft team. In some cases, there may be no clear-cut answers. But fortunately, there are ways to navigate these muddy waters. We can do our best homework, ask lots of questions, and try to make as careful a decision as we can—while remembering that the decision is ours alone to make.

> ## QUESTIONS ABOUT PRESURGICAL INFANT ORTHOPEDICS

Here are some questions to ask members of the cleft team:

- Which type(s) of infant orthopedics do you offer and why?
- Given my/our baby's diagnosis, can you describe possible surgical outcomes after using presurgical treatment X? Without it? How will treatment X affect the number of operations our baby will need later in life?
- Can you show us before-and-after images of lip-repair operations that you have performed? Did the babies in these images use IO? Which kind? Do these images depict ideal results or typical results?
- What is your opinion of other methods of IO?

Chapter 24

. . . .

Tips For NAM Treatment and Lip Taping

Ideas from Parents Who Have Been There

Are you considering pursuing NAM or lip taping for your baby? Or are you underway with one of these treatments at this very moment? Both *nasoalveolar molding* and lip taping require time and energy from caregivers as we bring our child to weekly appointments with members of the cleft team. But that is just the beginning. These treatments also require delicate handiwork as we arrange tiny webs of rubber bands and tapes. They occasionally demand patience and fortitude as we watch our child cry and fuss after her weekly adjustments (as much as I hate to relay that message). And then, of course, they call for problem-solving skills as we figure out what to actually *do* about that crying and fussing (we'll address the issue in this chapter). In short, these treatments can resemble a part-time job—a challenging, months-long period that can feel immensely rewarding for caregivers even as it may exhaust us and cause us to want to pull out our hair. Here are seven tips to help the experience go as smoothly as possible, the first three of which apply to both NAM and lip taping, and the remaining that relate to NAM.

. . . .

Tip No. 1: Line Up Your Ducks

When I asked parents for tips for success with NAM and lip taping, I noticed that their responses often began in one or both of two ways: with some mention of getting organized and with a surprising amount of enthusiasm. "I had this routine…" began one mother, her voice brightening as she described how she assembled her NAM supplies. Others shared similar ideas: "I set up a station," or, "It helped to have a system."

As these parents suggested, some simple organization and prep-work can help avoid a frantic search for supplies (that is, *prepped* supplies) while the baby is fussing and wiggling and threatening to roll off her changing table. "Every night I'd sit down in front of the TV and set up my tapes for the next day," said one mother, referring to the process of trimming and attaching each of the Steri-Strips™ to a tiny rubber band (see related descriptions, below). Another mother performed these duties during baby's naptime. Parents have acknowledged almost universally that NAM and lip taping require a lot of time, a lot of small moving parts, and in some cases, frustration. But many mentioned how much more positive, even enthusiastic they felt about the experience after getting systematized, both by organizing physical supplies and setting up daily routines.

Tip No. 2: Solve Problems with Tapes

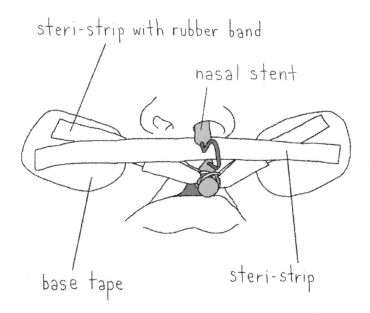

NAM treatment, unilateral

Tape! Tape! Tape! Of all the challenges parents have mentioned regarding NAM and lip taping, issues with medical tape seem to top the list. Not only do caregivers need to attach face tapes in a way that ensures the treatment is beneficial—through the use of Steri-Strips™—but in so doing, we need to do all we can to prevent skin irritation, through the effective use of base tapes.

Face Tapes: Basics. When a NAM or lip-taping regimen begins, members of the cleft team will give you a full explanation of what you need to know about your baby's treatment and may even give you some start-up supplies to take home. The protocol will vary from one treatment and baby to another, so, of course, it is best to follow the advice of the team for your child's specific needs. But common supplies often include two different types of tapes: large sterile bandages to apply directly to the baby's cheeks (called *base tapes*) to forestall skin irritation and thin Steri-Strips™ that (in the case of NAM) connect the acrylic mouth plate to the cheek tapes and, when applied with tension, engage the device. As mentioned previously, in many cases, some of the Steri-Strips™ need to be trimmed and connected in advance to a tiny rubber band—a daily task usually done by caregivers—in order to attach to the knob(s) on the NAM mouth plate. (Steri-Strips™ with rubber bands may or may not be used for lip taping.)

Base Tapes: Choosing a Brand. While pros on cleft teams often recommend applying a base tape of some sort on the cheeks for the baby to wear for several days at a time as a base tape (while changing the Steri-Strips™ daily or even several times a day), they generally can't predict which type or brand will work for your baby's skin—so you will probably need to do some shopping. A rule of thumb is that the best bandage is one that stays put on your child's face while minimizing irritation, a tricky balance that may require some trial and error on your part. The Cleftopedia site recommends looking for any tape that is "medical grade and allows the skin to breathe," specifically, a sterile bandage that is hydrocolloid and latex-free. The most common suggestions I've heard from parents and pros include Tegaderm™, DuoDERM˚ (available in thin and extra thin varieties), CVS Advanced Healing Adhesive Pads, and Band-Aids Blister Bandages (also produced as a CVS store-brand version, which some parents prefer to the name-brand product).

Remember that the first base tape you try may not be a match for your baby's skin. "We tried Tegaderm, and it did not work," said one mother about her experiments with that popular product during her son's early NAM treatment. But DuoDERM˚ did the trick, she found. This experimentation may take some time.

Base Tape Application: Tips and Tricks. Applying a base tape is not a complicated task; you simply remove the backing and apply the bandage carefully onto your baby's cheek(s). Yet several parents have offered off-the-beaten-path ideas to make the application as effective as possible. One mother mentioned applying *two* layers of base tapes onto her son's face during NAM treatment: one on the bottom, directly on her son's cheeks, and the other on top of the Steri-Strips™, like a sandwich. "It helped everything stay in place," she explained (and came recommended by the orthodontist on her son's team).

There is also a question of whether to trim the tape. While some cleft-team pros advise trimming the pad in order to reduce surface area (and potential skin irritation), another mother recalled hunting down the CVS version of the Band-Aids Blister Bandages (only available in certain retail locations) and *not* trimming the pads to fit her baby's small cheeks. "They have a large pad," she commented, "but I didn't cut it because it would compromise the seal." Experimentation, again, is par for the course.

Base Tape Application: Skin Barriers. Several parents have suggested applying a substance underneath the base tapes, if necessary, either to help them stay in place or to form a protective barrier. "Skin Tac Barrier Wipes were awesome," exclaimed one mother. The gluey substance, available from Amazon, needs to dry entirely before applying the base tape, she explained, but the glue can help the base tapes stay put.

The Cleftopedia site recommends spraying Cavilon No Sting Barrier Film on the surface of the cheeks to create a thin protective layer underneath the base tapes—or in dire situations when the skin is irritated, placing a thin piece of gauze underneath small areas of the base tapes. One parent even recommended applying an exceedingly thin layer of Aquaphor under the base tapes to serve the same purpose (an option that can cause the tape to simply fall off if applied too generously).

Base Tape Removal: Tips and Tricks. Parents uniformly recommend leaving base tapes on the baby's face for as long as humanly possible in order to avoid irritating her cheeks upon removal. "I could usually stretch it as far as two or three days if I was lucky," said one mother. When you do need to remove the tapes, the goal should be to peel them off as tearlessly (i.e., no crying), and *tearlessly* (i.e., no rips to the skin), as possible.

Aquaphor, Vaseline, and mineral oil are common aids. "I found that if I put a little Aquaphor on her cheeks when I removed the tapes, left it on for about fifteen minutes, and then peeled off the tapes SLOWLY, they would come off more easily," commented one mother. As she started to peel the tape, this mother noted, she would add even more Aquaphor. Then, she would wipe the whole area completely clean and start over again with fresh base tapes. The goal is to minimize the rip-rip-ripping of skin against tape. "I remember my son crying when I pulled off the tape and he bled," said another mother. "I felt like a horrible mom!" Fortunately, these easy-to-find supplies really do work.

Steri-Strips™: Purchase and Application. After applying base tapes to the baby's cheeks, it is time to deal with Steri-Strips™, the long, thin, relatively powerful adhesive bandages designed for postsurgical and other medical uses. These products are not manufactured in any real variety, thank goodness, so any brand will usually do the trick. You may be able to find these bandages for sale off-label at a drugstore or obtain them from your cleft team.

NAM treatment usually requires the use of both "adorned" and plain Steri-Strips™; lip-taping may use plain strips only or, in case of an elaborate taping regimen, both types. Caregivers create adorned strips by attaching a tiny rubber band to the end of a strip sometime in advance of needing them (as mentioned, during your "spare time"). The adorned strips then attach to the tiny knobs of the acrylic plate of the NAM appliance (for those using NAM) and then stretch and affix to the baby's cheeks. The orthodontist on the team may also recommend placing a single, unadorned strip of tape (no rubber band attached) horizontally across the baby's upper lip, in the location where a mustache would be.

Steri-Strips™, both adorned and plain, need to be applied in the correct position and with appropriate tension in order to ensure the treatment works. They can't be affixed too high or too low on the cheeks. And they need to be pulled tightly enough to work—but not so tightly as to smush and hurt the baby's face. These tasks may sound convoluted at first. And they are! Fortunately, they are doable. Many parents find that once they've figured it out—perhaps with some fumbling, at first, or even a lot of fumbling—the activity feels like second nature.

Steri-Strips™: Building Confidence. Since NAM treatment and lip-taping are individualized, the best way to learn to apply Steri-Strips™ correctly is to ask for a demonstration from an expert on the cleft team—and then, if you are up for it, to take a picture or video of your child (yes, right there in the office during a weekly check-in) to remind yourself what the whole thing should look like. As parents have mentioned, it is all too easy to feel confident during the team visit, where birds are singing and the details seem wonderful and doable and crystal clear—even fun!—but then to watch the information mysteriously drip out of our brains a few hours later, leaving us to fumble and sweat while, for the life of us, we can't figure out how to thread Strip A through Rubber Band B and over Body Part C. So, first of all, consider taking pictures— plenty of them—to act as an insurance policy. Next, take a look at the images in this book (and see the Cleftopedia site for some good examples too). While situations vary—and while treatment may evolve for a child over time—these images show proper alignment and tension of the tapes.

Steri-Strip™ Troubleshooting: The Mustache Tape. Several NAM parents have mentioned ideas for anchoring the "mustache tape," an affectionate nickname for the Steri-Strip™ that affixes horizontally to a baby's premaxilla. This tape can fall off the face extremely easily, especially after the baby cries or drools. The Cleftopedia site recommends spraying Cavilon No Sting Barrier Film (mentioned above) to the bare skin under the nose to prep the surface and help the tape stick. Another option, recommended by a mother of a particularly drooly baby, is to apply two strips of mustache tape, slightly offset, in order to cover as much surface area as possible. Still other parents mentioned cutting a small, additional strip to apply *vertically* in that spot, like train tracks, over the mustache tape, for extra oomph.

Special Tool No. 1: The Prep Board. Are you all thumbs when it comes to prepping your baby's Steri-Strips™? One mother constructed a cool, makeshift assembly board using a simple piece of wood and two small nails. If you hammer the nails into the board about a quarter of an inch apart, she explained, you can stretch the rubber band across the nails and then assemble the tapes easily, without having to monkey around too much with your fingers.

Special Tool No. 2: The Micro Brush. One mother, Denise, watched with wide eyes when the orthodontist on her son's cleft team laid out a NAM routine that seemed almost unachievable with human fingers. She was instructed to feed a tape through his two nasal stents and then direct it downward, like a rollercoaster, around a rubber band that stretched between the two buttons on the mouth plate. What to do? Fortunately, this orthodontist also recommended a threader tool called a *micro brush*. "It looks like a tiny, skinny, blue stick… with a white piece of cotton on the end, almost like a Q-Tip®," Denise explained. The idea is to get the Steri-Strip™ just the slightest bit stuck on the end of the stick, she said, and then to feed it through the NAM obstacle course. "It worked!" she exclaimed. The tool, called a Quewel Lash Disposable Micro Applicator Brush (available in diameters of 2.0mm, 2.5mm, and larger), can forestall a great deal of fumbling.

Special Tool No. 3: Loved Ones. Have your friends and family offered to help out with the baby? Now is the time to put them to work! One cleft-team orthodontist suggested enlisting loved ones to help prepare NAM and/or taping supplies since these tasks are eminently doable by others. The more help you can get during this time, the better.

Tip No. 3: Remember Sarah's Story and the Two-Week Adjustment Period

When I asked cleft parents about their experiences with their baby's NAM treatment, many mentioned how much easier the experience became with time. "At the beginning, it was really hard," commented one mother, Sarah, about the first two weeks after her son received the device. According to one cleft-team orthodontist, the adjustment period for the NAM varies from baby to baby, ranging from minutes or hours after treatment begins to as long as two weeks. But other pros suggest two weeks as the norm. "Our orthodontist told us that for almost everyone, this two-week period will be miserable," Sarah continued.

Indeed, Sarah's son did not have an easy experience starting out—and neither did his parents. "The first time I had to change the tapes I was a wreck," Sarah said, "a ball of nerves. I couldn't remember the directions." But the situation only worsened when her son wouldn't stop crying for forty-eight straight hours. "My husband and I were stressed out because we thought [the device] was causing him a lot of discomfort," she explained. At one point, her husband suggested they simply remove the appliance from her son's mouth during a feeding session—so they did. But then they remembered the advice from the orthodontist on the team and decided to see if he would get used to it with time. "I was beside myself," she continued. "I was heartbroken that our son had to endure it. He looked so pitiful with his face all squished up under the tape."

Around two weeks after their son received the NAM device—just the time when Sarah expected her son would have adjusted to it—she realized that, while he seemed slightly more comfortable with the appliance in place, he was still unhappy in general. Not only was he still crying a lot, but he was also sleeping fitfully and seemed to be suffering from gas. In desperation, she called their cleft-team orthodontist. "He told us that almost every baby has adjusted by this time," she said. So, they looked for another cause. Could it be colic? Another issue? Sarah's mother wondered whether the baby might have been suffering from a food intolerance. So, Sarah, who was pumping breast milk at the time, immediately cut dairy from her own diet. Within a few days, her son calmed down. Victory. Not only did NAM treatment smooth out from there, but Sarah remained dairy-free for seven months and her son seemed well-adjusted and content.

In Sarah's son's case, the experience improved with time, especially as he adjusted to the NAM *and* his mother solved problems with diet. But as time went by, Sarah and her husband also gained confidence using the NAM. The couple realized that despite their early concerns, their son eventually fed well with the device in place (note that recommendations vary regarding eating; see below for questions for the team). And during that critical first two weeks, the orthodontist himself ironed out the kinks of this personalized treatment. "You need to power through it and get to the other side," Sarah advised, "when your baby has adjusted, and you have more confidence in what you are doing." The meantime can be challenging and stressful. The key may be to stay in touch with the team and—if possible, amidst the pressure and exhaustion—to remind yourself, as Sarah did, why you decided to pursue this treatment in the first place. "I knew it was what I wanted, and the right thing for us," she said.

Tip No. 4: Make a Plan for Fussy Moments

While many NAM parents have reported that their babies calmed down measurably after the first two weeks of treatment, they also described additional ups and downs during the ensuing months, particularly following the weekly visits with the team. As mentioned previously, the acrylic plate of the NAM device needs to be modified each week (or so) by the orthodontist on the cleft team in order to manipulate parts of the baby's mouth before her lip-repair operation. (A baby may wear nasal stents as well, usually later on in treatment, which may also require adjustment). On the upside, these adjustments—when paired with consistent daily use of the device—are exactly what cause the treatment to work. Unfortunately, they can also be a source of discomfort for a baby.

As caregivers, you will probably not be surprised to hear that every baby will respond differently to these weekly adjustments. Some babies feel fine after the visit, more or less, and behave and sleep normally or near normal. Others, sadly, will be fussy or even downright upset. No one can know these responses in advance, for one baby or from one visit to the next. But a good way to tackle this situation may be to *expect* to have a difficult twelve-to-twenty-four hours following the appointment—and to make a solid contingency plan with the team and/or your child's pediatrician for that time (find some sample questions, below). This way, if the baby feels miserable after the visit, you will have made a plan. (Likewise, if she feels fine, you will enjoy a wonderful bonus.)

Fussy Baby? Weekly Troubleshooting. The best path to follow is always the one recommended by a professional. But it may help to know that troubleshooting after a weekly NAM appointment often relates to two common questions: assessing whether a baby's response stems from a concrete problem caused by the appliance—

for example, a sore that develops in the mouth as a result of the shape of the acrylic plate—or from a lack of acclimation to the new setup. If a baby has developed a sore or if the acrylic plate is rubbing against the mouth painfully, the team members may recommend you return to the office with the baby the next day or sometime ASAP for further adjustment to the device. If the fussiness seems to relate to the fact that the baby hasn't gotten used to the new setup, you may need to soothe him or otherwise wait it out.

QUESTIONS ABOUT NAM

Here are some questions to ask the dental/orthodontic specialists on the cleft team:

- What behaviors can I expect to see in my baby following the weekly NAM adjustment?
- If my baby seems to be uncomfortable, what should I do?
- Can you describe situations in which I should leave the NAM device in place or take it out?
- Should we remove the NAM during feeding sessions?
- Can I contact you to ask questions or troubleshoot during off hours?

Here are some questions to ask a child's pediatrician:

- Can I give my baby medicine for pain following the weekly adjustment of the NAM device? If so, which one can I administer and in what quantity/frequency?

· ·

Tip No. 5 : Older Baby?
Prepare for an Adventure

One of the most mystifying aspects of NAM treatment, according to parents who look back on their experiences, is the array of ways a baby may respond to it after several weeks or months have passed—specifically, the sneaky, creative, even ingenious methods some babies employ to pull the device out of their mouths. If your baby is very young, you may be pleasantly unaware of these kinds of antics. Perhaps your infant, in the dewy days of youth, has not fully awakened to the possibilities literally within her reach. But just wait. One day, she may not only discover the usefulness of her own hands but also detect the presence of a strange, intensely interesting, possibly bothersome interloper inside her mouth. On that fateful day, she may exclaim to herself with clarity, determination, and a command of language and medical jargon that belies her age: GET THIS DAMN NAM OUT OF MY MOUTH. And then, dear fellow parents, the NAM battle will have begun.

She may be clever. She will grow stronger and more charming with time. But fear not. You will win.

The first order of business is to get organized. *Just kidding!* You can skip the organization this time and simply do all you can to keep the device inside the baby's mouth. One mother was surprised one day to see her daughter reach up, grab the NAM, and rip it clear out of her mouth in the middle of a feeding session as if she had become an expert on the first try. Then, she did it again. And again. "She went in every chance she could get," she said. So, this mother bought one-piece outfits (she referred to them as *sleepers*) with fold-over mittens. "She could bat at it with them on," she commented, "but at least she was not ripping it out."

Another mother looked to the tools already available in her NAM kit—in this case the long Steri-Strips™ in their original length, before they'd been trimmed or prepped with rubber bands—to wrap around her son's nasal stents so many times that she very nearly mummified them. "We wrapped the strip around the prong to make it difficult for him to grab and pull out," she explained. "His finger couldn't get inside." Did the taping make the NAM device appear all the more noticeable to others? Sure, she said. But then she let out a laugh. "Really, how much more noticeable can you get?"

The method worked, deterring her son from pulling out the device and tallying one more victory for Team Parent.

Last, some parents go for the gold with a two-pronged approach of swaddling the baby *and* wrapping her arms in stiff, postoperative arm cuffs during sleep time. "We swaddled like we meant it," said another mother. "Otherwise, she would have pulled out the stents." As strange and over-the-top as it may feel to swaddle a five-month-old—or for that matter, to restrict her arms or cocoon her nasal stents with tape—parents have employed any and all inventive methods to ensure the success of NAM treatment, particularly after the baby has grown somewhat. Go, team!

Tip No. 6: Find Help

When Heather found out that another mother in her area had undergone NAM treatment with her daughter just a few months before her son Jack was born, she took the brave step of reaching out to her—and soon realized that, in so doing, she had found an informal teacher, a sounding board, and a friend. "The orthodontist shows you [how to do it], sure," Heather said, referring to the weekly appointments where parents learn how to perform the at-home tasks for the device. "But you're stressed. You need a tutorial after the fact. I'm [located] an hour and a half from the hospital. I can't just pop back in." So following Jack's weekly NAM appointments, Heather occasionally brought him to this fellow parent's house for an ad hoc help session. "It was huge," Heather commented about the relationship. "She was so generous. She said to me, 'Please do not hesitate.' It made all the difference." These kinds of peer-to-peer relationships can ease the burden, both logistically and emotionally. Plus, oftentimes, they're fun.

Of course, some parents don't happen to have a NAM family in the neighborhood. Moriah explained that at the time of her son's birth, she had never heard of this treatment, much less knew someone else going through it. While her husband had been born with CLP himself and had undergone operations and other treatments as a child, his early experiences took place during a different era, before NAM treatment had even come into existence. Moriah and her husband felt isolated—until they found a private Facebook group called "NAM Support (Nasoalveolar Molding)," which is devoted entirely to supporting caregivers during this treatment. "At two in the morning I'd have a question about tape," Moriah said. "By the time I woke up in the morning, I'd have six responses with suggestions and possible answers." The group felt like a welcome connection. "There are so many other parents going through the same thing!" she continued. "Without Facebook, I wouldn't have known that." While cleft-team pros emphasize that medical questions should always be directed to the team, online support can provide a springboard for questions—and feel reassuring, as well.

A final way to seek NAM-specific support is to communicate openly—and often—with the orthodontist (or pediatric dentist) on the team on any number of issues large and small. Of course, some pros are more accessible than others. But NAM parents have recommended taking practitioners up on their kind offer if presented. "We were lucky that Dr. X was not that far away from us, only twenty minutes from our house," commented another mother, Lexi. But the short physical distance between her home and his office, while convenient, was not the factor that Lexi most appreciated. "I could text him," she said. "I would send a picture and he would write back almost instantly." Lexi described instances shortly after treatment began in which she wasn't sure she had applied the tapes correctly to her daughter's face. "He would say, 'It looks excellent' or 'Try more of an angle next time,'" she said. That availability made all the difference. NAM treatment became easier and less frustrating for Lexi when she could get fast, reliable answers in the moment. And since she was beyond grateful for Dr. X's help, it was easy to develop a warm and trusting family-practitioner relationship as the weeks of treatment went by.

NAM treatment can be challenging for caregivers, not only because of the time commitment required but because of the steep learning curves all of us experience in order to understand how to use and maintain the device. So, the more NAM-specific help we can get, the easier the experience will be. When I've spoken with parents about the kinds of support they've found, I hear palpable relief in their voices.

. . . .

Tip No. 7: Relish the Moments without (and with!) the NAM

It is natural to learn about nasoalveolar molding and wonder whether a baby who undergoes this treatment will really need to wear the device *all the time*—as opposed to just most of the time or even, say, 90 percent of the time. This is a perfect question for the cleft team, since instructions will vary from child to child and team to team. But even if the pros advise that a child wear the device nearly 100 percent of the time (as my daughter's did), a baby will likely have moments when she won't wear it.

Some parents offer their baby a five-to-ten-minute break during the time each day when they clean the device. Others remove the appliance during feeding sessions, saying that the baby fares better without it. (Others find the opposite to be true: that their babies actually feed better with the NAM in place since it can function as a false palate). Still others change the base tapes every few days during the bath, giving their baby a thirty-minute reprieve from the device as her skin dries. In any case, these are moments to savor. "That was the best time for cuddles," commented one mother about her son's short daily breaks. Her advice? Maximize it! "Get as much as you can from that time off," she said, describing photo-ops and undivided attention. "Because it's got to go back on."

As heavenly as it may feel to see your baby's soft, sweet cheeks during those brief interludes, it is also important to note how many parents have relished—or done their best to relish—the time spent *with* the NAM in place. One mother described a conversation with her husband in which they debated whether to remove their daughter's appliance for an upcoming family wedding. While the couple did not feel ashamed or embarrassed about their daughter's CLP, this mother felt protective of her daughter in front of all of those people. "I wanted people to see her for the first time and see how beautiful she was not and not be distracted by this shocking NAM," she said. But they also knew the value of consistent treatment in order to make progress. And maybe just as important, her husband noted that the treatment represented the present moment. "He said, 'This is her. This is a chapter in her life. She needs it. Let's leave it on.'" As challenging as it may feel to accept the appearance of the NAM device, whether at home or in public, this father made a thoughtful point. Our time with our infant is fleeting, special occasions aside. The more we can do personally to enjoy what is happening right now, appliance or no appliance, the more content we'll be and, perhaps, the more readily we will bond.

Also, many parents do not mind the look of the device more generally. While I felt enormous relief during the moments when my daughter's face was soft and natural and free (as described in Chapter 22), others have readily accepted the appearance of the NAM. "Initially, I felt like I couldn't see her," commented one mother about the early adjustment period. "But now, it feels weird to see her *not* in the NAM. To see her *not* taped feels weird. It's become a part of her." As this mother looked ahead to her daughter's lip-repair surgery, she wondered out loud how that new phase would feel. "That will be a big adjustment, for sure," she said. Some of us feel just fine about the appearance of the NAM, as this mother did, even if we find it alarming or off-putting at first. With time, our child's taped-up appearance can feel like a new normal, just as we will also adjust to our child's new face after surgery and, for that matter, with growth.

Whether you love presurgical orthopedics or hate them—or both—the early weeks and months of treatment can be challenging for all kinds of reasons. But, hopefully, you will also find this time rewarding, not just as you envision long-term health benefits for your child, but also as you begin to experience the sheer magnitude of duties, in all their ridiculousness and absurdity, that a parent will undergo—voluntarily!—to benefit a child. You may be taping now. But someday, you may be spending four hundred hours driving your child to basketball games. Or fretting as she argues with her best friend. Our NAM- and taping-related moments—along with other moments, in all their glamor—are gestures of parental love.

Lip-Repair Surgery

Chapter 25

. . . .

A Second Smile

Lip Repair, Changing Faces, and Mama Geese

Lip-repair surgery can be a tender topic for parents. As the date approaches to close the gap in our baby's lip, many of us feel apprehensive. Any surgical procedure comes with risk, of course, and the idea of operating on a tiny, vulnerable infant can feel all the more nerve-wracking. When my daughter was a baby, I would leap out of bed at night to help her when she cried, barely able to stand the sounds of her everyday discomforts—much less imagine her enduring the pain of major surgery. Yet this procedure can feel momentous for other reasons too. Unlike an operation on the heart or the ears or the lungs (in fact, unlike palate-repair surgery and some of the other, later procedures for a cleft-affected child), lip repair permanently changes the look of a baby's gateway to the world—and a parent's gateway to a baby—her face. Many parents agree: emotionally, this one is a biggie.

Yet, while many parents feel nervous or anxious about this operation, our specific feelings about altering a baby's appearance seem to vary widely. Some welcome the change, eager to move forward (*finally!*). Others balk, mourning the loss of a unique appearance they have grown to love. "The night before the surgery," said one mother, "I took a picture of my son. It is not something special to anyone else, but it makes me cry. I can remember his first smile, ever." Whether you feel long-awaited relief, poignant loss, or both, these intense responses are normal and okay. What's more, these feelings may be illuminated, even clarified, by a body of scientific research based on the behavior of geese (yes, geese!).

Embracing Change, Resisting Change

When I asked Jenna, the mother of three, about her memories of her son Leo's lip-repair surgery, she recalled feeling nervous about it but also eager for it to be done with. "We just wanted it right," she said. While Jenna had noticed that other cleft parents described feeling sad about changing the appearance of their baby's face—she had seen many such conversations on social media—she was quick to point out that she did not share those sentiments. "We have never looked back and wished we had his CLP again," she said. "Is it vanity? Maybe. Pride?" Jenna did not want her child to have such a visible facial difference. "It is hard for a child," she said. Another mother also felt relieved, even upbeat, to see the process move forward for her daughter. "We were really, really pleased with lip repair," she said. "I thought my daughter looked great afterward. I was just excited to get the process going, to get it done." A third mother's voice wavered as she described an early incident in public when a waiter stared at her son. "We just wanted it to end," she said. "We wanted to bypass the stares and the questions. It was just too hard." Whether out of concern for their child's well-being or a strong desire to end what felt like a months-long, emotional holding pattern, these parents embraced the change that came with this procedure. Even in sharing their stories years later, they seemed palpably relieved.

Others feel loss, even grief. After weeks or months of bonding with their baby, they have fallen in love with her special, wide smile. "I know we need to have Ruby's cleft repaired for medical reasons and not just for appearance," commented one mother before her daughter's operation, "but I think she is beautiful and perfect as is." Another mother, Ashley, had such deep reservations about the operation that she hesitated to proceed with it at all. The health implications for her son Parker, who was born with an isolated cleft lip, were not as far-reaching as those for a child born with a cleft palate (whose parents and doctors may not see surgery as optional). Also, Ashley liked Parker's appearance. "I didn't want to go through with it," she said. "My husband didn't want to either, but he thought that it would be easier on our son to do it now rather than later. We were both terrified that something would go wrong in surgery. I thought he looked just fine!" Some parents question the necessity or ethics of a so-called "normalizing" procedure that occurs without a child's consent. But just as often, they have stared at their child's unique face over weeks and months and, in some cases, surprised even themselves when they find her face adorable as is.

A majority of parents express conflicting emotions. "I remember thinking of all the good reasons why we were headed into surgery but still dreading it," said one mother, "not just out of fear and anxiety, but because of the realization that my baby would look different afterward." Even years after the operation, many look back on the experience with special intensity, recalling uncanny details or speaking of it as an early yardstick against which they would measure other procedures. One mother started to describe her six-year-old daughter's upcoming bone-graft surgery but quickly compared it to her memory of lip repair. "This surgery isn't causing me nearly the anxiety the early ones did," she commented. "Back then, I was grieving the loss of what she looked like. It was really, really painful. I fell in love with how she looked. I thought, 'She will never look this way again. She will never have that smile again.'" Even as her pain eventually subsided, the idea of changing her child's smile felt enormously saddening.

Whether we embrace change, resist change or both, most parents believe that the moment is significant. It is a big deal, we seem to agree, to change the appearance of a human face. Of any of the procedures for a cleft-affected child, lip repair makes the most pronounced and lasting visual changes. The phrase, "My baby has a cleft lip" becomes past tense, even if other, related treatments take place many years into the future. We all confront change on a regular basis. Irreversible change to the face has special meaning.

Imprinting
Lessons from our Feathered Friends

Believe it or not, the strong feelings that parents associate with lip-repair surgery—whether we feel relief, loss, or some combination of the two—may be explained, in part, by the behavior of geese. In the 1930s, an Austrian zoologist named Konrad Lorenz conducted pioneering work on the behavior of geese and other species of birds, ultimately earning the titles "Father of Ethology" (*ethology* is the study of animal behavior) and less formally, "Foster-Mother of Ducks." He later won a Nobel Prize.

Lorenz observed the behavior of goslings during the minutes and hours after they hatched, during which time they would follow and attach themselves resolutely to their mothers, distinguishing her from other geese. He referred to the behavior as *imprinting.* One of the key elements of the discovery was that while these little birds usually imprinted on their mothers, in her absence they might just as easily follow and attach themselves to any bird—or even a human or another moving object that happened to be present during the early moments after birth (Lorenz earned the title "Foster-Mother of Ducks" because he allowed some little birds to imprint on *him*). At that point, scientists had already determined that infants had a "biological imperative"—meaning a hard-wired desire, sometimes called "instinct"—to recognize a caregiver. But Lorenz's work added evidence of an experiential impulse as well.

There's more. Further studies show that recognition of a caregiver occurs for humans as well, particularly shortly after birth—and that this behavior goes two ways. The infant sees and recognizes her mother (or father, or another caregiver, or whoever happens to be there), *and* a caregiver studies and memorizes the unique appearance of the child. From her side, our baby, like the little goslings, gazes up at us, takes in our looks and sounds, quickly memorizes us, and decides, "YOU are my person." Likewise, from our side, caregivers take in the appearance and other character-istics of our baby and conclude, "Yes, YOU are mine." Research published in the journal *Infant and Child Development* shows that while the exact timing and duration of this process is not yet clear—the studies attempt to distinguish among facial recognition that occurs seconds, minutes, and hours after birth—the human infant can differentiate and memorize faces very early on.

When I first read this research, I had a few small heart attacks. I thought back to the precious moments after my daughter was born—the moments when we were probably supposed to be imprinting on one another—when a small army of nurses and hospital staff whisked her away to a back room to examine her clefts, rule out further complications, and clean her up. For five or ten minutes—to me, a short eternity—she did not scamper after me blissfully in the sunshine like a gosling attaching to her goose-mother. Likewise, I most certainly did not identify her indelibly, saying, "YOU are mine." No. At that point, I couldn't even see her. She lay around the corner in a windowless room, having fluids sucked from her orifices while I waited, impatient, drugged, and stuck to a gurney. Also, at some point during that first hour or two, my husband and I turned away from the baby to call our parents to share the news. For that matter, I have spoken with several NICU parents, adop-tive parents, and mothers with their own medical complications who didn't even meet or hold their child, much less memorize her, until well after the geese-goslings test period had expired. Did my husband and I—and I assume a slew of other parents—lose our golden moments? Moreover, has my daughter imprinted on a labor-and-delivery nurse at Women & Infants Hospital?

Fortunately, the goal of discussing academic research in the context of real-life situations is not to put pressure on parents and babies to perform like birds in a *Planet Earth* documentary. The point is to say with some certainty that face recognition plays a role in the so-called attachment process. Even more, it is to say that, *of course,* some parents feel apprehensive about lip-repair surgery! This research shows that the unique appearance of the face—as well as sounds, smells, and the complex processes of nurturing and providing food—play key roles in our early relationships with one another. Studies on the reciprocal nature of imprinting may explain why, on some level, the idea of facial surgery can feel alarming to a parent, even existentially confusing. After weeks or months of bonding with *this* child with *this* face, we may reasonably wonder what else will change. And we may just as reasonably feel unsettled in the meantime.

As one mother prepared herself for the changes that would follow her daughter's surgery, she mentioned her uneasiness to the cleft-team nurse. "I was getting ready for surgery," she said, "and thinking about that smile that I've known since birth. I told the nurse, 'I'm not sure I am ready to see her a different way.'" Fortunately, the nurse responded, "'Every parent lives for a baby's first smile. You get two of them!'"

Whether we feel relief or loss about changing our child's face, our intense emotions are real. They are valid. And, perhaps, in an imitation of the enormous variability and adaptability of animal behavior that occurs in nature—whether guided by biology or by experience—parents also get more than one chance to imprint. As the nurse pointed out so astutely and reassuringly, we get two smiles. But maybe we also get two opportunities—or a string of them—to smell, hear, recognize, follow, and attach to one another, like geese.

Chapter 26

. . . .

Lip-Repair Basics

From Packing Your Bags
to Parking the Car

When Kim learned that her son's lip-repair operation would take place in less than a month, she started to feel nervous. Really nervous. "I was a mess," she wrote on her blog, *Cutest Little Cleftie*. The small, needling questions that came to mind seemed endless. "I hated that my baby wouldn't be able to drink after midnight," she started. "What would I do when he woke up, screaming in hungry anger? My drive to [the hospital] was about an hour and a half. Would he scream the entire drive?" Kim also worried about getting caught in traffic and finding a place in the hospital to pump breast milk. Practical questions flooded her thoughts. "Where would I eat?" she continued. "I was so scared for all the little details, I forgot to be scared for the actual surgery."

It was clear in talking to Kim that she did, indeed, feel strongly about her son's actual surgery, especially as she anticipated the loss of his beautiful, wide smile. But like many other parents, she worried about the choreography of the day. This chapter covers practical details, including a description of the procedure itself, tips on hospital protocols and logistics, the realities of rescheduling, ways to prepare the family, and what to bring to the hospital. Sometimes, it can be comforting to know what is going to happen, where to park the car, and how to find a cup of coffee.

What Happens on the Operating Table?

Some parents are more interested than others in learning what a surgeon actually does during a lip-repair operation. "I suddenly thought before surgery I'd really like to see what they do when they do a cleft repair," commented one parent in a study on parents' perspectives. YouTube offers near-instant access to footage of actual lip-repair (and other) procedures—for those who can stomach it. For everyone else, the following is a brief description of what happens during this operation.

Not Just the Lip. *Lip Repair* is an umbrella term that, depending on the circumstances, may include a collection of surgical procedures performed on the lip, nose, and gums, rather than just one operation on the lip. The exact procedures a child undergoes will depend on several factors including her unique diagnosis, a surgeon's training and opinion, and other considerations. But according to experts in the field, the most common procedures of lip repair for a person born with CLP include closure of the lip (called *cheiloplasty),* surgical reshaping of the nose (called *tip rhinoplasty,* or *primary cleft lip nasoplasty*), and sometimes closure of the cleft in the gumline (called a *gingivoperiosteoplasty* or "GPP").

Some surgeons opt to perform lip repair in two surgical sessions rather than one, particularly for children born with complete clefts or those who do not undergo presurgical orthopedics (like NAM or Latham treatment, as described elsewhere in this book). In these cases, the surgeon may start with a *cleft-lip adhesion* or *nose adhesion,* a surgical first step that involves narrowing the spaces in the lip/nose, essentially turning a complete cleft into an incomplete cleft. The second operation finishes the closure(s). All lip-repair procedures, whether done in one step or two, are performed under *general anesthesia* by a surgeon on a cleft palate or craniofacial team.

Cut and Paste? When a surgeon closes a cleft lip, she makes a sequence of carefully measured cuts to the skin, tissue, and muscle, which she will then move and reconnect, piece by piece, to neighboring pieces of skin, muscle, or tissue. As the surgeon cuts and connects, step-by-step and layer-by-layer, the lip comes together in a new way, like an elaborate origami. The work is intricate, painstaking, and highly skilled, but the surgical actions themselves, in their very essence, are actually understandable. Basically, the process goes like this: cut, rearrange, reconnect. Typically, for cleft-lip repair, no material is borrowed from other parts of the body.

When reshaping the nose, the surgeon similarly cuts elements inside the nose, reconfigures them, and holds them in place with stitches (called *sutures*). Some surgeons operate extensively on the nose during infancy, while others wait to do so later in childhood. But as one cleft surgeon suggested, a person's nose, unlike the lip, will change over the years, in any case; most cleft surgeons recommend a second nose operation in the teen years.

The goal for all of the procedures, according to authors Adelle Green, Ashley Salyer, and Dr. Kenneth E. Salyer in the family guide, *Comprehensive Cleft Care: Family Edition*, is to "reconstruct the aesthetic and functional aspects of the lip and nose so that they will look and function as normally as possible." The outcome, the authors continue, should involve excellent shape, symmetry, and muscle function of the lip and nose.

Surgical Techniques. Every cleft is different, but not so different that a surgeon starts from scratch when deciding how to close each one. A surgeon usually selects one of several standardized surgical techniques for a child's lip closure, based on the child's anatomy, the surgeon's training, the surgeon's projections about long-term growth, and other factors. Surgical methods are like road maps that detail where to make cuts and how to reconfigure the tissue. The methods have names—such as "The Extended Mohler Unilateral Cleft Lip Repair," "The Millard Technique," "The Dallas Protocol," "The

Mulliken Method" and others—which, in some cases, are named after pioneers in the field. All of these methods involve meticulous work—first, in measuring and marking the skin, then in making incisions and manipulating thin layers of skin, tissue, and muscle.

It can be confusing to learn about variations in surgical techniques. Suppose one surgeon states a preference for a particular technique while the surgeon on the team down the road says she would opt for another? (If you're in the process of searching for a cleft team, see more discussion on this topic in Chapter 8). According to experts in the field, a variation in technique from one surgeon to another is par for the course. Orthodontist Samuel Berkowitz writes that an overall increase in understanding of CLP over the years has led to surgical methods that are "different yet frequently successful." It is important to note that some surgeons are more experienced and qualified than others in applying these methods. In fact, parents might inquire about a surgeon's reasons for choosing one method over another during the process of choosing a cleft palate or craniofacial team (again, see Chapter 8 for more questions to ask). But the variation in methods need not be a warning sign, necessarily.

Logistics, Logistics, Logistics

I can't tell you the best place to park the car, pump breast milk, or find a cup of coffee—unless you are bringing your child to one of my home-team hospitals in Providence, Rhode Island, or Boston, Massachusetts. But others are here to help. Let's start with the team and the activities that lead up to surgery day.

Preparing for Surgery: Visits and Tasks. Cleft teams and hospitals typically distribute loads of information and instructions to parents prior to a child's operation. First, the team may instruct you to bring your child to presurgical appointments, starting (unsurprisingly) with at least one presurgical meeting with the surgeon/team itself.

According to the guide, *Comprehensive Cleft Care: Family Edition*, a baby's general health will play a large role in her readiness for surgery. So, the team may also ask you to take your child to the pediatrician to get sign-offs on weight gain, immunizations, and other questions.

Last, the team may give you information on the registration process at the hospital, a process that can be surprisingly involved. Procedures will vary. Some hospitals recommend early registration, while others do it on the day of surgery. In any case, the process typically involves signing consent forms, confirming insurance information, receiving ID bracelets, and (at the time of publication of this book) scheduling presurgical COVID-19 tests. Registration can last thirty minutes or, in some cases, quite a bit longer—so you may want to plan to stay a while. "We spent the day prior [to our daughter's operation] signing eighty-five pieces of paper," said one mother. "It felt sort of horrible, signing your life away. We were so nervous." Other parents said they felt relieved to get the process underway, however, and to feel officially signed in and ready to go.

The team should also give you information on where to go on surgery day, what time to arrive, what the baby should eat or drink beforehand (likely nothing), and where in the hospital you should wait during the procedure itself. This information is important to review and follow, as some parts—like the eating restriction—relate to the baby's safety during the procedure.

The team may also give you information on what you will need to do to prepare for your baby's recovery, such as purchasing over-the-counter pain medications and perhaps a syringe feeder (again, surgeons' instructions vary). At this point, you will probably also get a sense of what kind of life accommodations you will need to make with work schedules, sibling care, etc. Some parents need to make travel plans, depending on the location of the hospital. One mother noted that her son's hospital offered vouchers for nearby hotels. While not all hospitals offer discounts for lodging, some offer shuttle services, special parking, meal coupons, or other perks for caregivers.

The Dry Run. Most parents agree that once you've experienced a child's surgery—even once—the various routines and locations will quickly become clear and understandable. But it can feel daunting to enter the big, shiny, complicated maze of a hospital building for the first time, much less choose the correct bank of elevators to get to your destination. Thank goodness for the dry run. Many hospitals offer tours and/or information sessions to parents (and patients, depending on age) to lay eyes on the place and see where everything is located. A tour might include a visit to:

- the registration area (the place where parents/guardians fill out paperwork, either on the day of surgery or some time in advance),
- the preoperative area (a room where a child and family go just prior to surgery, often to dress the child in a surgical gown and meet briefly with the surgeon and anesthesiologist),
- the waiting room(s) for caregivers during the procedure itself, and
- the recovery space (the area where caregivers meet the baby right after surgery, and where she "wakes up" from anesthesia).

The visit might also include information about whether the baby will then move to a private or shared room for the duration of the stay (for questions to ask the team about specific location and duration of stay, see Chapter 28). Just like middle-school orientation, this kind of visit can provide useful information and feel surprisingly comforting. If you don't have time for an official tour, a simple walk through the hospital can accomplish many of the same goals.

Pullout Beds and (Many) Other Questions. At this point, maybe your cleft team has given you pertinent details about surgery day like where, when, and how to show up at the hospital (and by *how*, I mean, with a very hungry baby). All of this information is useful and important, even critical. It may not address, however, the concerns of my friend Liz, who pulled me aside before the birth of her child at our local hospital and smiled as she whisper-asked, half sheepishly, "Do you think I will need to bring a hair dryer?" Small questions may abound. While it may not be productive to ask your child's surgeon or speech-language pathologist, for example, whether you will need to pack your slippers for surgery day, these questions have a place. They deserve answers, especially if those answers will give you some peace of mind.

Many parents wonder about accommodations. While a recovering baby usually sleeps in a special crib-bed in a recovery room in the hospital, caregivers often have the option to sleep next to the child on a simple, transformable chair that folds out to a single bed. According to a few parents, such a chair-bed works perfectly well for one medium-sized adult but decidedly less well for two adults (think: sardines). Meals are typically included for children during the hospital stay following surgery but may or may not be offered free of charge for caregivers. The specifics vary from one hospital to another. These are perfect questions to ask on a hospital tour.

Fellow parents of cleft-affected kids can provide invaluable information about the specifics of a surgeon and hospital, ranging from what happens when handing over your baby prior to anesthesia to where to get food afterward. "We talked to parents who know the day-to-day stuff," said one dad. "They told us things like, 'You can stay here'…'There is a shuttle to the hospital'…'This place is expensive.' A team or doctor won't tell you that stuff." These conversations can fill in the blanks. "That dialogue with other parents was big for us," the dad continued. Cleft-team coordinators may be able to introduce you to others who use the same surgeon and hospital. Facebook and other social media can also be good places to connect.

FAMILY STORIES
Pop Quiz

MAJOR SURGERY?

A few weeks before her daughter's lip-repair operation, Haley took her daughter to the first of several routine, presurgical medical appointments, starting with a visit to the pediatrician. Midway through the exam, the doctor turned to Haley and asked her a pointed question: "What is the difference between a major and a minor surgery?" Haley heard the question and froze. "I was sure she was quizzing me on one of the million little bits of info that we had been bombarded with during our presurgery day of visits and paper-signing," she said. Had she learned this information somewhere? Haley scanned the recesses of her brain.

Then the doctor smiled. "She told me, 'Major surgery is any surgery happening to the little person you love.'" The doctor then went on to explain to Haley that even though a parent may know rationally that a surgeon possesses skills and plenty of experience—and may even see this operation as a routine event—it is all right to be anxious and afraid. "She reassured me that it was okay to feel like this operation was a HUGE deal," Haley continued. "It made me feel a little less neurotic to know I was normal."

Surgery can feel scary. While it may ease our minds to solve logistical problems like packing our bags and setting up child care for our other children—and while those details do matter!—it may also help to know that it is okay to feel nervous and overwhelmed.

Hospital Resources: Above and Beyond. Some hospitals offer special services that are not immediately obvious to uninitiated parents—or to those of us who have not read every word of the hospital website or taken an official tour.

The UCSF hospital (University of California San Francisco), for example, offers family-life coordinators who help caregivers solve problems and otherwise act as "friends on the inside" during a child's operation and subsequent hospital stay. Chaplain services are common in hospitals too, not only to provide a physical space for contemplation or prayer but to lend an ear and offer respite regardless of religious affiliation. Several cleft parents have also mentioned Ronald McDonald Family Rooms, which are offered in some children's hospitals for families of children going through surgery and/or hospitalization. Ronald McDonald rooms are comfortable lounges in a hospital where caregivers can rest and regroup (see Chapter 28 for more information). One mother described refrigerators filled with food, computers, showers, and nap rooms. "I breathed easy knowing we were going to be taken care of," she continued. All of these services are put in place specifically to relieve the caregivers' stress and burdens. Many are offered free of charge. They can be wonderfully comforting.

Save the Date!
Now...Change the Date!?
Rescheduling an Operation

Unfortunately, it is possible that a child's operation will need to be rescheduled. My blood pressure goes up just mentioning this topic. Like many parents, I spent weeks counting down to my daughter's lip-repair surgery. Her surgery date—I will never forget August 22—became a logistical and emotional anchor of sorts. My husband and I rearranged our work schedules, called in favors from grandparents, stashed meals in the freezer, and bit our fingernails, all with August 22 in mind. Our countdown resembled an old TV reel of a NASA shuttle launch, with huge numbers flashing on the screen (and in our minds) as the liftoff neared. Then, poof! With one phone call, we learned that our big day had been delayed a week because of a scheduling hiccup in the hospital.

These things happen. If a child's operation needs to be postponed—hopefully, an unlikely event—it usually occurs for one of three reasons: the child's illness, inadequate weight gain or nutrition, or hospital administrative issues. For your peace of mind, here is a brief rundown of each situation.

Rescheduling Due to Sickness. Occasionally, a doctor on a cleft team will postpone a surgical procedure if a child becomes ill. "We were supposed to have the surgery in January," said one mother about her son's lip repair. But on the morning of the operation, the anesthesiologist at the hospital noticed that her son was wheezing. "It was so stressful to get prepared," she said, "and to know that it was happening, and to finally arrive at the hospital, and then… nothing." Another parent remembered constant vigilance before surgery as she took special precautions at her daughter's day care, in crowds, and in other germ-laden settings (all of which occurred before COVID-19). "I remember thinking, 'She cannot get sick right now!'" she said. "It was nerve-wracking."

It is important to consult with the cleft team about specific health requirements for surgery in order to understand the particular thresholds and reasoning for delaying a procedure or proceeding as planned. Some *anesthesiologists* (the medical professionals who administer anesthesia to a patient prior to a surgical procedure) are especially concerned with breathing. "It is important that your child is not suffering from any other illnesses that will make it harder for him or her to recover from their surgery," writes the Hospital for Sick Children (SickKids) in Toronto. "A cold, cough, runny nose, or sore throat can become much worse after an anesthetic or make it harder for your child to breathe during or after the procedure."

There are a few simple ways to keep a baby healthy—and, hopefully, reduce stress for all involved. The University of Rochester Medical Center recommends sticking with basics, especially with schedules and sleep. "It is important to keep your baby's routine the same before the day of surgery," URMC recommends. "Make sure you, your baby, and your family are well-rested." Other everyday methods, like those commonly recommended by a child's pediatrician, can help stave off illness too. The Mayo Clinic suggests suctioning the baby's nose, using saline spray and running a humidifier. One mother, Anna, raved about antibacterial wipes. And of course, some parents wear surgical masks in public to stave off COVID-19. While no one can prevent all unforeseen consequences of living in the real world, clear communication and simple wellness techniques really can make a difference.

Rescheduling Due to Weight. A baby's weight can be another factor for proceeding with surgery or delaying it. A team may require that a child reach or maintain a minimum weight, often ten pounds, in order to proceed with the operation safely. Such a threshold can be stressful for parents. Every ounce of every bottle becomes a big deal (Drink up, baby!). If you're worried about weight gain—either because your baby was small to start out or because you're unsure whether she's gaining weight adequately—the best thing you can do is bring up the concern with your pediatrician and/or cleft team— sooner rather than later—and ideally, to stay in touch with these folks on a regular basis. Some pediatricians will schedule weekly weigh-ins and/or recommend changes in diet. Remember, weight gain is a goal but also a process—and these professionals are there to help.

One nurse on a cleft team advised parents to know about wiggle room. "We are not absolute with weight," she said. "If the baby weighs nine pounds, fourteen ounces rather than ten pounds, it does not mean that we will cancel the surgery. I think that is important to say out loud because parents worry about those kinds of things." The key, in some cases, is for the baby to fall within a desirable weight range rather than meet a single number on the scale.

Rescheduling Due to Administrative Reasons. Last, a child's surgery may be postponed if the cleft team runs into problems reserving an operating room or encounters other administrative challenges. Unfortunately, hospital booking systems don't always run perfectly, especially when it comes to scheduling an operation that is not considered urgent. "It really upset us," said one father when his son's surgery was delayed (as he described in a study in the *Cleft Palate-Craniofacial Journal*). "It makes a very difficult situation a million times more difficult. We had both booked time off work. You get quite emotional because you build yourself up to it." There is not much that can be done about administrative rescheduling other than to ask the team in advance about the possibility—and to simply know that it could happen.

Preparing the Family

Readying Siblings for a Child's Surgery. As Tammy looked ahead to her son Nathan's lip-repair operation, she felt especially concerned about how his older brothers, ages two and four at the time, would handle it. How would the siblings react, she wondered, when their parents left the house for two days? And how would she explain the changes to Nathan's appearance when they returned? Fortunately, Tammy started preparing early—by contacting a nonprofit organization, Cuddles for Clefts, which mailed her a CLP-related plush toy and a children's book. "That group was awesome," she said. Not only were the contents of the care package educational for her older children, she explained, but they were comforting.

While the care package helped orient the kids for the upcoming operation, Tammy had actually begun preparing her children weeks earlier when she was honest with them about Nathan's CLP. Right from the start, she used simple, accurate language to explain his condition. "They knew from birth," she explained, "when we said, 'He has a cleft; we love him; the doctors will fix it.'" In an interesting twist, Tammy prepared her older children in another, subtler way as well, when she took them along to his early visits with members of the cleft team. "They saw all the appointments," she said, "and ended up hearing a lot of cleft talk in passing." While Tammy described the time around Nathan's surgery as nerve-wracking, it was clear that these different types of advance preparation—both active and passive—went a long way in maintaining stability in her family.

Professionals go one step further. Parent and social worker Hope Charkins, author of the book, *Children with Facial Difference: A Parents' Guide*, advises parents to be honest with siblings about the physical changes they will see in their brother or sister, as Tammy did before Nathan's operation. But Charkins also suggests sharing specific information related to a baby's postsurgical appearance. "Let them know that their sibling's face may be swollen and discolored," she writes. If you know in advance that the baby will have stitches and/or dark-colored Dermabond at the surgical site (*Dermabond* is a glue-like substance that protects the repair), for instance, you might explain that information to a sibling—and indicate that the area can never be touched.

In some cases, it may be necessary to go back to basics with an older child—perhaps further than you might expect. Another mother pointed out that some young children, especially those of toddler or preschool age, may not know anything about surgery. "Kids tend to expect their brother/sister to come home looking the same," she commented, "when many times there will be a drastic difference." Norton Children's Hospital in Kentucky advises parents to explain what a hospital actually is. Some younger children may not have heard of a hospital, the group points out, much less know what will happen to their sibling inside. However you explain these concepts, it is always advisable to do so in advance of the event, so that a child will feel as comfortable and prepared as possible.

Readying Siblings for Changes at Home. While siblings in the family will benefit from knowing honest, age-appropriate information about a baby's operation, it is just as important that they learn about day-to-day events that affect their own lives, whether they will be going to the hospital on surgery day or staying at home (or somewhere else) with a caretaker. Child-development experts at

Stanford University advise parents to consider their child's point of view when thinking about how to teach them or lead them through a transition: How does the child see a particular situation? While a baby's operation may seem enormously important to a parent (as of course it is!), it may help to remember that from a young child's perspective, the changes in her own routine can feel even more momentous. Depending on their age, siblings will likely feel reassured to know in advance where they will stay, for example, who will take care of them, and when they will be reunited with their family members.

Simple cut-and-paste methods—literally—can help illustrate these changes for a sibling and in so doing help reduce the element of surprise when surgery day arrives. The Massachusetts Department of Early Education and Care recommends constructing a simple paper chain for siblings who are too young to understand how to read a traditional calendar (as is typical for toddler or preschool-age kids). This classic preschool learning tool, made of strips of colorful construction paper fashioned into linked loops, takes minutes to make and when fixed to a wall or refrigerator, allows older siblings to participate in the countdown as they remove a link each day. The exercise not only shows them how many days remain until their younger sibling goes to the hospital and, say, Grandma Susan comes to the house, but gives them a sense of awareness and control of events in their lives. Each day of the week before the operation, you might remove a link from the chain and remind a child of what is to come—by describing specifically what her life will look like during the few days when her sibling is in the hospital, and then reiterate that her life will return to normal afterward.

Readying Ourselves. And now, finally—us. Adults can prepare in advance for a child's operation, too, with logistics certainly—as discussed elsewhere in this chapter—but just as importantly, with our own stress reduction, even if we place ourselves near the end of our own priority list. "Don't be afraid to say 'no' to your usual obligations," suggest pros from the Children's Hospital of Philadelphia (CHOP). "Get lots of rest and eat right. Whenever possible, ask for help from family and friends." As easy and logical as it may feel to focus on the baby's health prior to surgery, it is just as important for primary caregivers—as well as the baby's older siblings—to feel as healthy, relaxed, and prepared as possible during this time.

Packing for the Hospital

If you are wondering what to bring to the hospital on surgery day, you may be pleasantly surprised by the resources that exist within reach. Packing lists abound online. CLP advocacy groups and individual bloggers offer a wealth of tips, tricks, and helpful ideas for a smooth and comfortable hospital visit. Below is a compilation of many of those lists—a "greatest hits" of sorts—culled from print and online resources and recommendations from parents.

PACKING 101
Things to Bring to the Hospital

Items for BABY

Essential Supplies for Baby. Must-haves for the baby include diapers, medications (e.g., reflux medication), bottles or sippy cups (per a surgeon's instructions), baby formula, and nursing supplies, if applicable. Also, don't forget to bring tools for washing baby bottles, (e.g., a stiff brush), which the hospital will likely not provide.

Clothing for Baby. Most babies and children wear hospital-issued gowns during the recovery period following an operation (they are adorable!). Still, some parents recommend bringing the baby's most comfortable PJs to the hospital, particularly if they open in the front rather than over the head. "It's helpful to have sleepers that have snaps (not zippers!)" noted one mother. Remember, your baby will probably be hooked up to an IV and/ or monitors after the operation, both of which connect to the baby via tubes and wires. "Sleepers with snaps allow all the lead lines to go where they need to go," this mother explained, "and let your child have a little freedom of movement."

Useful Items for Baby. When I asked parents about surprises they encountered during their baby's recovery from this operation, some mentioned topics like pain management and parental advocacy (which we will discuss in Chapter 28). Others mentioned drool. Lots of drool. "Our son drooled like crazy," said one parent about the period directly following his operation. The baby's stitches, she explained, plus the limited use of his mouth were probably to blame. "Whenever we would hold him on our shoulder," she said, "there would be a trail of massive drool down our back." Burp cloths can absorb spit-up and general messiness coming from the baby's mouth during the early hours and days of recovery. Traditional cloth diapers work well too since they are exceptionally absorbent and easy to find online or in the baby section of retail stores.

An oatmeal bath can be useful for some children, as well. "Some babies wind up with a rash from the after-effects of anesthesia," another mom writes. "An oatmeal bath helps soothe it. Aveeno makes one."

Comfort Items for Baby. Of all the recommendations I heard from parents and professionals about things to bring to the hospital, comfort items for the baby were probably the most common. "Recovering from anesthesia when you are that tiny is not enjoyable," commented one mother. "My son was out of it. He would doze fitfully and wake screaming and could only be comforted by being held and nursed. Blankies, favorite stuffed animals, can really help." Some parents report that their little ones preferred old, special toys and playthings to anything newly purchased for the occasion. Also, keep in mind that these items may become soiled quickly because of occasional blood and ooze near the wound site.

Items For CAREGIVERS

Essential and Useful Items for Adults. Insurance cards and IDs (like a driver's license or passport) are essential for the registration process prior to surgery. Medications, glasses/contact lenses, toothbrushes, etc. are additional must-haves. Also, unsurprisingly, a tablet computer and charger can come in handy for many purposes. Last, don't forget to bring a phone/camera and charge to communicate with family members and take pictures.

Clothing for Adults. When parents describe their own clothing choices for the hospital stay, two themes arise: keeping comfortable and dodging errant bodily fluids. Many parents recommend bringing loungewear or other casual clothing for 24/7 use. While caregivers will usually sleep alongside their child during the one- or two-day recovery period—and while hospital staff might dim or turn off some lights at night—patient rooms are usually shared with another patient/family and visited often by hospital staff. Don't expect a lot of privacy (or a lot of sleep!). An eye mask may come in handy. Also, slippers can be comfortable for walking around on institutional floors.

Also, keep in mind that blood, goop, and other bodily fluids abound. "Do not wear white!" one mother commented. "My son was drooling and bloody. I had blood all over my white shirt! What was I thinking?!"

Comfort Items for Adults. In retrospect, many parents say they wish they had taken some extra steps to make their own experience at the hospital a little bit more comfortable. Distractions like books, magazines, blank journals, and small inspirational items can reduce stress. "You need to be at your best," commented one mother, "because it is all-consuming to take care of an infant who cannot communicate other than by crying." This mother remembered bringing travel-size shower gel and lotion. "Seems petty and silly, but let me tell you, having something that smelled nice for the ten-minute shower was a huge relief and pick-me-up, instead of that institutional hospital smell." Parents also mention bringing favorite snacks, a water bottle, and anything else that feels comforting.

People. Friends or family members, if available, can help with running a quick errand when parents are in the hospital. "My son wanted his mommy and daddy when he was still recovering," said one mother. "That meant that we traded turns holding him, and even when I wasn't holding him, I wanted to be in the room. It was nice to have my mom, who was willing to run down the road and get us our favorite coffee (I'm kind of an addict) and good food."

Coatroom? Bonus Tips. Most hospitals offer families a shared room for one to two nights following surgery. During the surgical procedure itself, however, parents might not have a place to store bulky coats and bags. Some prefer to leave all but the essentials in the car until the surgery is over.

Cwir J. *I Wish I'd Known...How Much I'd Love You.*; 2018.

Your Child's Surgery: What to Expect. www.ucsfbenioff-childrens.org. Accessed January 11, 2022. www.ucsfbenioffchildrens.org/your-stay/your-childs-surgery-what-to-expect

Cleft Advocate – What Should We Bring to the Hospital? Accessed August 8, 2020. www.cleftadvocate.org/hospital.html

Pelligra AR. What to Bring to the Hospital. Children's Craniofacial Association. www.ccakids.org/assets/one-sheet_take2hospital.pdf

Whether we are reading and following the materials issued by the cleft team, asking questions large and small, or preparing other family members (and ourselves) as best we can, the homework we do before a child's surgery can go a long way toward easing our minds and reducing stress for all involved.

Chapter 27

· ·

The Handoff

Hand Over My Baby? I Don't Think So!

When a baby is born with CLP, medical people sometimes say, "Every cleft is different." As mentioned elsewhere in this book, families learn early on that variations in type, severity, and complexity will require different treatment paths. "My daughter has had more surgeries than I can count," commented one mother of a young adult. Another patient might undergo a few operations over the years—and that's it. Each person has her own story to tell.

Yet from a parent's perspective, every operation is marked by a short, universal experience: a single moment at the outset when we hand over our child to the doctors and staff. One minute, she's there, in our arms. The next, she's off to the operating room. It's a moment that parents mention again and again, across diagnoses and age groups. "We trusted the surgeon," said Michelle about her son's recent lip-repair surgery, "and I'm glad we did. But it was gut-wrenching and scary to hand our son over to the nurse and see him being carried to the OR. They take your baby away." The goal of any operation is to make a person's life better and easier. But handing over an infant can feel frightening and, on some level, wrong. It goes against a powerful urge to protect her from harm. Does it have to be this way?

Surgery day often begins with a very early wakeup for parents and baby in order to arrive at the hospital in time to fill out paperwork, dress for surgery, and review with medical people—one final time—what is going to happen. Typically, parents receive instructions not to feed the baby during this time, a directive that can mean, of course, that these early activities may be soundtracked with hysterical crying (WHY AREN'T YOU FEEDING ME?), or in some cases, with unusual calm or even sleeping. Our child, at her first surgery, went with crying. A lot. Loudly. I was right there with her, crying too, though for different reasons.

When the time comes, a parent usually hands the baby to a nurse or another professional, who will then carry her to the OR. For many of us, this moment symbolizes a tremendous leap of faith. Sometimes, the medical people sympathize. "We were so nervous," said one mother about the morning of her daughter's operation. "I kept thinking about them taking the baby from me while she was awake. I was imagining the big cold table, and the little, tiny baby, and that she would be scared, and I wouldn't be with her. Then, the surgeon actually came out himself—I was surprised!—to get her. At that point, I was trying not to cry. I started to ask him, 'How are you going to get her to sleep?' He knew. He said, 'I will hold her until she is asleep.' That meant the world to me."

Parents who hand over a child generally trust their surgeon and the need to have surgery. Otherwise, we wouldn't do it. And when we do our homework beforehand by interviewing surgeons and asking lots of questions, we can usually solidify trust and reduce our overall stress. Yet even as our rational minds tell us that surgery is the right thing to do, our gut might disagree. One doctor spent her career leading patients (and their nervous families) through medical procedures but did a double take when her own child needed ear tubes. "I have an M.D. and Ph.D.," she writes in *Slate* magazine, "but when my son had a minor procedure, I was terrified." With new eyes, she describes, "the frightening bargain of uncertainty, as [parents] entrust their children to the medical system." Other medical professionals, in fact, acknowledge *pre-surgery anxiety* as a normal and common phenomenon. Of course we feel nervous! There is sedation involved! And cutting! Surgery involves risk, as low or as tolerable as that risk may be. And just as much, it involves loss of our own control.

To intensify matters, the very idea of an operation sometimes lands in our laps during a sensitive time: new parenthood. It is one thing to anticipate our own surgery but quite another to imagine it for our child. When a baby arrives, so does a new awareness of everyday dangers—and an urge to safeguard our baby against those dangers, often in very small ways. We insert outlet covers. We cut grapes in half. Barely thinking, we move hot coffee away from the edge of the countertop. Protecting a child from physical harm is a big part of parenting, especially during the early years. Even if we have decided that surgery is a sound decision, that little voice might say, "I don't think so."

Fortunately, these feelings are normal. One study published in the journal *Biological Psychiatry* concludes that specific areas of the brain govern "diverse and complex maternal behaviors for vigilant protectiveness." Our neuroanatomy, it seems, plays a role in our interactions with our child, whether we are bonding with her or shielding her from harm. Other research into animal behavior shows that humans are not the only ones to resist handing over our young. Anthropologist Sarah Blaffer Hrdy studies humans and nonhuman primates like chimpanzees and langur monkeys. Certain mother animals won't hand over their young to anyone, she says. Others may acquiesce, depending on the species and the situation. But the bottom line, she says, has to do with the trust "that her infant will be returned to her unharmed."

This research not only highlights the importance of trust but brings to mind the question of scale. It is one thing to hand a baby to a friendly fellow langur monkey for a routine favor—or let's say, in our case, a favorite aunt or close friend standing sock-footed in our kitchen—as if to say, "Can you hold her for a sec while I stir the chili?" It is quite another to hand her to a group of masked near strangers who will take her away and operate on her face. With this context in mind, it seems reasonable to wonder who *wouldn't* resist handing over a child! It's a sign we are doing our job. Whether the urge to protect comes from hard-wiring or learned behavior (or both), the feeling is real. The little voice is not crazy. Our rational minds tell us that surgery is the right decision. But it is also valid and normal for everything else about it to feel wrong.

As the years go by, parents learn to hand over a child to many people in all kinds of situations. It is our job, after all, to teach our child to eventually fend for herself in a world full of risks. Bit by bit, event by event—ever so carefully—we oversee an eighteen-year-long series of firsts that begins with total dependence and continues into adulthood. The first babysitter. The first day of school. Driving! Surgery preempts that careful journey. It barges in, too much too soon. It scares us. And it leaves us standing there in a hospital hallway, empty-handed and wobbly.

So now, what? At the moment of the handoff—and perhaps similar moments to come—all we can really do is breathe. Some will turn to their faith. And hopefully, we will think of the instinct of the langur monkeys, the element of trust, and our rational decision based on risks and rewards. "It's good to remind ourselves that we have such good doctors and nurses," said one mother, Lisa, as she anticipated her daughter's lip repair. "As much as you know it, it never hurts to keep thinking it." It may help to remember, too, that soon enough, a child will be lying in a recovery bed, waking up. Surgery will be over. And if all goes according to plan, her life will be better and easier for having done it. "Afterwards, in post-op," Lisa said later, "I could hold my daughter and feed her. That calmed her down." It probably helped Lisa calm down too.

Chapter 28

. . . .

Lip Repair:
Recovery in the Hospital

Staying Comfortable, Resuming Feeding, and Speaking Up for Your Baby

Lip-repair surgery is over! For some parents, this moment marks a joyous new beginning. For others, it is hard to see a new face where a familiar face had been. Everyone confronts the immediate challenge of recovery.

Recovery begins in the hospital and continues at home. Below, you will find basic information and ideas on what to expect in the hospital, principles of managing pain, tips for resuming feeding, and perhaps most important, ideas about advocating for your child immediately after surgery. While these topics—and also the material in the following chapter on a child's continued recuperation at home—relate primarily to a period of several days following lip-repair surgery, the concepts can be applied to recovery after palate repair as well, or to any other cleft-related procedures that take place during infancy.

Surgery Is Over. Now What?

How'd It Go? When a child's lip-repair operation has ended, two events will probably occur from a caregiver's perspective. First, the surgeon will probably give you the lowdown on what happened in the operating room and describe the results. Personally, I was more than a little bit eager to hear these conclusions following my daughter's first operation, especially after pacing around the hospital nervously for several hours wondering how she was doing—not to mention pacing nervously through life for several months waiting for the procedure to take place. Even before I saw our baby, I felt reassured to hear a summary of the outcomes from a trusted professional (and in our case, enormously relieved that the procedure had gone well).

Following this conversation (timing may vary), someone will probably escort you to a recovery area—at long last—to join your child.

Not Your Average Wake-Up. When Leah met her son after his lip-repair surgery, she realized that she had not been emotionally prepared for the sight of his new lip and nose. "I almost didn't recognize him," she said. While Leah was immediately pleased with his appearance and later praised the surgeon's work, the first sight of him took her aback. "It was a shock getting back a different face," she said. "Nobody tells you. They should have said, 'This will be hard.'"

Meeting a child after lip-repair surgery can feel momentous. And as explored in the next chapter, parents' responses can vary widely in this situation. Some feel stunned when they actually do not recognize their child. Others identify her easily but have myriad strong feelings about her new appearance. Such reactions may be difficult to predict. But if you're reading this book in advance of the experience, it may be helpful to ready yourself—by simply knowing that for other parents, these moments have been emotionally intense. This is not your average wake-up.

There's more. A baby's face will look different from before because of the surgical changes, of course, and because of visible stitches or a postsurgical dressing placed on her upper lip. But some parents are surprised when the postsurgical trappings do not end there. A baby will likely have the typical, temporary facial swelling that follows this surgery. She may also have soft tubes in her nose, called nasal stents, to support the nostrils, and in some cases, she may have a U-shaped splint called a Logan's Bow taped to her cheeks to take pressure off of the sutures. Some cleft teams wrap a child's arms in stiff splints to prevent her from bending her elbows and touching the delicate surgical area. And of course, she will have an IV that she received prior to surgery. What a scene! Even her behavior may seem out of the ordinary. Some babies sleep as the anesthesia wears off and, at some point, simply open their eyes. But most cry at some point in the recovery room, one surgeon noted, even if they are not in pain. And a few children respond adversely, sometimes acting loopy, squirming, or even crying out as they awaken.

One mother, Karine, was surprised by her son's behaviors at wake-up. "The worst part, both times, was when KJ woke up after surgery," she said about his lip- and palate-repair procedures, "because he was screaming and wouldn't stop." KJ looked disoriented, upset, and even frightened, she recalled, as if he were fighting the feeling of coming out of anesthesia. To Karine's relief, KJ's response ended after a few minutes both times. Yet she was eager to warn other parents of the possibilities.

Experts at the National Institutes of Health (NIH) label the wake-up from anesthesia the *recovery* period, also called *emergence*. These pros explain that up to one-third of children experience "lingering confusion" for a few days after undergoing surgery and anesthesia. Cleft-team anesthesiologists writing in the book *Comprehensive Cleft Care: Family Edition* describe a less-common occurrence called *emergence delirium*, which occurs in approximately 10-to-15 percent of children and involves "extreme irritability, combativeness, and inconsolability," perhaps resembling the symptoms Karine saw in KJ. This type of delirium, if it happens, will go away in about fifteen minutes, the pros explain. Other doctors state that these behaviors may be alarming to witness but do not indicate that a child is in pain. Moreover, the cleft-team anesthesiologists in *Comprehensive Cleft Care* remind families that a majority of infants "do very well after anesthesia and surgery and have no residual effects."

So it may be helpful to keep in mind that a child can have a surprising response to anesthesia. Be sure to ask the team and/or the anesthesiologist about it in advance if you are concerned. It may also help to remember that you can help your baby by soothing her and trying to stay calm. "Babies are sensitive to emotion in the parent," one surgeon commented. Every parent, too, will respond in his or her own way to the array of circumstances that occur when reuniting with a child postoperatively.

Moving Upstairs: Locations, Goals, and Duration. Once a baby wakes up following surgery, the caregiver(s) and child will typically go to a hospital room for the remainder of the hospital visit (as mentioned elsewhere in this book), so that the medical staff can monitor the baby and give her medications for pain. Specific locations, however, can vary. According to one cleft surgeon, some babies go to a pediatric ward (a regular hospital room) while others might stay in the ICU (Intensive Care Unit), where they will be monitored especially closely. This determination relates to the characteristics and health history of the baby, he said, how the baby experienced surgery (or wake-up from surgery), the ability of the hospital to provide certain levels of care, or simply the surgeon's preference (see related questions, below, to ask the surgeon and team in advance).

The goals for the rest of the hospital stay and even its length will also vary by cleft surgeon, cleft team, and/or hospital. As time passes and a baby's pain starts to ease, professionals usually look for the resumption of certain bodily functions before giving parents the okay to take a baby home from the hospital. While these criteria will vary, the cleft team at the Children's Hospital of Pittsburgh, the American Cleft Palate-Craniofacial Association (ACPA), and the UCLA Mattel Children's Hospital offer the following examples: showing stable vital signs, eating/drinking well (or at least holding down liquids), urinating normally, breathing easily, and feeling relatively comfortable pain-wise.

A two-to-three-day hospital stay (including surgery day) tends to be the norm in order to achieve these goals after lip repair; in fact, it is the length of stay described by a majority of parents and professionals I spoke with. Yet recommendations and situations can vary. The cleft team at the Children's Minnesota health system states that postoperative children "almost always go home the morning after surgery," but sometimes stay longer to overcome troubles with eating or to take extra time to control pain. And other cleft teams recommend going home on the same day of surgery (called an *outpatient stay*), with no trip to the pediatric ward or ICU at all.

It is important to ask your child's surgeon and team about goals and time frames in advance of the operation so that you can know what to expect, particularly if your child will go home at the early end of the range—possibly placing a larger burden on you for her continued recovery at home. And as one surgeon noted, in a case when a team recommends same-day discharge (officially leaving the hospital), you could even ask for an inpatient stay. "If [parents] feel uncomfortable with outpatient," she said, "they can request to stay."

QUESTIONS FOR THE TEAM

Locations, Goals, and Time Frames for Hospital Stay

- Where in the hospital might our baby stay following surgery? A regular hospital room? The ICU? What are the circumstances for each scenario?
- What are your goals and benchmarks for a child during the hospital stay following surgery?
- What is a typical duration of stay in order to meet these goals? If I/we feel uncomfortable with this duration, can we request to stay for a longer time? How and when can we make that request?

The First 48 Hours

Principles, Tips, and Questions to Ask after Surgery

Pain Management—With a Twist. There is good news and bad news regarding the recovery from lip repair. The bad news, perhaps unsurprisingly, is that this operation causes pain. The good news is that the pain is manageable with medication and that it will lessen with time. The twist? It may be useful to know that relieving pain and resuming eating can go hand-in-hand when a baby has had surgery on the mouth—since the point of contact for a baby bottle is precisely that of the procedure (an unfortunate coincidence). We will explore this issue in more detail later in this chapter.

While we know that the pain of surgery is both manageable with medications and will lessen with time, it is important to keep in mind that surgeons, teams, hospitals, and even individual staff members can vary in how they recommend handling it. It is beyond the scope of this book to give advice on particular protocols or decisions. Yet the parents I spoke with mention certain themes they feel passionately about passing on to others. These topics are described below, along with related questions to ask the team. First, however, let's make a brief stop at Pain Management 101.

PAIN MANAGEMENT 101
How Does Pain Management Work?

What about Addiction?

The pain after surgery often starts at its worst and lessens with time. So, medical professionals usually recommend that a child start with powerful medications for the worst pain, downgrade to less potent ones as the pain lessens, and then stop altogether as recovery concludes. This process often begins with a *narcotic*—also referred to as an *opioid* or *opiate*—directly following surgery to ease the earliest, strongest pain. Morphine is a common example used for babies, but there are several others.

After an infant takes strong pain relievers for a certain period, doctors often recommend stepping down to an everyday pain reliever like baby Tylenol (acetaminophen) or Motrin/Advil (ibuprofen). Some teams don't recommend ibuprofen—or only allow it after a certain age—because of an increased risk of bleeding. Other teams recommend babies take a combination of these two pain relievers (ask your team for more information).

Many parents wonder, reasonably, about the risk of addiction to opiates. Several major children's hospitals offer articles on this topic such as UCLA Children's Hospital, Children's Hospital of Philadelphia (CHOP), and the SickKids hospital in Toronto (see the reference section for details). According to CHOP, "Children who take narcotics for pain relief rarely experience addiction." Still, it is important, as always, to talk with your child's doctors if you have any questions about pain management in general or about the use of these strong medications in particular.

TOPIC for the TEAM: When to Ramp Down? About twenty-four hours after Baby B's lip-repair surgery, his mother Kim felt pleased with the state of his recovery. The opioid medications he was taking seemed to be keeping his pain at bay, and Kim was happy to see that he had had a good night's sleep following surgery. "After the first night, he seemed to be doing a little bit better," she wrote on her blog, *Cleftest Little Cutie* (where she does not describe her baby by name; *Baby B* is a pseudonym). At that point, B was not yet eating from a bottle—he was still receiving fluids from an IV drip—but his eyes had started to brighten, a few times even becoming animated. Kim felt hopeful about the possibility of taking him home sooner rather than later, maybe even by the evening of that second day. In a consultation with the hospital staff, Kim agreed that they should transition B from the oxycodone to everyday pain relievers.

As the morning of Day Two progressed, however, B showed signs of increasing discomfort. Instead of appearing calm and somewhat alert as he had at wake-up, he started to cry and fuss. And when his mother held him, he seemed downright inconsolable. Kim was understandably alarmed—and wondered whether the decision to move off the strong pain relievers had been overly optimistic. By midday, the situation had only worsened; B was clearly in pain. "He desperately needed medication," she said, and she immediately called for help. The staff re-administered the strong pain relievers, and the medications kicked in after several minutes. But by that point, Kim felt rattled. "I realized I didn't want to risk it again," she said.

After consulting with the surgical assistant on the cleft team, Kim decided to continue giving B the opioid through the remainder of that second day. "The doctor said that it was perfectly fine to keep [patients] on [the opioid]," she said, "...since their mouths have been through so much trauma. So, I didn't feel bad about it." By the morning of Day Three in the hospital, B had had another night of restful sleep. Again, he appeared comfortable and somewhat alert—as he had the previous morning. But this time, his IV had also been removed and B was starting to drink liquids on his own (from a bottle) in small amounts. And this time, he seemed to be acting more like his normal self. After consulting with the hospital staff and members of the cleft team at a morning visit, Kim agreed to switch B to a combination of acetaminophen and ibuprofen. It worked. B seemed content with that regimen. And Kim felt enormously relieved. B was released from the hospital that day.

While it may be clear to parents that their child is experiencing pain—as it eventually was to Kim during B's second day in the hospital—it can be challenging for a nonprofessional to know how aggressively to treat that pain. And paradoxically, it can be hard to know how to respond when a child appears to feel comfortable (as B did after his first night in the hospital). The point of telling this story is *not* to advise parents to simply keep a child on strong medications—necessarily. Rather, it is to encourage you to find out as much as possible about the surgeon and team's particular approach to these situations in advance of surgery, if possible. You might ask about types of medications recommended for a particular situation and child, their effectiveness for managing pain, potential side effects, a recommended period to stay on a particular medication (hours? days?), and perhaps most important, what signs and signals indicate that a baby should continue a current medication or move to a different one (see questions for the team, below).

Other parents have reported similar difficulties reading their babies' signals—again, particularly when deciding to move from opioid medications to everyday pain relievers like acetaminophen and/or ibuprofen. According to the FDA, children can experience side effects, such as constipation and/or drowsiness, with the stronger medications. These responses can be puzzling to read and react to—and they can be compounded by the fact that drowsiness can lessen a child's appetite. "He couldn't tell us anything!" commented one mother. "We thought, 'Is it pain?' It was very hard to decipher."

Another mother described her son's recovery as relatively easy overall. "He bounced back pretty quickly," she said. "But coming off the opioid was really hard. We didn't know if he was in pain and uncomfortable or if things were just new and different. Once he was off the hydrocodone and past constipation, the recovery was easy for us. He went straight to Motrin." While it may be difficult to read a child's responses at this stage, the key is to speak up if you think your child is in pain and to communicate as specifically as possible with the team and with the hospital staff when questions arise, however small they may seem.

It is also important to keep in mind that children respond in their own ways to both pain and pain medication. "There are clear biological differences between people in how much medicine they need and how well it works for them," writes Charles Berde, MD, PhD, of Boston Children's Hospital. This doctor recommends tailoring pain control to a particular surgical procedure, a child's history with pain (if known), and her individual biology. As we saw with Kim and B, it is important for parents to be aware of these differences and to speak up when a child seems uncomfortable or if the situation feels at all puzzling.

> **QUESTIONS FOR THE TEAM**
> **PAIN MANAGEMENT FOLLOWING SURGERY**

- What types of medications do you typically recommend after surgery?
- What are the side effects to know about?
- For what purposes and for how long (hours? days?) do you typically recommend a child take each type of medication?
- What signs and signals can we look for to determine when a child should continue a medication or switch to a different one?

TOPIC for the TEAM: Stay Ahead of the Pain? The parents and professionals I spoke with about recovery from cleft surgery frequently mention the idea of "staying ahead of the pain." This approach involves administering medicine in a timely manner. While it is beyond the scope of this book to give specific recommendations, it may be helpful to know about this idea in advance, so that you will be able to explore it with the professionals who treat your child (see questions for the team, below).

According to the American Cancer Society, pain medications work best when taken right away as a pain emerges—before the pain becomes severe. "You'll want to treat pain when it first starts and regularly after that," the group writes. So, let's back up and talk about timing. When a medication wears off after a certain number of hours, a recovering patient can start to feel pain. According to Minnesota Children's health system and the instruction labels on prescription and over-the-counter medications nationwide, medicines must be administered within certain time frames and not sooner. We've all seen instruction labels on over-the-counter medications that direct us, for example, to "Take one caplet every four-to-six hours as symptoms persist." But what happens if the pain reemerges before the clock runs out?

Let's say, for example, it is noon, and the baby takes a dose of ibuprofen that calls for a six-to-eight-hour wait between doses. Now let's suppose that 5:20 p.m. or 5:30 p.m. rolls around and—here it comes!—the baby starts to fuss and cry, a likely signal that the pain has reemerged. At this point, she will have to wait through thirty or forty minutes of discomfort before receiving the next dose, a period that can feel endless to a sympathetic parent. "It was not bad, really," commented one mother about such a situation with her daughter. She noted that once her daughter received the meds, her pain seemed to ease. "But the wait felt endless while it was happening."

Cuddling and physical comforts can go a long way in reassuring a baby who feels uncomfortable during this time. But a theme to remember, according to numerous parents and professionals, is that while we must follow the parameters noted in the instructions for medications, it can be helpful to administer them promptly when the next appropriate moment comes—therefore allowing the baby to "stay ahead of the pain." Some professionals sidestep this issue by administering two analgesics (like acetaminophen and ibuprofen) at the same time—and by staggering the start times of each medication, so that when one wears off, the other continues in full force. Clever, right? But recommendations vary. As mentioned above, some teams don't recommend ibuprofen to babies of a certain age because it can increase the risk of bleeding (again, ask your cleft team for more information).

One mother, Lisa, recalled an unfortunate situation following her son's lip repair. "The first time our son had surgery, the nurse said to us, 'Maybe we should lay off of the medicine,'" Lisa said. "So, we said, 'Okay, let's just lay off and see what happens.'" The plan, as Lisa understood at the time, was to wait and see whether her son felt pain before medicating. "Well, that was the wrong advice," she continued. "Then, we were just chasing the pain." When her son's second surgery came around to repair his palate, Lisa had learned from the first experience. "We took them up on all the meds," she said. In the meantime, Lisa sought additional recommendations from another professional on her son's team. "We realized that we shouldn't listen to that advice again," she said. "It is important to stay on top of the pain."

Again, "staying ahead" does not mean jumping ahead of the time frame indicated on the printed instructions; it means administering medication when a baby feels pain and then giving the next dose promptly when the time arrives.

It is worthwhile to reemphasize that I do not offer this information to serve as advice, but to use as a springboard for asking informed questions—hopefully in advance of surgery—so that you can learn as much as possible from your child's doctors about managing her pain.

> ### QUESTIONS FOR THE TEAM
> ### STAYING AHEAD OF THE PAIN AFTER SURGERY

- What is your approach to assessing and alleviating pain?
- What is your recommendation for alleviating pain that reemerges before a prescribed time limit has expired, both in the hospital and at home?
- Do you recommend staggering acetaminophen and ibuprofen?

TOPIC for the TEAM: Who Takes the Lead? It may be reassuring to know that a recovery ward nurse can be a parent's best friend when it comes to managing a child's pain and helping her resume eating after surgery. Many nurses and other staff have extensive experience and expertise with pain management and will work closely with the parents and baby to make decisions.

It is also important to know, however, that a nurse may *not* become your best friend during the recovery period and not necessarily for lack of commitment or friendliness. As mentioned above, we know that pain-management routines can vary from one surgeon, team, or hospital to another, particularly with regard to deciding which medication(s) to use and when. But routines can also vary regarding who takes the lead in a child's recovery and to what extent a nurse provides guidance and advice.

Let's look at a lesson in contrasts, starting with my own daughter's case as an example. When my daughter underwent lip- and palate-repair surgeries, her recoveries could only be described as team efforts led by the nurses in the recovery ward. My husband and I discussed our daughter's situation with the nurses every few hours; we assessed her pain levels together and decided what to do when the time came for another dose of medication. My husband and I offered input since we knew our daughter best and were familiar with her physical cues. But as novices, we were glad to follow the nurses' lead—and they seemed ready and willing to guide us. They kept track of the timing for medications, visited us without prompting, shared their recommendations, and administered medication at the appropriate moments. Our daughter's surgeon checked in regularly too, along with other members of the team, to oversee the whole process. I wouldn't say that the entire recovery was stress-free. I felt especially nervous following her first operation since I was new to the experience and hated to see my daughter in pain. But my husband and I felt supported throughout and were grateful to rely on the advice of the staff and team.

Another mother, however, described quite a different situation following her son's lip repair. As soon as Kara arrived in her son's recovery room following his operation, she learned that the hospital had assigned her, as parent/caregiver, complete responsibility for her son's medication. "Every few hours I was supposed to tell them, 'He needs his medication now,'" she said. The nurses kept track of timing during the first day, she said, but thereafter asked her to take over that task. "This is not a good method!" Kara exclaimed. "If the parents don't know what they are doing, then all heck breaks loose." While Kara kept accurate notes on her son's medications and recalled the nurses responding to her inquiries in a timely manner, she clearly felt nervous shouldering this burden of care, particularly during the sensitive period directly following surgery.

As we can see from these two stories, it is important to find out who will be expected to take the lead with a child's recovery in the hospital, whether it be a recovery ward nurse providing guidance or a caregiver holding the reins (see questions to ask the team, below). Situations can vary widely depending on the hospital, team, and individuals involved.

> ### QUESTIONS FOR THE TEAM
> ### ROLES OF STAFF AND TEAM

- What is the role of the recovery ward staff in terms of attentiveness and guidance during my child's recovery from surgery? Who will monitor and administer pain medications? Who will decide how that process plays out?
- What role will the cleft team play during my child's recovery?
- Whom should we speak with if we have questions while in the hospital?

MILLION-DOLLAR TIP: Advocate. If there is one piece of advice that came up again and again among the parents I interviewed for this book, it relates to the role of parents during a child's recovery from surgery. Regardless of who takes the lead with the recovery process officially, parents need to take charge of their child's care unofficially. Put another way, it is our job as parents to be our child's chief advocate.

Let's say the hospital nurses and staff step in with confidence, kindness, and expertise following your child's operation—as they did, fortunately, in the case of my daughter. And let's say that they act with a spirit of collaboration so that you feel comfortable discussing your child's pain management with them and agree with their choices. Wonderful! This situation is ideal. But it is important for you to take charge of your child's care *as well.*

Advocating for a child simply means that as a parent or caregiver, you need to keep track of what is going on with your child's condition and to speak up on her behalf, even if someone else, a professional, is also on the job. This responsibility starts in advance of the surgery and continues into the recovery room and beyond (in fact, it could be said that advocating for a child is a central role in parenting, starting most prominently during infancy when she cannot speak for herself).

By way of examples, during the days or weeks before surgery, you could learn about a surgeon and team's approach to pain management. You could ask about the nurses' roles in the hospital—and about any other concerns you may have. You could also read books (like this one) and seek other reliable sources in order to learn as much as you can about a given procedure and recovery. Then, as the recovery begins, it will be important to keep track of the timing and dosage of medications (even if someone else is performing the same task), have conversations with staff, stay in touch with members of the cleft team, ask questions, and speak up for your child, especially if you think she is in pain. The key is to participate actively in the entire process. It is a never-ending job.

It is worth noting that as chief caregivers, we can read our child's signals better than anyone else. It is our job to speak up when something seems not quite right and, as one mother advised, to "stick to our guns" if we have a concern that we feel is not being addressed. While nurses in the recovery ward may or may not be in charge in terms of guiding us through this experience, it is our job to take tenacious charge of our child's care anyway.

HOSPITAL TIP: *Smooth the Transitions.* During a child's recovery in the hospital, a nurse or other staff member(s) in the recovery ward may be assigned to attend to your child for several hours at a time. As mentioned above, many parents feel pleased with the resulting relationships and even deeply appreciative of a nurse's friendliness, warmth, and expertise during a sensitive time. It is important to know, however, that the parent-nurse connection can end abruptly—or change in nature—when nurses change shifts.

Parents occasionally describe inconsistencies from one professional to the next with regard to how he or she reads a baby's signals or recommends medications. One mother described a decision, in consultation with a nurse, to ramp down from morphine to Tylenol with Codeine, only to find that the next nurse recommended resuming Morphine—ramping back up!—just a few hours later. It is beyond the scope of this book to determine how well that particular decision worked for that child (in fact, as we saw with Kim and Baby B, such a decision can be appropriate, if surprising). But crossed signals between staff and caregivers can feel frustrating and confusing, particularly when the baby is crying, and the parents are tired.

Sometimes, abrupt changes like these are unavoidable. Other times, you may be able to circumvent the issue, at least in part. When a nurse comes into the recovery room for the first time, you might ask about the timing of the next shift change. It can't hurt to introduce yourself in a friendly way while you are at it, even if you feel exhausted and stressed out. Remember that it is in everyone's interest for these relationships to proceed as smoothly and constructively as possible. In a few hours, the outgoing nurse may be able to introduce you to the incoming person and have a conversation about where things stand, sort of like passing the baton. The more you can do to smooth this transition—and to foster positive, friendly working relationships—the better.

Resuming Feeding

Goals: Drink Up! While it is critical to manage a child's pain following surgery, it is also important to help her resume eating. As mentioned above, many cleft teams want to see that a child has resumed feeding and is urinating normally before they give her the okay to leave the hospital.

Resuming feeding is important for a baby's nutrition, of course, but this recommendation often relates just as much to staying hydrated. According to two doctors of pediatric emergency medicine writing in the book *Pediatric Dehydration*, babies and young children are generally susceptible to *dehydration* (a lack of necessary water in the body) because of their metabolic rate and their inability to communicate. Unfortunately, this susceptibility can worsen for postoperative cleft babies since the surgical site doubles as the point of contact for the baby bottle. Simply put, the baby may not feel inclined to drink (who would blame her?). And dehydration is a serious concern. No one wants a baby—or anyone, for that matter—to become dehydrated because the body doesn't function properly without enough fluids. The American Academy of Family Physicians suggests that moderate-to-extreme dehydration requires medical intervention.

So it is important to make sure that the baby gets enough to drink. And the key for us as caregivers is to make sure that she is on the road to drinking normally *before* she leaves the hospital so that her recovery will go as smoothly as possible at home. While we can say with confidence that the risk of dehydration is low while a baby is still in the hospital—since for much of that time she is receiving fluids from an IV drip—we can also say with confidence that most of us do not have an IV drip available at home (at least I don't!). If the baby refuses to drink at home and eventually becomes dehydrated—I have heard a few anecdotes about such a scenario with postoperative babies and experienced it firsthand with my daughter—she may need to return to the hospital to receive fluids, a trip that no one wants to take.

Resuming Feeding: First Steps. Some parents wonder—as is more than reasonable when a baby has had surgery to the mouth— whether resuming feeding will harm the baby's delicate sutures or cause pain. Unsurprisingly, surgeons vary in their answers to these questions and in their subsequent recommendations for how a postoperative baby should take in liquids. Some surgeons recommend resuming feeding with the very same cleft-palate bottle the baby used prior to surgery (for babies using bottles), asserting that the baby's contact with the bottle will not compromise the surgical outcome. Others recommend syringe-feeding at first, followed by regular bottle-feeding or breast-feeding (if applicable).

Many parents report that their babies resumed feeding fairly easily, if slowly, using their previous cleft bottle. "We went back to the bottle right away," commented one mother about her son's lip repair. "We were kind of scared of him bumping the nipple," she said, "or of us being too rough with the bottle." It can be tricky, she added, to gauge how firmly to place the bottle in the baby's mouth during feeding. "You have to relearn things," she said. But overall, her son's recovery was so smooth that he started to behave like his normal, energetic self just three days after arriving back home.

Parents who syringe-feed after surgery often recommend the TenderCare™ feeder, a very thin, funnel-shaped tube that attaches to a soft, squeezable, TenderCare™ bottle or to the body of most standard cleft bottles (see Chapter 30 for more information). While, technically speaking, the TenderCare™ is considered a nipple, its tube is so thin that the baby can't really suck on it. A complaint that arises with the standard syringe and the TenderCare™ is the time required to feed the baby. While these methods will get the job done—and may be necessary based on a baby's comfort levels and/or a surgeon's instructions—parents never fail to mention their inefficiency.

Resuming Feeding: Pacing and Tips. As important as it is to resume feeding in the hospital, the process itself may not be more complicated, nuanced, or different than it was before—just slower. One mother noted that her son eventually drank normally after surgery, but only after his pain had largely subsided. "Overall, the recovery went much better than we thought it would," she said. "The only problem was having to get used to eating again. It took a while."

As this mother saw with her son, a delay in resuming feeding can occur for a variety of reasons: discomfort in the mouth, side effects from medications (such as constipation and drowsiness), or as other parents and pros have noted, a baby's lack of thirst when receiving fluids from an IV drip.

While patience and persistence are generally the best ways to help a child resume eating, parents have also mentioned a few tips for moving the process along. One mother asked the nurses in the hospital to remove the IV drip during her son's last half-day in the hospital, not only to simulate conditions at home but also to encourage him to drink (see questions for the team, below). Other parents relax their baby's feeding schedule, offering small amounts of liquids in between "meals" in order to maximize the intake of liquids.

Other types of liquids can also come in handy, as can other feeding methods (ask your pediatrician and/or surgeon to approve both. Also see the story, below). If you are feeding your baby formula with her regular bottle, for instance, you could offer "snacks" of Pedialyte in between feedings using a syringe feeder. These extra bursts of liquid can go a long way toward helping a baby stay hydrated. As one mother mentioned, "every little bit counts." Small amounts really can go a long way.

FAMILY STORIES
POSTOPERATIVE FEEDING

A New Setup?

Kara had expected that her son might need a day or two to resume feeding with his trusty Dr. Brown's bottle after his lip-repair operation. So, she was patient with him as he fed from a TenderCare™ Feeder for the first couple of days. She didn't anticipate, however, that by the fourth day after surgery, she would still be feeding him this way. "We were at home and my son wasn't interested in taking a bottle at all," she said. Not only did he refuse the bottle, but he also he fussed and whined, acting hungrier and unhappier by the day. "I was at wits' end," Kara said.

Then, as luck would have it, a fellow cleft parent visited the family, saw Kara's frustration, and asked if she had considered offering the baby a different type of bottle. This mother happened to have brought a Haberman bottle with her to the house. The baby had never fed with anything other than a Dr. Brown's, but Kara thought, Why not? She knew that the Haberman bottle had been approved by her daughter's surgeon. "She gave it to me, and he took it instantly!" Kara's excitement was palpable. "We went from him not eating to using the Haberman full-stop. AAAAH!"

In retrospect, Kara reasoned that the Dr. Brown's bottle may have put too much pressure on her son's tender, postsurgical upper lip. "The Dr. Brown's doesn't require a lot of sucking on the baby's part," she said, "but it requires some. The Haberman requires zero. He could just munch it." After starting with the new bottle, Kara and her son never turned back. "I never really had to squeeze it," she added, "and I love the fact that it has three flows [settings]. It worked out really well for us."

The best-case scenario after surgery is a seamless return to eating. But recovery can be unpredictable. It can never hurt to be open to new ideas, as Kara was, and to even stash a few different bottles in your hospital bag (pending a surgeon's approval, of course). The more ways you prepare, the better.

QUESTIONS FOR THE TEAM
STAYING HYDRATED AFTER SURGERY

- How much liquid should my child consume in order to stay hydrated?
- When is the best time to remove an IV drip? Will I be able to request that my child's IV drip be removed in order to stimulate thirst?
- What feeding methods do you approve for postsurgical use?

Leaving Las Vegas?
Finding Respite in the Hospital

Whether you are managing a child's pain, speaking up on her behalf, or helping her resume feeding, escorting a child through surgery can feel nothing short of exhausting for parents, both physically and emotionally. If you happen to get any sleep during the night before the surgery (I stared at the ceiling), you can practically count on losing one or two subsequent nights during the hospital stay afterward.

The atmosphere of a hospital can also feel somewhat static as if reality has been temporarily suspended and sunrise and sunset no longer take place, like being in a Las Vegas casino (minus the smoking and gambling…). "This morning I am recounting the past day," writes one parent on her blog, *The Jennings' Jabber*, "and then I suddenly realize that it hasn't even been a whole day…not even twenty-four hours since [my son] was wheeled out of surgery! No wonder he was still a mess! Time seems to just poke along. Less than twenty-four hours seems like a week!" This environment can feel disorienting.

Self-care may be more important than ever when you are living from moment to moment. One mother recommended taking plenty of breaks while in the hospital in order to eat and rest whenever possible. "You'll be far more able to take care of your child if you're able to take decent care of yourself," she advised on the Kids with Cleft Utah site.

Fortunately, hospital resources can be ample for caregivers— even if you need to search them out. Some hospitals offer a separate lounge just for parents. Many offer a Ronald McDonald House (or wing), as mentioned in previous chapters, either for free or for a small donation per day. Chaplain services can be comforting too, regardless of religious affiliation. The key is to actually use these services. Whether you are taking a break to eat a warm meal, look out the window (to remember whether it is day or night!), or simply get a cup of coffee, this respite can make a big difference in your stress levels, stamina, and ability to help your child.

Lip-repair surgery can involve a momentous experience for a baby and her parents; some characterize it as one of the most intense parts of the cleft journey. The subsequent recovery can also feel exciting, draining, hopeful, confusing, exhausting, and even strangely static. With the right information in hand—and the courage to ask questions and speak up for your child—the experience can also feel satisfying (for a parent) and comfortable (for the baby). Recovery may not be over when you leave the hospital. But hopefully, you can take a moment to pause, take in some fresh air, and celebrate the fact that you are almost out of the woods.

Chapter 29

. . . .

Lip Repair:
Recovery at Home

Asking Questions, Massaging Scars, Managing Strong Feelings, and Saying Yes to No-Nos

When Terri and Jeremy returned home with their son after his lip-repair surgery, their first feelings were exhaustion and relief. After months of anticipation for the procedure itself (which had gone well), followed by an intense and sleepless hospital experience over several days, they felt enormously comforted to set foot in their own, familiar space. Yet just at a moment when the adrenaline rush of the hospital experience had started to fade, the couple realized—as do some other parents who arrive home with their baby after surgery—that their son's recovery had not ended. The baby was fussing at lot, Terri said, and hadn't started acting like his normal, happy self. Terri and her husband also felt stressed about decision-making without the help of 24/7 nursing care and in-person input from the cleft team. Most of all, both parents were processing strong feelings about their son's new appearance.

In this chapter, we will explore ways to manage a child's continued recovery at home, starting with staying in touch with the cleft team when questions arise, then turning to the ever-popular topic of arm cuffs, a.k.a. "No-Nos," and a brief discussion of postsurgical scars. Finally, we'll look at ideas for seeking help and managing our own strong feelings during a sometimes-trying time. While the period after surgery can be bumpy for babies and caregivers—as it felt initially for Terri and Jeremy—fortunately, there are lots of ways to get through it and cope.

Welcome Home

Guidance from the Team (Not Facebook!). When members of the cleft team give families the okay to leave the hospital after surgery, they usually do so after determining that a baby's worst pain has passed, that she is on her way to eating and urinating normally, and that she does not have a fever, as discussed in Chapter 28. In most cases, the process of hospital discharge also involves lots of paperwork. There will be sign-offs, to start. But the team should also give you detailed instructions on how to care for your baby.

While information from the team should provide critical guidance on administering medications and navigating other aspects of recovery, many parents find that once they've returned home, other questions arise. It is natural to wonder whether a certain amount of pain (or drooling, fussing, bleeding, etc.) is normal—and it can be tempting to turn to cleft-related social media groups for answers. While such groups can be a wonderful outlet for a collective, postsurgical sigh of relief, cleft professionals emphasize the importance of staying in touch with members of the team for medical questions, for the sake of your baby's well-being and your own reassurance. Unsure? Contact the team!

Now What? It Depends. Recovery from surgery—and in particular the period of recuperation that typically takes place at home—can vary from child to child. For some families, the process of helping a baby recover is fairly straightforward, requiring time, attention, and patience more than anything else, especially with the slow-going process of resuming feeding. Some parents noted that while the period may have taken longer than they expected, the process itself went relatively smoothly. Phew.

Other families feel stressed or confused by their baby's behaviors and/or the decision-making that can come with administering medications—including deciding when to stop them altogether. "The big fear was that if he was looking comfortable and I backed off the meds, he would be in pain," commented one mother. "[A few days in], I finally felt comfortable enough to think he probably was not in pain," she continued. But the situation wasn't crystal clear. "There weren't any cues," she said.

If you are unsure about a detail of your child's recovery, however minor, it is always advisable to pick up the phone and call the team, especially regarding decisions about pain management. It may also help to remember that recovery can last for several days after arriving home, that resuming feeding can require patience as well as vigilance, and that the concept of "staying ahead of the pain" may continue beyond a child's time in the hospital (see Chapter 28 for information).

QUESTIONS FOR THE TEAM
RECOVERY AT HOME

- What signs and signals should we watch for at home during a baby's recovery?
- How much liquid intake and urination should take place at home?
- Should we wake our baby to administer medicine?
- How will we know when to stop giving our baby medication for pain?
- How can we contact you if we have questions? During non-business hours?

*For Future Reference...*When I asked parents of cleft-affected children about their child's recoveries from surgeries during infancy, many had forgotten the specifics. Well, naturally! Months later, the experience can feel like an intense, sleepless blur. "I can't tell you the details of my son's recovery," joked one mother, "because I think I blocked it all out!"

As fresh as this information may feel in the moment, it may be helpful to jot down a quick record of your child's experience with regard to pain management and eating, both in the hospital and at home. You might note how long the child spent on particular medications (hours or days), roughly how much liquid she consumed each day (and with what feeding method), and any other observations during particular stages. Research shows that children respond individually to pain and to medication (as mentioned before), so this information may come in handy for future surgical procedures, not just for your baby's comfort, but for your own peace of mind and planning.

Saying Yes to No-Nos

Arm Cuffs, a.k.a. Braces, Elbow Splints, No-No's. Some cleft surgeons require a baby to wear padded arm cuffs during the days and weeks following surgery (as mentioned previously). These removable braces, worn 24/7 and popularly called "No-Nos," prevent a child from bending her elbows, so she will not harm the delicate surgical area with her hands following the procedure. I remember learning about these arm cuffs before my daughter's first operation and finding the overall concept and simple design sort of clever, especially since the team assured me that my daughter would not be harmed or traumatized by their restrictiveness (which can initially seem weird and mildly torturous). At first glance, the cuffs can even appear kind of charming, as we imagine our sweet, loveable, postoperative baby transformed by soft, colorful, robot arms. But here's the rub. Initially, the No-Nos may appear to be a nonissue, even a breeze to manage, while the baby is still in the hospital after surgery and barely eating, much less moving her arms. Once she arrives home, however, she will likely regain some of her regular spirit and strength. This is when some caregivers—but not all—find the arm cuffs slightly less charming than before.

No-No or Yes-Yes? Parents generally describe two ways their children respond to postsurgical arm cuffs: by adapting or by squirming. Adaptable babies don't appear to be bothered by the cuffs and generally speaking, seem pretty amenable to wearing them. If this is the case for your child, congratulations! Problem averted. You may skip forward in this book. While you're at it, make yourself a nice cup of tea. It is important to celebrate small victories.

Babies who squirm, in contrast, somehow defy all odds when, Houdini-like, they decide that they *will* get their arms out of those cuffs. Squirming babies often do their best work at night. "We made it through our first night at home!" exclaimed one mother—with tongue in cheek. She had spent the majority of the previous night on hands and knees, searching for her son's No-Nos. "Every time I found Michael awake," she said, "one of his splints was off." By the next morning, she discovered that one of her son's cuffs had traveled clear across his bedroom. Another baby responded so negatively to the No-Nos that her mother felt truly frustrated—and unsure of what to do next. "We've been giving [our daughter] long breaks from the cuffs, and also watching her like a hawk," she said. "She just hates them. I can never tell if it's better to give her a break and then have to put them back on, or if it's less bad to just leave them on."

If you are at a similar impasse with the No-Nos, be sure to contact your child's team (also see some potentially useful ideas from parents, below). But it may also help to simply know in advance that responses may vary. For whatever reasons, some babies have no problems whatsoever with the cuffs, while others find them uncomfortable or even intolerable.

Arm Cuffs: Tips. Parents mention several tricks of the trade for keeping a baby comfortable in arm cuffs, ensuring they remain in place, and finding doable day-to-day activities during this time. One mother recommended buying baby-size, sleeveless sweater vests, since the padded arm cuffs can be bulky and overly insulating (a variation is to buy low-cost sweaters or sweatshirts and cut off the arms). Another parent suggested the opposite approach: buying large-fitting, long-sleeve sweaters or sweatshirts that the child can wear *over* the cuffs, using the sleeves to keep them in place. "My daughter would shake her arms wildly until the restraints came off," this mother explained. The long-sleeved outfits kept the cuffs in position amidst her daughter's most valiant efforts to bat the hem off (a small victory!).

Another mother offered a creative and fun variation: she bought several pairs of fashion leg warmers to hold the cuffs in place. "Every day, we had a different pattern," she said. "We had leopard print, zebra, polka-dots…it took my mind off it and hers too." Still another mother, the blogger Elizabeth From Scratch, suggested securing the cuffs to the baby's clothing with athletic tape (in fun colors, no less). So, there are lots of options. The sleeveless route, which offers freedom of movement, may be most appropriate for a Yes-Yes baby. A No-No baby, especially one who shakes her arms wildly, may need any and all kinds of assistance to keep the things in place.

For activity time, certain toys may come in handy during the first few weeks after surgery. One parent resurrected the floor gym her daughter enjoyed during infancy, saying that the little dangly toys were both fun and physically reachable by her daughter. An ExcerSaucer can be a good option as well, as would a drawing easel with dry-erase markers (particularly for an older infant recovering from palate repair). One mother mentioned blowing bubbles and simply playing music to distract and soothe her son. While some toys and activities can be out of reach (literally) during this time, creative options abound.

Some parents report taking off their child's arm cuffs during bath time and clearing the tub of toys. One dad thought to fill the tub with whiffle balls following his daughter's palate-repair operation, noting that the balls were fun to play with while being too large to fit into her mouth. It is important to note that while this trick worked well following palate-repair surgery, it may not be advisable following lip repair. If you have questions, be sure to consult with the team.

Postsurgical Scars

When Gina first learned about her daughter's CLP prenatally, one of the first things she wondered was whether she would have a postsurgical scar. "What would it look like?" she wondered. "I was worried." It is reasonable to think of the permanence of a scar, as Gina did, not to mention its metaphorical heft, and shudder at the possible long-term implications for our child, especially socially and emotionally. How will a child feel about her scar as she gets older? When she notices how insensitively scars are portrayed in popular films? The mind races. But Gina and her husband were surprised to learn from their surgeon that the appearance of their daughter's scar would likely change over time—and that they would need to care for it immediately after surgery.

Short Term versus Long Term. As concerning as the question of scarring felt to Gina and her husband during their baby's infancy, the truth is that no one can predict how a child will feel about a scar or even her overall appearance down the line. That self-awareness occurs slowly and incrementally—and individually—with growth. Moreover, it may be illuminating (or perhaps ironic) to learn that the appearance of a surgical scar—the look of the actual, physical entity—will likely change in the meantime. According to Philip Kuo-Ting Chen, MD, in the book *Comprehensive Cleft Care: Family Edition*, a scar is dynamic during the first six months after surgery as it heals. Some scars can even be altered later on, whether through surgery (called a *revision*) or other kinds of treatment. So, while it is true that a scar will never disappear entirely, we can't know how it will look, in terms of physical appearance, for some time after a baby's initial operation.

Meanwhile, the ACPA informs parents that a postoperative scar may appear to become more prominent before it recedes. One cleft surgeon explained that the scar will become "red, raised, and hard" during the weeks that follow surgery. Others from Seattle Children's Hospital go on to say that a scar will become softer to the touch and lighter in color as time passes, in a healing process that can last from six months to two years.

Homework: Sun Protection. While cleft professionals vary in how they direct parents to care for a scar—or leave it alone—following lip-repair surgery, a near-universal initial recommendation is to protect a baby's scar from sun exposure in order to avoid permanent darkening as it heals. According to parents, applying sunscreen is easier said than done with a wet, drooly infant—but it may help to remember that other methods may come in handy to help block the sun, such as a stroller shield (or blanket), a sun hat, or as the cleft team at Seattle Children's recommends, even a Band-Aid placed over the surgical site.

Homework: Massage? Instructions for scar massage seem to vary significantly from one team, surgeon, and situation to another—as do parents' strategies for carrying them out. One mother, Ally, received directions from her son's surgeon to massage his postoperative scar several times a day starting a few weeks after surgery. While this mother had heard of other cleft parents who massage the scar while the baby sleeps in order to sneak in the activity slyly under the cover of night, she decided to make the activity fun and distracting to her son by turning on her favorite music during massage sessions while he was awake. "I put on Maroon 5 and let him watch the video while I held him and we danced," she said. "Then I massaged his scar. We did it for the duration of the song." Ally used shea butter as a massage cream and applied a moderate amount of pressure to the scar, gradually building up to five or six total minutes per day. (Note that while shea butter worked in this case, a few cleft teams recommend sticking with a simpler cream or oil such as vitamin E or Vaseline. Be sure to ask your team for advice.)

In contrast, some cleft teams don't recommend scar massage at all or suggest doing it in small amounts. Another mother, a former professional massage therapist, felt comfortable dealing with scars and had even begun to massage her son's upper lip with some vitamin E oil after his operation. But she soon stopped touching it altogether. "The doctor didn't recommend it," she said. "With the healing, he didn't want the area to be touched." The Cleft Lip and Palate Association (CLAPA) explains to caregivers that circumstances can vary widely from one patient to another—and reminds us that it is always best to follow the instructions of our child's surgeon. "What works for one child [with regard to massage] may not be appropriate for all," the group writes. Each baby and circumstance are different.

Accepting Strong Feelings... and Accepting Meals

Second Impressions: A Baby's New Smile. The first time Rachel saw her son in a hospital recovery room following his lip-repair operation, she felt a rush of frantic energy. "For twenty-four hours, I was crazy," she said. While this mother recognized her baby literally—that is, she could identify him in the bed—she admitted that she felt deeply unsettled by his new appearance as if she couldn't see the son she had grown to love. For a day, she fought back tears. She even wondered, "'Can we undo it?'" Rachel couldn't see a way to move forward.

Still disoriented when she returned home from the hospital, Rachel phoned a fellow cleft parent who had been in her shoes. "She told me, 'I know you are suffering now, but it will get better,'" Rachel said. This other mother reassured her that her son's features would become familiar with time and that Rachel's feelings were normal. As the days wore on, Rachel found, indeed, she slowly began to recognize her son, even wondering if his features had physically settled somewhat after surgery, reminding her of his previous appearance. Rachel also felt better when she spoke with her own mother. "When my mother saw [my husband and me and the baby] on the day we got home," she said, "her reaction was all positive. That really helped. She said, 'He looks beautiful.'" Sometimes, it can feel reassuring to hear supportive responses from trusted friends and family. But just as often, we simply need time to adjust to a new situation—perhaps in the same way we did when we first met our newborn.

Some parents feel comforted when they recognize other, nonfacial features in their baby: a hand, a toe, a chubby arm. "One of the biggest things for me," one dad shared, "was hearing my daughter's voice." This father joked that he never thought he would feel so happy to hear his baby cry. But the moment he heard her familiar wails, he relaxed. "It's the same baby," he continued. "I realized it was going to be okay."

Perhaps most of all, parents say they find comfort in seeing their baby smile. One mother, Kerri, felt disappointed, initially, to think that her son's new grin might not be as bright or as wide as the first one had been. "To be honest," she said about the early days after the operation, "I wasn't thrilled about his new mouth." His features seemed forced together and small, Kerri recalled, nothing like the rainbow that had lit up his face during his early months before surgery. But when Kerri's son experienced his first, real, genuinely happy moment a few days later, Kerri realized that while she had taken in the appearance of her son's new lip and nose, she hadn't actually seen him smile. "I was wrong," she declared. "[His new smile] reached all the way up to his eyes."

Arriving home can be challenging, especially with regard to pain management and other medical decisions. The period can feel shaky. But the comfort of familiar surroundings—not to mention additional time and support from loved ones—may allow you to process your feelings and move forward. "Once we were in our own atmosphere," another mother commented, "when the baby was not so swollen, and the shock wore off…we were so appreciative [of our surgeon's work]."

Could You Please…? Just at a moment when many of us parents are coping with intense feelings about our child's new appearance (not to mention exhaustion and stress from the ups and downs of her continued recovery), it can be easy to forget about one more responsibility: ourselves. Fellow parents, it is time to ask for help! The baby is crying. An older sibling is pulling at your sleeves. You've been wearing the same pants for six days. It is time for someone— anyone!—to bring over a spare quiche (or three). Yet the act of asking for assistance is not always easy. It can feel uncomfortable to impose a burden on others.

As awkward as it may feel to ask others for help, it may be encouraging to know that people are usually more willing to lend a hand than we realize. A Cornell University study on how individuals ask for and receive everyday assistance from others shows that people asking for aid "underestimated by as much as 50 percent the likelihood that others would agree to a direct request for help." In other words, as a *New York Times* journalist states succinctly, "People want to help you. But you have to ask." Several cleft team professionals and parents have recommended accepting help during the recovery period after a child's surgery or asking for it in advance—even if we chafe at the idea initially. "Have friends provide some meals," advised one mother. "Then, you can focus on your child." It may not be easy to bring up this subject when talking with family, friends, neighbors, or members of a religious community—but it can be even less easy to care for a postoperative baby when you are exhausted, frazzled, emotional, and at wits' end.

FAMILY STORIES
Overwhelmed?

About a month after her daughter's lip-repair surgery, Meredith* found herself crying nonstop. This mother realized long after her daughter's recovery ended that she, herself, had not completely healed from the experience.

Fortunately, Meredith had the wherewithal to pick up the phone and schedule a visit with a therapist. "I was told that I was depressed, and the worst was over," Meredith said. Her therapist explained that it is common for parents to suffer from post-traumatic stress following a child's operation. "The reason I had begun to cry after a month had passed was because I felt I had to be strong for my family," she continued. "I had repressed all my feelings."

As other cleft parents have experienced, this therapist provided a valuable perspective that Meredith was unable to see for herself. "It took a few sessions," she continued, "before I finally worked through it."

Quote drawn from Charkins, H. *Children with Facial Difference: A Parents' Guide.* Woodbine House; 1996. *Name assigned by the author.

While it is natural to focus on the baby before, during, and after surgery, it is important not to underestimate the impact of surgery on the mental health of a parent or caregiver. Professional treatment, if appropriate and feasible, can be an important part of our own recovery from this experience. In some cases, it can even give us a framework for handling operations or other challenges down the road.

No one knows how a baby will respond to surgery, especially the first time around. We can't know how she will react to anesthesia, how she will experience pain, or when she will find a desire to resume eating. We can't know whether she will say "Yes-Yes" to No-No's or squirm like crazy. And who knows how *we* will respond to any of these events? But we can do our best to shore up our resources, honor our own feelings, and if possible, accept help, whether it's with child care, a home-cooked meal, or more formal assistance. We can also take a moment to celebrate this large victory (in addition to the small ones) knowing that our child—and we ourselves—have made it through a major milestone in our family's journey.

Palate-Repair Surgery

Chapter 30

. . . .

A New Challenge: Cups!

A Start-to-Finish Guide on the Transition from Bottles to Cups
PLUS: A Primer on Starting Solid Foods

Midway through a baby's first year, parents of children born with cleft palate usually receive an assignment from the surgeon and team. Due date: palate-repair surgery. The job: transition a baby from bottle-feeding to drinking from a cup. The goal is to teach the baby to drink out of a vessel that will not make contact with—and potentially harm—the delicate palate area following surgery. The special, long-nippled baby bottle that enabled her to drink during her early days will become Enemy Number One following palate repair. "This is a technically challenging operation," remarked one craniofacial surgeon. A surgeon can close the gap in the palate in the operating room, she continued, "but the area is fragile." So, a caregiver's job is to be ready to protect the newly repaired palate immediately after surgery—by teaching the baby to use an appropriate cup beforehand.

When it comes to making a transition from bottle to cup, the specific assignment will vary from one team to another. A few lucky parents will skip this task entirely in instances when their child's surgeon gives permission to continue using a particular bottle following surgery. Most will be instructed to teach their child to drink from a short-spouted sippy cup or a regular cup. Yes, you read that last part correctly: the team may recommend a regular, open cup. For a six-month-old. With a cleft palate. (Please read on! It's not as difficult as it sounds). The instructions will depend on a surgeon's ideas about which materials and levels of contact will threaten a particular repair.

One mother felt particularly daunted by this assignment. "This is the surgery I have dreaded the most since my daughter's birth," she said. "The fear of her not being able to eat or have her bottle back afterward—those are my main concerns." The good news is that this task will help a child resume eating as smoothly as possible following surgery. Also, it is doable! Below, you will find tips for choosing a cup, methods and tips for making the transition, information on a possible sidestep, a short primer on introducing solid foods, and hindsight from other parents for staying clear-headed—and perhaps most important, relaxed.

Choose a Cup
Sippy Cups, Open Cups, and Hybrids

Choices, Choices. First, you will probably need to choose a cup. While sippy cups seem to be the most commonly recommended type of vessel these days for the transition from bottles to cups, cleft teams tend to vary in their specific instructions. Some teams recommend a particular brand and model for postsurgical use, occasionally even giving parents an actual cup to take home. One mother responded almost gleefully when an Early Intervention professional gave her daughter a cup at an intake appointment. "We thought—great!" she said. "It's sanctioned." More often, however, a team will give you general recommendations for the type, shape, or material of the cup—and in particular, the length of the spout—but leave you to your own devices to face The Wall of Cups at Target, Walmart, etc.

The first time I went to Target and saw The Wall, I was completely unprepared for its sheer magnitude, with dozens—hundreds?—of different kinds of cups on display, stretching up to the fluorescent heavens. If I hadn't lost my breath, I would have laughed. Each cup has different features, proportions, and materials. There are *systems*. Parents of kids with special feeding needs can't just grab one and throw it in the basket. For those parents, The Wall is something to contend with. It's worse than buying jeans.

Sippies. One way to manage this initial choice, while also bringing down your own blood pressure, is to follow the instructions from the team and pretty much forget about the other details. Sippy cups are common recommendations from cleft teams. Over the last several years, parents and professionals have mentioned cups by Tommy Tippy, Nuby, Playtex, Tupperware, and Philips Avent, all with short, soft spouts that meet the requirements of many teams. These spouts measure about a half-inch long, though it is hard to know where to start measuring. (For detailed brand information on all the cups described here, see the list at the end of this chapter.)

Another thing to keep in mind is that sippy cups seem to vary quite a bit from one to another, but only really differ in a few ways (let's set aside spoutless sippies, for now). The spout of a traditional sippy cup might be soft or hard. It might be long or short. That's about it. Soft spouts seem to be popular among cleft parents and babies. But if you think your child might tolerate a hard spout—and some parents have been pleasantly surprised in this regard—Playtex makes a classic, short-spouted sippy cup that has been around for years, as does Tupperware. It is also important to remember that all of these cups will need to be modified before use by a baby with CP in order to remove the suction (see How to Perform Sippy Cup Surgery, below, for instructions).

Specific brands and models for sippy cups come in and out of production frequently, certain mainstays aside. It is hard for anyone, whether parent or professional—or book writer—to stay on top of these changes. The team will give you instructions, of course. But an online forum can also provide up-to-the-minute information. Facebook and *BabyCenter* groups are helpful places to start.

Open Cups. If your baby's cleft team instructs you to teach her to use a regular, open cup before palate-repair surgery, it is important, first, not to panic and run out of the office. This task can be surprisingly manageable. The team may direct you to specialty companies that manufacture products intended for this very purpose. One example—the FlexiCut Cup, manufactured by AliMed and North Coast Medical and sold online—has a U-shaped cutout that allows the caregiver to see the child's mouth and regulate flow. These cups are amazingly easy to manipulate—nothing like the stiff baby cups that you might think of from decades past. The team may also direct you toward one of several amazing, new-fangled open cups that allow a caregiver to control the flow of liquid. The Reflo Smart Cup, for instance, is a plastic, open cup that looks just like a regular, adult water cup but has a cool, removable insert that limits spillage.

One mother had wonderful luck teaching her daughter to use an open cup, remarking that the U-shaped cutout made all the difference. "These cups are the best," she said. Another mother chose open cups, in part, because she disliked—shall we say, strongly disliked—the other options. "I loathe sippy cups!" the mother of six exclaimed. "They are such a pain with all of their parts. You lose one and find it a week later." Expense played a role too. She didn't want to invest in sippy cups only to find out that none of them would work for her child. Whether you receive instructions to use a particular cup or have strong preferences as this mother did, it can be reassuring to have the open cup option in your back pocket as a simple, low-cost method, whether you try it right away with your baby or wait until later.

If you are shopping for an open cup, you should know that the cups with the U-shaped cutouts come in a variety of sizes. One occupational therapist (a professional who helps with feeding, also called an OT) recommended starting with a four-ounce cup, the smallest available of this type, indicating that it fits most babies well. One parent described using small Dixie cups in the same way—she cut the U-shape herself—but ended up using and throwing away a lot of cups.

Hybrids. An alternative to the traditional sippy cup and regular cup is a spoutless sippy cup, a simple hybrid that resembles a portable coffee cup and allows a baby to release liquid by pushing against the rim of the cup with her upper lip—while also mimicking her hip, on-the-go parents drinking vanilla lattes from matching vessels. Sunglasses are optional.

While spoutless sippies are generally straightforward to choose and use, cleft babies seem to go one way or the other with them, either embracing them happily or rejecting them flat-out. If a baby has had recent lip-repair surgery, it is of course possible that the pressure required to emit liquid will cause pain or discomfort to her upper lip. The list at this chapter's end includes a few models popular among cleft babies (though there are a lot of other hybrids commercially available). These favorites may be gentler on the upper lip than other options.

Too Many Options? If your child's team directs you to choose any kind of cup—a sippy cup, regular cup, or a hybrid—the soft-spouted sippy cup may seem like the easiest and most obvious choice. There's a reason why The Wall of sippies exists in the first place: these contraptions are conveniently sized and shaped for little hands (and little physical coordination), clefts or no clefts. But if you are willing to try other options—and you happen to have a Dixie cup lying around the house—you might consider cutting a U-shape and giving the regular cup a try.

The prospect of teaching a six-month old to drink from a grown-up cup may seem ludicrous, at first, as if by some twist of logic, you are actually asking your child to spill formula or precious breast milk all over the floor and then giving her the tools to do so. But I was surprised, personally, when my daughter's first attempt to use the open cup was not a complete disaster. She spilled formula all over the floor, of course. But she didn't do so immediately. And with a regular, open cup, you've saved yourself some cash, a few trips to the store, and the larger task of making another transition down the line. Every option has trade-offs (don't forget the hard-spouted sippy as another underdog option). It can be useful to approach this choice with an open mind and even a sense of adventure. Cleaning products will come in handy too.

The Transition
Three Methods

Have you purchased a cup? Are you ready to dive in? It is time to roll up your sleeves and get started. We will begin, below, by exploring three approaches for structuring your baby's transition—all of which, with no particular agenda on my part, bear titles related to deli sandwiches. Then we will look at variables such as positioning, timing, and type of liquid in the cup. This way you can mull over your options and devise a plan that makes the most sense for you and your baby. While you're mulling, grab a sandwich.

The Double-Decker Sandwich Approach. The Double-Decker Sandwich Approach is based on the premise that practice makes perfect and that a gradual transition—with some trial and error—can be an effective way to facilitate change. Some specialists on cleft teams suggest that parents introduce the new cup as a bonus feeding method that either precedes or follows a regular feeding session with a familiar bottle—then gradually replace the bottle during the day and eventually, switch to the cup for nighttime feedings too. As the process plays out, you will be able to read your child's signals and experiment with variables while also giving her time to adjust to a new cup.

You might think of one of those stackable BLTs: experiment for a short time (bread) + acclimate for a longer time (BLT fillings) + experiment again (bread) + acclimate again (fillings). Continue.

You could introduce a new cup on Day 1 and spend a short amount of time—let's say for five or ten minutes—making adjustments to meet the needs of your baby, say to increase the flow of the cup with a knife if the baby is straining, or try another cup. Then you can stop experimenting and spend time practicing, say for a few days in a row. Then repeat.

If a baby rejects the new cup, keep trying. "Don't give up," one parent wrote on a *BabyCenter* cleft forum. Remember that babies can be idiosyncratic. Experimentation, repetition—and patience—are key.

HOW TO PERFORM SIPPY-CUP SURGERY AT HOME

Removing the Suction

Attention, parents! It is time to operate! If you have decided to use a sippy cup or hybrid for the transition from bottles to cups, it will need to be modified before presenting it to a baby with cleft palate in order to remove the suction—because as we've discussed before, a child with CP cannot suckle. Do you have a small paring knife in your kitchen? Excellent. Let's prepare for surgery.

The first step is to examine the cup to figure out the mechanism that creates the suction. It could be a plastic plug, or more likely, a small vent. You will need to remove the plug or slice into the vent to free up the flow of liquid. You may also want to slice into the spout itself. If you turn the cup upside down, the liquid should pour out pretty quickly (you can test it out with water and drink from the cup yourself to check the flow). While it is always advisable to start conservatively and make small cuts, you should know that many of these cups require an astonishing amount of suction right out of the box. The valve itself may need major modifications.

One minor drawback to cutting into the spout of a sippy cup is that with time and wear, the hole will become too large to use without flooding the baby (you may remember this common occurrence with the nipples of cleft bottles, as well). Once you've chosen a cup, spares may come in handy.

> While these alterations may feel unconventional at first, especially as you are standing in your kitchen ostensibly destroying a perfectly good cup with a paring knife, they have become the norm before surgery and really do work.

The Cold-Turkey Method. Now let's suppose that your slow, patient, methodical Double-Decker Sandwich attempts don't seem to lead anywhere or feel frustrating, annoying, unproductive, or generally burdensome to the poor soul in your household who washes dishes or cleans stray liquids from the rug. Enter Option B. As often as professionals and parents recommend a gradual transition (and even as I offer the advice "repetition is key" above), it is true that some caregivers simply throw their hands in the air, skip the patience, and opt for a cold-turkey method. "We picked a cup," writes one parent in a *BabyCenter* forum, "...and on Friday night packed up the bottles and put them away. By Monday morning it was like the bottles never existed."

A cold-turkey approach may feel awkward in the moment (to say the least) when your sweet, unknowing baby expects to see his familiar bottle at mealtime and finds a strange, oddly shaped interloper instead, with no evidence of the previous bottle in sight. "Yes, he threw a fit," this mother continues, "Several of them. But eventually, the tummy wins." Sometimes, a parent's gotta do what a parent's gotta do. If you have the energy for it—and perhaps a spare weekend—you may discover that a sudden, full-on change can be swift and successful, in some cases trading weeks of time, effort, and painstaking experimentation for a short, possibly loud, probably frustrating, but ultimately victorious few days.

The Warm-Turkey Method. The cleft parent and blogger Elizabeth From Scratch has offered a clever variation on the cold-turkey method. When Elizabeth's daughter switched from her trusty Dr. Brown's bottle to a hard-spouted sippy cup, Elizabeth made the swap all at once. There was no wiggle room, no looking back; it was classic cold turkey. Yet before she made the switch, Elizabeth prepped her daughter by gradually increasing the flow of liquid in her Dr. Brown's bottle. Over several weeks, she attached larger and larger nipples to the Dr. Brown's, ultimately reaching the Dr. Brown's No. 4 nipple. Once her daughter became accustomed to the faster flow using the old bottle, the cold-turkey change went smoothly. What's not to love about a warm Thanksgiving sandwich?

The Transition
Variables to Consider

Have you considered a method for the transition from bottles to cups? Now let's look at other variables such as positioning, timing, and type of liquid in the cup.

Positioning: Start Upright. You will probably not be surprised to learn that cleft team pros recommend that a baby born with a cleft palate sit up straight when trying a new feeding method prior to palate repair—just as she did in early infancy. But one occupational therapist also stated that a caregiver should probably hold the new cup at first during feeding, then pass it to the child as she becomes more comfortable (depending on age and development, of course). Some kids crave the independence. "Riley loves being able to try to feed herself!" exclaimed one mother a few weeks after her daughter's transition. While Riley started with a conventional, soft-spouted sippy cup, the adult-led feeding (at least initially) and upright posture will be useful for any type of vessel.

Positioning: Try the Finger-under-the-Chin Trick. According to one feeding specialist on a cleft team, many babies (cleft or no cleft) move their chin up and down a lot initially while drinking from a bottle. While these motions may work just fine with a traditional baby bottle or special cleft palate bottle, she said, they don't lend themselves to smooth, efficient drinking from a cup, especially an open cup or hard-spouted sippy. One trick to consider, at least at first, is to place a finger or two under the child's chin as she drinks from the cup, to help her keep still while she drinks. Not only will your fingers limit the baby's range of motion, but they can prevent a hard spout from banging against her lips.

While the physical positioning of an open cup may feel odd at first for a caregiver, some babies take to it—or to a hard-spouted sippy—amazingly well. Just don't forget to limit the amount of liquid, stay physically involved with the baby's movements, and practice, practice, practice.

Consider Timing (for a Gradual Transition). Several parents and professionals have recommended introducing a new cup as a bonus following a daytime feeding, then gradually working up to evening and nighttime feedings. But you might also consider the timing within a feeding session itself. Some parents appeal to the power of their child's hunger by offering a new cup at the outset of a feeding session when the baby is most hungry. Others opt to start the session with a familiar baby bottle and wait five or ten minutes before introducing the cup—until a moment when the baby has satisfied her initial cravings and seems calmer than before. A third option is to offer water in a cup during another time of day—apart from a feeding session—as one mother did successfully with her son. The goal, she said (which was based on advice from the team), was to treat the transition like a game, apart from meal times, as a gentle introduction to the cup. Eventually, she put formula in the cup and gave it directly to him following his regular feeding sessions. The process, she said, took a few weeks.

None of these ideas is necessarily better than the others; decisions about timing depend on the baby's responses, personal preference, and of course, the input of the cleft team. In any case, it is okay for this entire process to take a while. A baby may need weeks or months to get used to a new setup before using it as a primary feeding method.

Purchase Cups Strategically. While the transition from bottle-feeding to cup-feeding oftentimes benefits from some experimentation with different styles of cups and setups (while following instructions from your cleft team, of course), it is important to remember that most babies are highly adaptable. Some parents end up investing a lot of time in this process, if not money, with several trips to the store or online to search for different models. "I've purchased sooooooo many dang cups" one mother writes in a *BabyCenter* forum, "it's not even funny." While such an investment in cups *can* lead to pleasant surprises (as I hope it did for this mother), it is not necessary to spend a small fortune—or much of a fortune at all—on this transition.

The key is to follow your surgeon's instructions, your household budget, and your instincts. If you are looking to spend strategically, you might invest in different types of cups—but one of each—rather than buying say, several types of similar, soft-spouted sippies. As mentioned earlier, the underdog cups—i.e., the open cup and the hard-spouted sippy cup—can sound challenging at first but may be worth a try.

Consider Flavor and Consistency. Whether a child moves to a soft or hard-spouted sippy cup, a hybrid, or an open cup prior to palate repair, the liquid will likely flow faster than it did before. Cleft bottles like the Haberman or Pigeon generally dispense milk or formula in a relatively slow, predictable way. With the new method, the liquid usually pours out in one big gush, making a big mess.

One way to ease up on the gas is to look for a cup that regulates the flow of liquid (see the list, below). But another option is to thicken the liquid itself, pending advice from a medical professional. An occupational therapist, nutritionist, and/or speech-language pathologist (SLP) may recommend thickening breast milk or formula with rice cereal or some pureed baby food, like the jarred Stage One fruits or vegetables. A thicker liquid will slow down the flow and as a bonus, add some bulk and flavor, creating a sort of smoothie. As the child gets used to the new system, the caregiver can gradually reduce the number of add-ons. A nutritionist will tell you what proportions to use (and again, professional input is a must).

Sidestep?
The TenderCare™ Option

When Marina began teaching her son, Wyatt, to use a sippy cup, she wasn't surprised to see the process start slowly. When he swatted the cups playfully with his hands, she laughed. When he examined a cup with initial interest—as if to momentarily raise his mother's hopes—and then swiftly dumped all of its contents onto the floor, she showed patience. Yet Marina never anticipated that these antics, however charming, would continue unabated over weeks and months. She presented new cups at moments of obvious hunger. She varied the types of cups. She focused on FUN. And yet. "We have every sippy cup in the universe in our house and he doesn't like any of them," she said. So, with no time to spare before surgery, Marina made a bold and admirable decision to simply move on. She wiped her hands clean of the situation, ended the cup journey altogether, and opted for an escape valve: the postsurgical syringe feeder.

Known by the trademarked brand name TenderCare™ Feeder, the postsurgical syringe feeder is a transitional method of feeding (as discussed elsewhere in this book). Some parents, like Marina, use this method directly after palate-repair surgery, sidestepping the cup transition altogether and returning to a previous special-needs bottle once the surgical site had healed.

I know what you're thinking: If the TenderCare™ Feeder works so well after surgery, couldn't I plan to use this sidestep method exclusively, skipping the cup ordeal altogether? Well, sure, you could. But the syringe comes with possible downsides too, depending on your situation. First and foremost, your child's surgeon/ team will have an opinion on which kinds of feeding method(s) are acceptable after surgery and will give you specific instructions on the dos and don'ts. Some surgeons don't want a spout of any kind to enter the child's mouth after surgery.

But just as important, syringe-feeding can be inconvenient. Since the TenderCare™ Feeder is designed as a transitional method, by definition it is slow-going, emitting only small amounts of liquid through a thin tube. As several parents have noted, this path can feel frustrating and inefficient, especially with an older baby who demands more calories than before. It is possible, as well, that your child's surgeon will want to know that the baby has learned to use a sippy cup or open cup prior to the procedure, even if she starts out with a transitional method postoperatively. As always, it is important to consult with the team. If this option is on the table for your child, it may be helpful to keep it at the ready as a viable and possibly stress-relieving sidestep if necessary.

Bottles to Cups
Hindsight from Parents

When I asked parents of cleft-affected children about their experiences preparing for palate-repair surgery and whether they would do anything differently if they could rewind the clock, three main ideas emerged.

TIP No. 1: Find (Free!) Help. The parents who sought professional help with feeding raved about it, describing their experiences as almost universally helpful if not instrumental to their baby's transition (I count myself as one of the ravers). What's more, the services of feeding specialists are often available free of charge. Specifics will vary from team to team and state to state, particularly in terms of the types of professionals to seek out. In some cases, a feeding specialist on the cleft team fills this role. In other instances, the best match might be an occupational therapist (OT) or speech-language pathologist (SLP) whether he/she comes from a cleft team or an Early Intervention program. EI programs are state-run services (the exact name of the program will vary by state), designed to help individuals with special needs. Many make house calls for babies.

TIP No. 2: Expect More "Process." In looking back on their experiences with their babies, some cleft parents were also surprised when they had to undergo a certain amount of trial and error with feeding *following* their child's operation. Sure enough, the hours and days after this procedure are just the moments when all of the presurgical practice—and perhaps a few cup options—will come in handy. But even then, you may end up tinkering here and there. "We are trying to find the best way to get Sklyar to eat comfortably," explained one mother on the day after her daughter's palate repair. "We tried the soft sippy, which was okay, but she would push it out and made a mess. Then we used the 10 cc syringes pretty well, but she wasn't taking in a whole lot."

While many parents recall that their baby drank readily from her familiar sippy cup immediately after surgery, some children, like Skylar, need time to find a comfortable vessel. This stage, like the one before surgery, can also involve a process.

TIP No. 3: Aim for a B-Plus. Last and most important, some parents wished they hadn't fussed so much with feeding—and gone easier on themselves—during the weeks and months before their baby's palate surgery. However you choose to navigate the transition from bottles to cups, it may be useful to try not to let this task take over your life. After the baby has become *reasonably comfortable* with a new cup, you have probably reached the promised land. That's it! You're there. Now is the time to go with it—to go with a solid B or B-plus. This assignment often arrives on the heels of lip-repair surgery, after parents have devoted several months to the demands of a NAM or other treatment. It can be easy to let this new, smaller task fill that time and emotional space. Feeding a baby is very important, of course. But so is parental sanity.

BONUS SECTION

Starting Solids 101
Is It Possible? Is It Painful?

During the lead-up to palate-repair surgery, around the time when a baby with a cleft palate is learning to drink from a cup, many parents wonder how to introduce her to solid foods—and it is reasonable to wonder whether this endeavor is even possible. Will the baby feel satisfied with solids? Or will rice cereal, prune puree, and variously shaped puffs simply emerge from her nose, causing frustration, dissatisfaction, physical pain, potential embarrassment, and (provided the baby is not in pain) possible amusement from her parents?

The short answer is yes. It is possible, doable, and common to start solids with a cleft baby, more or less on the same schedule as any other baby (pending advice from the pros on the cleft team, as always). Here are a few tips to keep in mind, all related to CP. (For general information on solids and nutrition, see traditional sources.)

Timing during Infancy. Pediatricians generally recommend introducing solid foods to babies with a cleft palate approximately at the age of six months, around the same time as other babies, and when they are showing signs of readiness like sitting up on their own, leaning toward their food, and showing general interest. Cleft-team pros writing in the *Cleft Palate-Craniofacial Journal* recommend starting with traditional purees, followed by "meltable/soft solids" at age seven-to-nine months, then "easy table foods" at age nine-to-twelve months.

While many babies with CP are developmentally ready to take this new step and do so with few problems, the timing can be tricky if the baby's calendar is full. Many teams recommend scheduling operations (and recoveries) during the window of age six-to-twelve months. What to do?

As always, it is important to ask the feeding expert on the cleft team for guidance. Research shows that delaying the introduction of solid foods as late as age nine months can cause decreased consumption of certain food groups later in childhood. But some pros and parents describe minor postponements as harmless. The feeding expert may be able to evaluate your child's development, preferences, schedule, and other factors.

Nasal Regurgitation. When a baby with a cleft palate begins to eat solid foods, in most cases the food will come out of her nose more or less immediately, bringing to mind the geography of the face and the close proximity of the nose to the palate. The first time this happened with my daughter, I realized that these two body parts are so near one another that I might as well have been putting the food directly into her nose.

As surprising as such regurgitation may seem, it might be reassuring to know that this occurrence is common and usually normal and okay, especially at first (See Chapter 14 for a more complete discussion). One mother admitted she found it a little nerve-wracking to see globs of rice cereal emanating from her son's nostrils so shortly after receiving the food, but she was quick to note that he showed no signs of discomfort. Another mother was confused to see an odd, sneezing-coughing response from her son. "There was an occasional time when it almost seemed like he was choking," she said, "but he wasn't. It freaked me out at first." The feeding specialist on the team advised thickening the food a little bit, in this case stirring in a small scoop of pureed peas and carrots. "That helped with the choking," she said, "so he wasn't having to clear it out."

According to cleft experts at Seattle Children's Hospital and Children's Hospital LA (and others), everyday nasal regurgitation is not painful or dangerous. Sneezing, too, is typical and can help empty the nose (always check in with your child's team if you have concerns about choking). Fortunately, nasal regurgitation usually lessens with time as the baby learns to push food back with her tongue.

Aspiration. *Aspiration* occurs when something like food or liquid accidentally ends up in the airway or lungs. Aspiration is important to know about because some babies with cleft palate, especially those who have trouble swallowing (called *dysphagia*), are more likely to experience it than non-cleft babies. Professionals explain that the occurrence is usually harmless in small amounts but can become dangerous in large amounts or with repetition. While some aspiration is silent, you can identify it by looking for signs such as stopped breathing during feeding, a red face and watery eyes, frequent coughing or choking during a swallow (or afterward), and a wet-sounding voice (or breathing) during or after a meal.

Aspiration can be frightening for caregivers. But a pro on the cleft team should be able to help you learn to distinguish between this occurrence and the common sneeze-coughing (and regurgitation) that occurs among cleft babies. Be sure to touch base with the team with any concerns.

Positioning and Tools. When Tara first introduced solids to her daughter, Olivia, at around age five months, she noticed that Olivia swallowed more easily when she ate from the right-hand side of her mouth. "She showed me where to go," Tara explained about this discovery, "just as she did with the bottle." Sure enough, one glance inside Olivia's mouth confirmed she had a little ridge of palate intact on the right-hand side. Like Olivia, many babies with a cleft palate seem to favor spoon-feeding on one side.

Several parents report that regular, commercially available spoons work just fine for feeding their babies, but others use special tools. One OT recommended using a special, flat spoon called an EZ Spoon (see the list, below, for brand information). My own daughter, born with bilateral-complete clefts, had wonderful luck with this spoon, which resembles a doctor's tongue depressor. Some parents find that the flat surface of this spoon helps deliver the food precisely, cleanly, and easily, like a tiny pizza peel going in and out of an oven.

BRAND INFORMATION
for the Transition from Bottles to Cups

Popular Products Recommended by Parents and Pros

Popular Sippy Cups
(Valve Must Be Disabled)

Sippy Cups with Short, Soft Spouts

- Bell Tumblers by Tupperware
- Click-It Soft Spout Cup by Nuby
- First Sips Transition Cup by Tommy Tippy
- No-Spill, Super Spout, Easy Grip Cup by Nuby
- Sipsters "Stage 1" soft-spout sippy cup by Playtex
- Spout Cup by Philips Avent

Sippy Cups with Short, Hard Spouts

- Disney Mickey Mouse Insulated Hard Spout Sippy Cup
- Gerber Graduates Advance Developmental Hard Spout Sippy Cup
- Playtex Sipsters Stage 2 Sippy Cup (Hard Spout)
- Playtex Sipsters Stage 3 Spout Cup
- The First Years Take & Toss Spill-Proof Sippy Cups

Popular Open Cups
Open Cups

- Doidy Cup by Bickiepegs
- Dixie Cup (generic, wax-coated paper cup)
- EZPZ Tiny Cup
- Flexi Cut Cup by North Coast Medical
- Flexi-Cut Cup by AliMed
- Medicine Cup (generic plastic cup packaged with liquid medicines)

Open Cups with Restricted Flow

- Infa-Trainer Cup

- Provale Regulating Drinking Cup (Combo Open/Sippy Cup)
- Reflo Smart Cup
- The First Years My First Open Spoutless Cup

Spoutless/Hybrid Sippy Cups

- Munchkin Miracle 360 Sippy Cup
- My First Big Kid Cup by Philips Avent
- No-Spill 360 Wonder Cup by Nuby

Syringe Feeders and Spoons

- The TenderCare™ Feeder
- EZ Spoon Firm

Chapter 31

. . . .

Palate-Repair Surgery

New Concepts and Transferable Lessons

W hen Filomena met her son, Ricky, in the recovery area after his palate-repair operation, she half-expected that he would act mildly fussy but relatively calm, as he did after his lip repair a few months earlier. Not so. "He was crying a lot," she said. "He seemed very uncomfortable." Filomena said she didn't feel as apprehensive about this operation as she had the first time around. As she shared the story, she spoke matter-of-factly about it. But the experience seemed harder on her son, she noted, in terms of pain.

Ricky's recovery from palate repair lasted longer than the previous operation and involved more discomfort. Yet as other parents have discovered with their babies, the overall process looked like a variation on a theme—it was more similar to lip repair than it was different. And also, like other parents, Filomena handled the process more comfortably, since she had done it before and knew the ropes.

This chapter offers five tips related to a baby's palate repair, but it is important to note that the material builds on transferable lessons. If this is your first time helping a child through an operation or if you would like to take a moment to review themes on managing pain and advocating for your child, see Chapters 28 and 29. Many of the concepts in those chapters apply to palate repair (as well as to other procedures during infancy and beyond).

· ·

TIP No. 1. Expect Some Pain (But Remember That It's Manageable). Several of the parents I spoke with regarding palate repair saw signs of increased pain or discomfort following surgery, as Filomena did, especially as compared to their baby's recovery from an earlier operation. Indeed, a couple of cleft surgeons suggested that palate repair *can* be more painful than lip repair (though not always). Closing a cleft palate is a major endeavor, one surgeon explained. The roof of the mouth is a sensitive area in the first place, and then a surgeon moves around the tissue and muscle to repair the cleft.

As daunting as the idea of increased pain may sound, it is important to keep a level head (or as level as possible) in the moment. "There are many reasons for infants to cry after palate surgery," explained another cleft surgeon. A baby could cry from pain, he reasoned, but also from other discomforts such as nasal congestion, hunger, anesthesia, or fatigue. What's more, postoperative pain is manageable.

A cleft team's protocol for pain management following palate repair may resemble the regimen that followed lip repair: a multifaceted approach that may include several possible types of medications, depending on the purpose, the level of pain, and other factors. A surgeon might prescribe narcotics, for instance, for intense pain, followed by everyday pain relievers. It is important to administer medications as prescribed, both in the hospital and later, at home, in order to "stay ahead of the pain" (a concept discussed in Chapter 28) and to ask a professional and/or contact the cleft team as recovery plays out, whenever questions arise. But it *is* possible to manage a baby's pain following this procedure.

Also, if you've already ushered a baby through surgery and recovery, the process of pain management may be familiar to you this time around. Cara reported that her ten-month-old son did not resume playing or even sit up for a full week after his palate-repair operation. Yet while she described that period as nerve-wracking and interminable, she also trusted the process. "I knew what to expect," she explained. Her son's recovery, from her perspective, was more about forging through a challenging time, she said, than about discovering *how* to forge through.

PALATE REPAIR 101

Why Palate Repair? Cleft-palate repair, also known as *palatoplasty*, is a surgical procedure to close an opening in the roof of the mouth (a *cleft palate*). Closing a cleft palate improves a person's ability to eat and speak. Many of us know from experience that a baby with a cleft palate usually *can* eat and drink. In many cases, she gains weight during infancy and does amazingly well as is, either with the help of special bottles or as the result of her own inventiveness as she pushes solid food through her mouth with her tongue. Even so, closing the space will make those processes infinitely easier, both now and over time. Food and liquids will not come out of her nose. Her life will be far less burdened each time she eats a meal.

Closing a cleft palate is also invaluable for a person's speech because in order to form certain sounds in English (and other languages), we need the roof of the mouth to be sealed off from the nose. We also need the *levator veli palatini* muscle, a horseshoe-shaped muscle located in the roof of the mouth, to work properly. While the name of this muscle sounds like an incantation from Harry Potter's Charms class (go ahead, say it out loud: *levator veli palatini*), its function is actually just as otherworldly and cool. Under normal circumstances, the levator functions like a valve: it moves the back of the palate in an upward and backward direction during speech in order to seal off the back of the mouth while making certain sounds. When a person is born with a cleft palate, that muscle may be split in two. It is important for this muscle to function properly, so that air doesn't escape out the back of the mouth during speech, causing a nasal tone of voice and making a person difficult to understand.

What Does the Surgeon Do? When a surgeon closes a cleft palate, he or she does not borrow material from elsewhere in the body. Usually, the surgeon makes a series of incisions into the existing tissue of the roof of the mouth to either "relax" the tissue—so that it can be stretched or released and then attached elsewhere with stitches—or to create a sequence of flaps, which are then brought together to close the space. (If you have ever seen a paper Advent calendar during the Christmas season, you might think of its flap-like doors.) The surgeon also reconstructs the *levator* muscle "sling."

As with lip-repair surgery, a surgeon usually chooses a particular surgical technique based on a baby's anatomy, his or her training and/or personal preferences, and other factors. If you are curious about how your child's surgeon will close her cleft palate, be sure to ask for details.

* * *

TIP No. 2. Ask the Team about Pain Management, Feeding, and Lessons Learned. As similar as the recovery from palate-repair surgery may look to a baby's lip repair and/or a previous surgical experience, it is important to ask the cleft team about differences. Will any protocols change based on the advancing age of the baby, particularly regarding pain management?

Some hospitals don't administer ibuprofen, for example, to babies under a certain age (sometimes age three months), a policy that may rule out its use for lip repair but bring it into the equation for palate repair, to many parents' relief. Intravenous Tylenol, which enters the bloodstream through a child's IV, may also be available in the hospital for fast-acting pain relief. "IV Tylenol is nice for palate repair," commented one OR nurse, "because you don't have to wake up a kid to administer it. If you are trying to get a kid to drink, and they have a rough night with lots of interruptions, they won't want to drink." With an IV-administered medication, she continued, the child can get a good night's sleep and may wake up feeling refreshed—and therefore more likely to recover at an optimal pace. While these changes in hospital procedures may seem small, they can help enormously when a baby is in pain following this operation.

You could also ask the team how to feed the baby directly following surgery (if you don't already know that information). And you might take this opportunity to ask about any lessons learned from a previous procedure. If there were aspects of a recovery that you think could have gone more smoothly, be sure to ask the team for advice. It is always advisable to contact the team after surgery if you have questions or concerns, however small. But communication *beforehand*, if feasible, will allow you to ask all your questions, learn from any past experiences, and feel as comfortable as possible about what will happen.

> ### QUESTIONS FOR THE TEAM
> ### PALATE-REPAIR SURGERY

- What protocol will you prescribe for pain management following palate repair?
- How will your recommendations for pain management vary from those that followed a previous operation (based on expected levels of pain following this operation, the baby's age, lessons learned from a previous experience, etc.)?
- How do you recommend I/we feed the baby after surgery?
- What is the best way to contact you with questions, particularly after we've returned home after surgery?

TIP No. 3. Cultivate Patience and Flexibility with Regard to Eating. Did your child's surgeon instruct you to teach her to drink from a sippy cup or another kind of drinking vessel prior to palate-repair surgery, as discussed in Chapter 30? If so—or if you plan to use a syringe feeder or a previous baby bottle following the operation—you may wonder how to employ this new method after surgery and navigate the resumption of eating more generally.

When parents of children with CP describe their experiences with feeding after palate-repair surgery, it is clear that situations vary. But generally speaking, their advice tends to fall into two categories, which at first glance may seem incompatible with one another: to have patience and to be open to experimentation.

Let's start with patience. It is important to keep in mind that while the pain of palate repair is manageable, it can take time to resolve. One cleft surgeon estimated that the most intense pain tends to last forty-eight hours following this procedure. Anecdotes from parents suggest an additional few days for the entire recovery. We also know that pain management goes hand-in-hand with resuming eating when a baby has had surgery to the mouth (an unfortunate coincidence we've explored in previous chapters). So simply put, resuming feeding may take time. Patience—or your best attempts —will go a long way.

Experimentation can come in handy too. One mother, Anna, described palate repair as one of the more challenging procedures her son experienced. "[Our son] did not eat post-palate for about thirty-six or forty-eight hours—a long time," she said. While he took in very small amounts of formula from a syringe feeder in the hospital, Anna grew worried when he had not taken in enough liquids after they returned home. Even as she encouraged him to drink, he acted fussy and uninterested. No matter how she adjusted his position in her arms and played with the location of the syringe in his mouth, he would not be convinced.

Feeling desperate—and increasingly aware of the risks of dehydration—Anna thought outside the box. "We're going outside!" she declared. Anna carried her son onto her back porch, where the New England temperature was well below freezing. Sure enough, it worked. "He took the syringe like a champ," she said. In retrospect, Anna wondered whether her son's sudden desire to drink occurred because of the change of scenery, the frigid winter temperature, his general thirst, or because of her own persistence—she couldn't tell. But at that point, she was so happy to see him drink that she didn't much care why.

Anna not only did her best to be patient with a slow-going transition, but stayed on her toes. The key, as mentioned in Chapter 30, is to know that this this period may involve a process.

. . . .

TIP No. 4. Trust Your Experience with This Child. When I asked Jen about her son Dylan's recovery following palate repair, she explained that he acted fussier than he had following his lip repair, but that the second experience went smoothly overall. "I think he is just tough," she said. Jen described Dylan's temperament as easygoing and flexible in situations that other babies might find difficult. "[The doctors] sent us home with oxycodone," she continued, "but we felt he didn't need it." Jen not only knew her son's disposition and signals but trusted her ability to read them.

You know your baby best. Even if you have never set foot in a children's hospital with your child, you *have* probably seen her respond to a common cold, for example, or cry out from the discomfort of gastrointestinal reflux, or for that matter, fall down in the sandbox. "The important thing to remember," advises Professor Alice Roberts, PhD, on the informational website *My Child is in Pain,* "is that you will probably be very good at knowing if your child is in pain.… Knowing how your child has responded to pain in the past, you'll be able to spot if your child is in pain because of treatment or surgery." You can rely on this awareness to help your baby as she recovers from this procedure.

. . . .

TIP No. 5. Advocate: "Wait a Minute!" When cleft parents have looked back on their experiences helping their children through surgical procedures, one theme that comes up, again and again, is the importance of speaking up. As stated in previous chapters on surgery—and is worth repeating—it is a parent's job to advocate for a child. One mother, Molly, described a shift in mind-set that occurred with the birth of her son. During her early adult years, she recalled, she responded passively each time her primary care doctor offered a diagnosis regarding her (own) health. "I would simply say, 'Okay,'" she said, no questions asked. "Then Tyler came along," Molly continued, "and I started to say, 'Wait a minute!'"

While doctors and hospital staff may offer advice before, during, and after a child's operation (and in other medical settings as well), it is never wrong to ask as many questions as necessary to make sure that A), you understand what they are saying, and B), you feel comfortable with the information and/or advice. Does your child appear to be in pain? Is there something about treatment that seems not quite right? Do you fully understand what is happening? Not only is it okay to speak up when these kinds of questions arise, it is our job as parents to speak up. Ideally, the conversations with medical professionals would be friendly and constructive. In perfect circumstances, the pros would ease our minds each time by answering our questions fully and clearly. But it is always our duty to pay attention to what is going on with our child's care and to participate actively.

Any operation can be nerve-wracking. Palate repair may involve more discomfort (for our child) than before, not to mention moments of surprise (for her concerned parents). But fortunately, you can lean on the team, as always. And you can rely on your keen awareness of your own child's behaviors and needs. You've got this. Now is the time to be brave, take charge of your child's care, and speak up with a strong voice.

Beyond Year One

Chapter 32

. . . .

Conclusion: Now What?

Outlooks beyond Year One

Kyle was not surprised to learn that his daughter's surgeon requested she come to the office for a postoperative exam shortly after her palate-repair surgery. When he heard the team's instructions for the timing of her subsequent appointment, however, he was floored. "They told us to come back in a YEAR," he exclaimed. "A year! I couldn't believe it." After helping his daughter through cleft treatment on a near-constant basis for her first year of life, Kyle felt stunned to see it end.

As Kyle knew well, his daughter's treatment hadn't ended; there would be more to come as she grew. But the first phase felt so intense for him and his wife, as it does for other families, that its completion—and the subsequent period of relative inactivity—felt like a major shift.

If you are in this position, you may wonder: What now? In the short term, it is time for a sigh of relief! But it may also be helpful to shift gears in terms of outlook, both for your own sake and the sake of your child. Looking ahead, you may also want to consider issues and themes that can come up with an older child, including some that may be new to you and others familiar. Fortunately, fellow parents have offered ideas on ways to handle these challenges. And just as important, you have probably already developed some tools of your own.

A New Mind-Set
Moving beyond "Cleft Mode"

Take a Breath of Fresh Air! (For Parents). Kyle is not the only cleft parent who has noticed a shift after year one. "It was a huge relief," commented Kara about the days and weeks after her son's palate-repair operation. And for two years since then, her family's life has been relatively calm, cleft-wise. "Now we only go to the dentist and the pediatrician," she said, "and the annual visit with the cleft team. That's nothing." Another mother admitted that while the early months with her baby felt special, they also felt like a never-ending roller-coaster ride. "It was so hard," she said, "when I was in the thick of it, to see that there was a light at the end of the tunnel." The new chapter, to her, felt like a breath of fresh air.

Now, it is true that every cleft—and circumstance—is different. While many babies complete the first phase of treatment in one year, some undergo treatment into the second year of life due to their diagnosis, their adoption, a move to a new area or cleft team, or for any number of other reasons. And of course, some babies born with syndromes or other complex conditions continue the go-go-go nature of treatment unabated. While other health issues may persist—as may other life issues for that matter—now might be a time to celebrate *this* victory, in whatever form feels best.

Move beyond Cleft Mode (For a Child). As meaningful as it can be to celebrate the end of a period that one mother character-ized as, "a constant state of *cleft mode*," it may also be useful to consider a shift in mind-set about the role of CLP within family life—and in a child's identity. *Cleft mode* can be a very real frame of mind for us as caregivers during the baby's first year. But it is important to remember that the condition is only one part of a whole person. "It is time to forget about the clefts and treat your child like any other kid," one oral surgeon (also a family friend) advised my husband and me at a holiday party a few months after our daughter's palate-repair surgery. As consuming as it may have been from our perspective to deal with special bottles, NAM treatment, and major operations, he reminded us that our child didn't—and needn't—see the experience that way.

So, as you usher your one-year-old into the world, as you speak about her with friends and family, as you narrate your own experiences as a parent, and most of all, as you speak directly with her, it is important to try to turn another corner, too: to send the message that while CLP is a part of a child's experience and identity—and at that, a meaningful one to talk about and be proud of—it is but one piece of her identity. As fifth-grader Logan Bristow wrote so simply and wisely about her experience with CLP, "It's not the most important thing."

New Challenges after Year One

Now, what about the years to come? When I spoke with parents of school-aged children and young adults born with CLP, they mentioned two ideas about the period directly following year one. The first point relates to communication, the second to independence.

Let's Talk about It. Parents of older children emphasized the importance of speaking about CLP in an open, honest way with a child. While our explanations about the condition should be age-appropriate, they say (as cleft professionals advise as well) we should not withhold information from our child in the interest of trying to protect her. In other words, as important as it is to take pictures of a baby (as discussed in Chapter 18), it is equally important to *show* them to her and talk about them—because in so doing, we normalize the condition.

Liza remembered pulling out some old photos with her two-year-old daughter, including a few of her very early months of life, before surgery. "She saw the cleft, pointed to it, and said, 'Boo-boo,'" Liza said. "I told her it was a cleft lip," she explained, reasoning that she wanted to address the topic early on. Liza used simple, accurate language to teach her daughter about the condition rather than pretend it wasn't there. "I want her to feel okay about who she is," she continued, "and how she was born."

Professionals concur. Three cleft-team psychologists write about the importance of creating an environment of positivity—you guessed it—by talking about CLP and being honest as we do. "The child's difference should not be a forbidden topic," they write in the book, *Comprehensive Cleft Care: Family Edition*. The more openly we talk about this subject, the easier it becomes to help shape a positive mind-set for our child. As the author and cancer survivor Meg Rosoff points out so astutely in *The Guardian*, "Give a child an unpalatable truth and she will figure out a way to process it. But 'protect' her and the ghosts will whisper in her ear."

Let's Pass the Torch. Parents of older children go one step further, not only recommending we communicate openly with our child about CLP, but suggesting we eventually include her in decisions about her own care. When I first talked to Emily about her experiences raising her daughter Kayla, who is now in her mid-twenties, she mentioned how proud she felt of her daughter's sense of confidence over the years, even as she underwent upwards of thirty surgical procedures related to CLP and two other health issues. "We didn't hide her condition," she said.

When I spoke with Kayla directly, she described some ways her parents included her in decision-making as the years passed. At around age five, for example, Kayla recalled some of the members of the team sharing comments and information with her mother, but not much to her. "My mom would turn to me and then ask the doctors to tell *me* what they had just said, but in a language that I could understand," she said. Those conversations were a team effort between the family and the pros, she noted, but also between Kayla and her parents. So, by the time she was a teen and now as an adult, Kayla felt comfortable taking the reins. "I think it was very natural for me to go ahead and take charge," she continued, "and it's because as soon as I was old enough to understand, they would always involve me as much as possible, even from a very young age."

Professionals echo these recommendations. "Promoting the development of autonomy," explained Ruairidh Gallagher in the *Cleft Palate-Craniofacial Journal*, "really prepares children for lifelong management of their condition." Even now, as Kayla's treatment has extended into adulthood, the parent-child teamwork continues. "I always, always get my parents' input" she added— perhaps because they always sought her input, too.

Three Tools
Looking Ahead While Looking Back

Then there is Glinda, the Good Witch. As familiar or even cliché as *The Wizard of Oz* may feel to those of us who watch it year after year, the 1939 film sends a message of empowerment that might help us—and even reassure us—as parents. You may remember the near-final scene when Glinda descends from the sky inside an ethereal, pink (and wonderfully low-tech) bubble to find Dorothy pleading for help returning home from Oz. Glinda smiles and informs Dorothy that no, she doesn't need any help. "You've always had the power to go back to Kansas," she says.

It is also true that *you* possess the power to go back to Kansas— in this case, to make the best decisions you can as parents because you've learned some lessons from your journey. The advice you'll hear from cleft-team pros will be indispensable, of course. But after finishing your baby's first year of treatment, you have likely developed much of what you need to move forward—in this case, three tools for your parenting toolbox.

The Power of Homework. When Sarah first learned the news of her daughter's CLP (as mentioned in Chapter 6), she threw herself into researching clefts, not only to learn more about the condition but to reduce her own stress. When Megan and Mark had misgivings about their son's first surgeon after seeing the results of their son's initial lip-repair operation (see Chapter 7), they realized that they needed to find a team to treat their child rather than an independent plastic surgeon. They eventually moved forward confidently, but only after making tireless phone calls with professionals and other parents. And when Heather felt befuddled by her son's NAM device one night after a weekly appointment with the team (Chapter 24), she texted two people—her son's orthodontist on the team and another mother in her area who had been through the same experience. Other parents mention seeking out ACPA booklets and fact sheets, which are penned by professionals in the field.

All these families did their homework, in whatever form that took. While the tasks themselves may change over the years, the research skills—not to mention the scrappy determination—will not.

The Power of Teamwork. Then there is the question of where to direct that homework. First stop: the cleft team. As the ACPA states in a booklet for parents (see Chapter 7), the team should be a family's primary resource for information and advice. Parents concur, in large part because they have seen positive results with their children over the years. "Your relationship with these people is crucial," advises one mother (see Chapter 7). "Ultimately, how comfortable your child becomes with them will be a direct outcome of your belief in them and your relationship with them as parents." One dad sang the praises of his daughter's cleft-team care not only for the quality of outcomes but for the sake of his own peace of mind. "[The team] makes a world of difference in terms of a parent's comfort level," he says in Chapter 7. "I can't emphasize that enough."

Fortunately for families, this relationship is designed to last years. Whether we are shifting gears when our child starts speech therapy during the preschool years, pivoting for orthodontics and bone-graft surgery a few years later, or sending our young adult out into the world, the team will always be there for information and support.

The Power of Advocacy (and Courage). Finally, there is the ever-important matter of speaking up, mainly by asking questions—all of them, large or small—that arise about our child's condition and its treatment. "No question is a stupid question," advises Valerie (in Chapter 20) about her interactions with the team during her annual visits with her daughter. It is our duty as parents to take charge of our child's care by asking for help, leaning on the team, and acting as our child's chief advocate.

As cleft professionals say again and again, parents are members of the team too. Whether we are asking questions about pain management after surgery, looking for a clarification from a specialist, or having the courage to say to a medical person, "Wait a minute—I'm sorry—I don't get it. Can you explain that idea again?" it is not only okay to speak up; it is our job. And while this role begins during our child's infancy, it may continue or even intensify as the years go by.

Postscript

My Story: Neighborhood Walks
and Cleft Babies

About six months ago, my family got our first dog. Coco is an affectionate black Lab-mix whom the kids and I adore (and who is slowly winning over my husband). Coco also has a lot more energy than I realized when I first met her and exclaimed, "Let's do it!" to the friendly adoption person at our local shelter. As a result, Coco enjoys two long walks a day. Also, as a result, I end up seeing a lot of other people on the sidewalks walking their dogs—and a lot of other people walking with their babies.

My baby years are behind me. But I continue to crave conversations with other cleft parents. Each time I walk our dog through the neighborhood and spot a tired-looking, youngish adult pushing a stroller, I feel a tiny spark of anticipation, a flicker so small that it almost doesn't qualify as a feeling. I can't help but wonder whether the baby inside the carriage will have a sweet little rosebud cleft. Here I am, years beyond the stroller, still hoping to talk to that parent in order to share, learn, and feel reassured about a journey that few families understand. The sense of community, especially a community of caregivers, is meaningful to me. It lifts me up.

And so, I hope that by meeting other parents in this book—and of course, a bunch of professionals as well—that you have felt lifted up too, not only by the awareness that other parents are out there in the world with their thoughts, feelings, and responses to this experience but by the knowledge that, with some information and some pluck, you will have the resources you need to feel empowered to navigate a challenging time—and beyond.

Acknowledgments

Just as raising a cleft-affected child requires a team of supporters, so does writing a book about it. This project would not have been possible without the generosity of seventy-six parents of children born with CLP and fifty-nine cleft-team professionals who took the time to share stories, insights, and expertise through anonymous phone interviews. When I first initiated these conversations, I wondered whether anyone would respond at all. I was a stranger to most of them, a cold caller. I remain overwhelmed by their thoughtfulness, candor, and eagerness to help. Their input forms the backbone of this book.

In addition to conducting interviews, I sought specific feedback from cleft-team professionals. Starting during the earliest stages of this project, I leaned on Tricia Bender, Margaret Byrne, Noreen Clarke, Elena Hopkins, Margaret (Peg) Langham, Dawn Leavitt, Dorothy (Dottie) MacDonald, Marsha Ose, and Carole Reilly on matters related to feeding, nursing, and navigating aspects of early infancy. I also relied on cleft-team orthodontists for input on pre-surgical infant orthopedics, including Dr. Patricia Beals, Dr. Sandra Kahn, Dr. Serena Kassam, Dr. Megan McDougall, Dr. Pedro Santiago, Dr. Lindsay Schuster, and Dr. Ivy Yu. Several surgeons, including Dr. Seun Adetayo, Dr. Sharon (Ron) Aronovich, Dr. Oksana Jackson, Dr. Rohit Khosla, Dr. Richard Kirschner, Dr. Martha Matthews, Dr. Joyce McIntyre, Dr. John Mulliken, Dr. Stephen R. Sullivan, and Dr. Helena Taylor offered generous conversations and detailed feedback regarding cleft-lip repair, palate repair, team care, and more. Dr. Sarah Blaffer Hrdy, Dr. Nicola Marie Stock, and Dr. Ronald P. Strauss provided thoughtful, honest input, particularly on bonding and attachment. Speech-language pathologists Paul Austin,

Liza Catallozzi, Bridget Harrington, April Johnson, and Deborah Redfearn helped me understand the intricacies of speech and language. And Dr. Catherine Nowak and Lynn Schwartz offered detailed feedback just as this work was nearing a close.

I met most of the above-mentioned cleft-team professionals through my research for this book. A few of them have also treated my daughter. I am grateful to these individuals for their help with this project. But I thank them too—and others on the teams in Providence, New Haven, and Boston—for modeling a level of expert and compassionate care that I had never experienced before my daughter's diagnosis. Their examples have contributed to this book, indirectly and enormously.

Cleft advocates have lifted the lives of others, including mine. Anna Pileggi, of AboutFace, helped shape early chapters. Hugh Gillard and Zack Rodetis-Urenda offered lively conversations and ideas. Alyssa Hotes of the Global Smile Foundation, Kara Jackman of CCA Kids, and Pat Chibbaro of myFace/NYU Langone were generous with support and encouragement.

The American Cleft Palate-Craniofacial Association (ACPA) entered my life in 2012 when my daughter received an adorable stuffed bear in the mail. My appreciation for the organization ballooned in 2015 when I began working with cleft-team professionals on informational texts for families. The dedication and congeniality of the ACPA community is inspiring. Adam Levy offered thoughtful, thorough help with this project and a true sense of team spirit. And I am enormously grateful to Lynn Fox. Ever since I phoned Lynn to say, "I have an idea for a book," she has been a sounding board, mentor, enthusiastic lunch partner, reader, and friend (she's also the one who sent the bear).

I appreciate the good humor and warmth of cleft parents who have become friends, especially Meg O'Neil, co-conspirator in NAM taping, as well as Kenny Scott Guffey, himself a writer on this topic, and Tiffanie Guffey. Jen Gold provided thoughtful input at critical junctures.

Nickie Osborne at Hal Leonard and Megan Lanzotti at Sony/ATV helped secure permission to use material by the Beatles.

Maria Fong created the immaculate, thoughtful illustrations. And Jim Cooke's cover expresses the reassuring idea: that when things don't appear as expected, we can still find beauty and hope.

The staff at Luminare Press, including Patricia Marshall, Kim Harper-Kennedy, Sallie Vandagrift, and Kristen Brack, paid thoughtful and rigorous attention to this project every step of the way. And Catherine Rourke provided impeccable copyedits and kindhearted encouragement from afar (any errors that remain are my responsibility).

I am grateful to all of my extended family; I especially appreciate Bernard Mendillo, Tina and Steve Pollock, Jodi Lane, and the late Nancy LeClaire for their encouragement. And Dr. Emily Spurrell and the members of the "group" have been generous and supportive from the start of this project. I couldn't have started, continued, or finished this work without them.

Finally, Susan Dearing has read every word of this book and many more. She is a meticulous, curious, and astute developmental editor and a consummate grammarian, but also the kindest and gentlest of advisors. I cannot thank her enough.

I am grateful beyond words to my parents and sister. I am delighted beyond words by Zachary and Nadia. But while a parenting book undoubtedly reflects a writer's relationship with her parents and children, this one would not exist, nor would its journey have been nearly as fun or meaningful to undertake, without Ethan. I created this book to help other parents; I dedicate it, with love, to him.

References

Chapters 1–32

Interviews with Parents. Quotes and extended stories in this book that are not attributed to other sources draw from seventy-six anonymous, one- to two-hour phone interviews conducted by the author between June 2013 and September 2020. Interviewees were selected based on their self-identification as parents of children born with cleft lip and/or palate (CLP). Interviewees learned about the project via direct email inquiries from the author, unpaid inquiries by the author through private Facebook groups, word of mouth, recommendations from members of ACPA-approved cleft teams, and through the website www.parentsandclefts.com; all participated on a volunteer basis. Some interviewees participated in second, third, and fourth follow-up interviews during the interview period. All interviewees and the people they mentioned have been assigned pseudonyms to ensure anonymity; some genders of children have also been changed.

Interviews with Professionals. Quotes from professionals in this book that are not attributed to other sources draw from fifty-seven anonymous phone interviews and/or email correspondences conducted by the author between May 2013 and November 2021. Participants were selected based on their identification (via team websites) as members of ACPA-approved cleft teams in the US. Participants specialized in the fields of audiology, dentistry/ orthodontics, nursing, psychology, social work, speech-language pathology, surgery, and team coordination. Some participants engaged in second, third, and fourth follow-up interviews and/or correspondences during the research period. All were contacted initially by the author via phone or email. All participated on a volunteer basis.

Interviews with Others. A few quotes and stories in this book draw from anonymous, one- to two-hour phone interviews conducted by the author with individuals who self-identified as grandparents of children born with CLP as well as individuals born with CLP who were parented by a participant (a parent-interviewee). A few quotes in this book draw from anonymous interviews with professionals located outside the US and/or those who identified as specialists in fields outside cleft care, including perioperative nursing and advanced-practice registered nursing. All participated on a volunteer basis.

Chapter 1. Learning the News

ACPA Family Services Prenatal Diagnosis.pdf. Accessed February 26, 2020. https://cleftline.org/wp-content/uploads/2019/03/ACPA_booklet_prenatal.pdf

Costa, B., Williams, J. R., Martindale, A. & Stock, N. M. Parents' experiences of diagnosis and care following the birth of a child with cleft lip and/or palate. *Br. J. Midwifery* **27**, 151–160 (2019).

Cwir J. *I Wish I'd Known…How Much I'd Love You.*; 2018.

Flasher LV, Fogle PT. *Counseling Skills for Speech-Language Pathologists and Audiologists*. Cengage Learning; 2012.

Ford MD. Prenatal Diagnosis and Consultation. In: *Comprehensive Cleft Care: Family Edition*. Family Edition. CRC Press/Taylor & Francis Group; 2015:51-56.

Foundation for the Faces of Children. Videos. Understanding Cleft Lip and Palate: A Guide For New Parents. Foundation for the Faces of Children. Accessed February 26, 2020. https://facesofchildren.org/resources/videos/

Maier, S. F. & Seligman, M. E. P. Learned Helplessness at Fifty: Insights from Neuroscience. *Psychol. Rev.* **123**, 349–367 (2016).

McDonald-McGinn DM, DiCairano L, Mennuti M. Prenatal Genetic Counseling. In: Losee JE, Kirschner RE, Smith DM, Lawrence CR, Straub A, eds. *Comprehensive Cleft Care: Family Edition*. Family Edition. CRC Press/Taylor & Francis Group; 2015.

Miller AM. Children's Craniofacial Association: A Parent's Journey to Acceptance. http://www.ccakids.com/assets/one-sheet_journey2acceptance.pdf

Munabi NCO, Swanson J, Auslander A, Sanchez-Lara PA, Davidson Ward SL, Magee WP. The Prevalence of Congenital Heart Disease in Nonsyndromic Cleft Lip and/or Palate: A Systematic Review of the Literature. *Ann Plast Surg*. 2017; 79(2):214-220. doi:10.1097/SAP.0000000000001069

Philadelphia TCH of. The Comprehensive Prenatal Diagnostic Workup for Cleft Lip/Palate. Published June 4, 2020. Accessed June 9, 2021. https://www.chop.edu/news/comprehensive-prenatal-diagnostic-workup-cleft-lippalate

Sharp, Helen, PhD, CCC-SLP. Expecting the Unexpected. *ASHA Lead*. 2013;18:44-49. http://leader.pubs.asha.org/article.aspx?articleid=1788314

Stock NM, Costa B, Williams JR, Martindale A. Breaking the News: Parents' Experiences of Receiving an Antenatal Diagnosis of Cleft Lip. *Cleft Palate Craniofac J*. 2019; 56(9):1149-1156. doi:10.1177/1055665619830884

Stock, N. M., Costa, B., White, P. & Rumsey, N. Risk and Protective Factors for Psychological Distress in Families Following a Diagnosis of Cleft Lip and/or Palate. *Cleft Palate. Craniofac. J.* **57**, 88–98 (2020).

Chapter 2. Cleft Lip and Palate: Basics

ACPA Family Services: For-Parents-of-Newborns_2019.pdf.

ACPA Family Services: Your Baby's First Year_2021.pdf.

Chibbaro PD, Breen M. Nursing and Perioperative Care of the Child With Cleft Lip and Palate. In: Losee JE, Kirschner RE, Smith DM, Lawrence CR, Straub A, eds. *Comprehensive Cleft Care: Family Edition*. Family Edition. CRC Press/Taylor & Francis Group; 2015.

Gallagher R. An Exploration of Carers' Perceptions of Children's Well-Being During Treatment for Cleft Lip and/or Palate in the United Kingdom. In: Vol 58(4S). The Cleft Palate-Craniofacial Journal; 2021:86-87.

Gosain AK, Hollier LJ. Submucous Cleft Palate. In: Losee JE, Kirschner RE, Smith DM, Lawrence CR, Straub A, eds. *Comprehensive Cleft Care: Family Edition*. Family Edition. CRC Press/Taylor & Francis Group; 2015.

Kummer AW, Baylis AL, Bartley CK. Speech Assessment for Children With Cleft Lip and Palate. In: Losee JE, Kirschner RE, Smith DM, Lawrence CR, Straub A, eds. *Comprehensive Cleft Care: Family Edition*. Family Edition. CRC Press/Taylor & Francis Group; 2015.

McDonald-McGinn DM, DiCairano L, Mennuti M. Prenatal Genetic Counseling. In: Losee JE, Kirschner RE, Smith DM, Lawrence CR, Straub A, eds. *Comprehensive Cleft Care: Family Edition*. Family Edition. CRC Press/Taylor & Francis Group; 2015.

Chapter 3. Hindsight for New Parents

AboutFace Words That Work 2014.pdf.

Losee JE, Kirschner RE, Smith DM, Straub AE, Lawrence C, eds. *Comprehensive Cleft Care: Family Edition*. Family Edition. CRC Press/Taylor & Francis Group; 2015.

Stock NM, Martindale A, Cunniffe C, VTCT Foundation Research Team at the Centre for Appearance Research. #CleftProud: A Content Analysis and Online Survey of 2 Cleft Lip and Palate Facebook Groups. *Cleft Palate-Craniofacial J Off Publ Am Cleft Palate-Craniofacial Assoc*. 2018;55(10):1339-1349. doi:10.1177/1055665618764737

Chapter 4. Why Did This Happen?

ACPA Family Services Your Baby's First Year.pdf.

Brender Jean D., Weyer Peter J., Romitti Paul A., et al. Prenatal Nitrate Intake from Drinking Water and Selected Birth Defects in Offspring of Participants in the National Birth Defects Prevention Study. *Environ Health Perspect*. 2013;121(9):1083-1089. doi:10.1289/ehp.1206249

Cedergren DM, Källén DB. Maternal Obesity and the Risk for Orofacial Clefts in the Offspring: *Cleft Palate Craniofac J*. Published online December 15, 2017. doi:10.1597/04-012.1

Cleft Palate Foundation Genetics and You_2008.pdf. Accessed March 30, 2020. https://cleftline.org/wp-content/uploads/2018/05/GEN-01.pdf

E-cigarette aerosol exposure can cause craniofacial defects in Xenopus laevis embryos and mammalian neural crest cells. Accessed March 30, 2020. https://journals.plos.org/plosone/article?id=10.1371/journal.pone.0185729

Facts about Cleft Lip and Cleft Palate | CDC. Accessed March 30, 2020. https://www.cdc.gov/ncbddd/birthdefects/cleftlip.html

Folic acid supplements and risk of facial clefts: national population based case-control study | The BMJ. Accessed March 30, 2020. https://www.bmj.com/content/334/7591/464

Genetic Testing - NFED. *National Foundation for Ectodermal Dysplasias* https://www.nfed.org/learn/diagnosis/genetic-testing/.

Gestational diabetes and risk of orofacial cleft birth defects and fetal programming of obesity and diabetes mellitus in offspring – Utah State University. Accessed March 30, 2020. https://portal.nifa.usda.gov/web/crisprojectpages/1009718-gestational-diabetes-and-risk-of-orofacial-cleft-birth-defects-and-fetal-programming-of-obesity-and-diabetes-mellitus-in-offspring.html

Glow K. I Have a Son With Autism, and I Sympathize With the Anti-Vaccine Movement – SheKnows. Accessed March 30, 2020. https://www.sheknows.com/parenting/articles/1117211/robert-de-niro-vaccine-movie/

Hughes S, Grote L, Kaye A. Genetics 101: A Primer in Cleft and Craniofacial Genetics for the Non-Genetics Provider. In: Vol 58(4S). The Cleft Palate-Craniofacial Journal; 2021:90.

Hutson MR, Keyte AL, Hernández-Morales M, et al. Temperature-activated ion channels in neural crest cells confer maternal fever–associated birth defects. *Sci Signal.* 2017; 10(500). doi:10.1126/scisignal.aal4055

Kutbi H, Wehby GL, Moreno Uribe LM, et al. Maternal underweight and obesity and risk of orofacial clefts in a large international consortium of population-based studies. *Int J Epidemiol.* 2017; 46(1):190-199. doi:10.1093/ije/dyw035

McDonald-McGinn DM, DiCairano L, Mennuti M. Prenatal Genetic Counseling. In: Losee JE, Kirschner RE, Smith DM, Lawrence CR, Straub A, eds. *Comprehensive Cleft Care: Family Edition.* Family Edition. CRC Press/Taylor & Francis Group; 2015.

Reference GH. What does it mean to have a genetic predisposition to a disease? Genetics Home Reference. Accessed March 30, 2020. https://ghr.nlm.nih.gov/primer/mutationsanddisorders/predisposition

Reference GH. What is a Chromosome? Genetics Home Reference. Accessed April 26, 2020. https://ghr.nlm.nih.gov/primer/basics/chromosome

Stock MNM, Rumsey DN. Starting a Family: The Experience of Parents with Cleft Lip and/or Palate: *Cleft Palate Craniofac J*. Published online July 1, 2015. doi:10.1597/13-314

Chapter 5. Early News: Gift or Burden?

Adisen's Financial Assistance Testimonial. Children's Craniofacial Association. Accessed March 31, 2020. https://ccakids.org/adisen.html

Aspinall, Cassandra L. Dealing with the prenatal diagnosis of clefting: a parent's perspective. *Cleft Palate-Craniofacial J Off Publ Am Cleft Palate-Craniofacial Assoc*. 2002;39(2):183-187. doi:10.1597/1545-1569(2002)039<0183:dwtpdo>2.0.co;2

Deramo P, Biaggi-Ondina A, Cepeda A, Nguyen P, Greives M. Survey of Maternal Post-Partum Depression in Infants with Cleft Lip and/or Palate. In: Vol 58(4S). The Cleft Palate-Craniofacial Journal; 2021:20.

Grollemund B, Dissaux C, Gavelle P, et al. The impact of having a baby with cleft lip and palate on parents and on parent-baby relationship: the first French prospective multicentre study. *BMC Pediatr*. 2020;20(1):230. doi:10.1186/s12887-020-02118-5

Sreejith VP, Arun V, Devarajan AP, Gopinath A, Sunil M. Psychological Effect of Prenatal Diagnosis of Cleft Lip and Palate: A Systematic Review. *Contemp Clin Dent*. 2018; 9(2):304-308. doi:10.4103/ccd.ccd_673_17

Tierney, S., Blackhurst, M., Scahill, R. & Callery, P. Loss and rebuilding: A qualitative study of late diagnosis of cleft palate. *J. Spec. Pediatr. Nurs. JSPN* **20**, 280–289 (2015).

Chapter 6. Early News: What's Next?

Bright Horizons Family Solutions. Helping Children Deal with Change and Stress. Accessed April 2, 2020. https://www.brighthorizons.com/family-resources/helping-children-deal-with-change-and-stress

Peck C, Parsaei Y, Lattanzi J, et al. Accessing Cleft Care in the United States: A Nationwide Geospatial Analysis of 1-Hour Access to ACPA Certified Cleft Teams. In: Vol 58(4S). The Cleft Palate-Craniofacial Journal; 2021:34.

Transitions for Children: Helping Children Change Activities. Raising Children Network. Accessed July 3, 2020. https://raisingchildren.net.au/preschoolers/behaviour/behaviour-management-tips-tools/transitions

Videos – Foundation for the Faces of Children. Accessed April 2, 2020. https://facesofchildren.org/resources/videos/#vid1

Chapter 7. Team Care: The WHAT and the WHY

Chibbaro PD, Breen M. Nursing and Perioperative Care of the Child With Cleft Lip and Palate. In: Losee JE, Kirschner RE, Smith DM, Lawrence CR, Straub A, eds. *Comprehensive Cleft Care: Family Edition*. Family Edition. CRC Press/Taylor & Francis Group; 2015.

Chibbaro PD, Breen M. Nursing and Perioperative Care of the Child with Cleft Lip and Palate. In: Losee JE, Kirschner RE, eds. *Comprehensive Cleft Care*. Second Edition. Thieme Medical Publishers, Incorporated; 2015:57-82.

Fox LM. Fundamentals of Team Care. In: Losee JE, Kirschner RE, Smith DM, Lawrence CR, Straub A, eds. *Comprehensive Cleft Care: Family Edition*. Family Edition. CRC Press/Taylor & Francis Group; 2015.

Peck C, Parsaei Y, Lattanzi J, et al. Accessing Cleft Care in the United States: A Nationwide Geospatial Analysis of 1-Hour Access to ACPA Certified Cleft Teams. In: Vol 58(4S). The Cleft Palate-Craniofacial Journal; 2021:34.

Philadelphia TCH of. Feeding Your Baby with Cleft Palate. Published May 5, 2014. Accessed May 9, 2020. https://www.chop.edu/health-resources/feeding-your-baby-cleft-palate

Chapter 8. Considering a Cleft Team?

ACPA Family Services Paying-for-Treatment.pdf. Accessed May 5, 2020. https://cleftline.org/wp-content/uploads/2019/11/Paying-for-Treatment.pdf

ACPA Family Services Preparing for Surgery_2019.pdf. Accessed May 6, 2020. https://cleftline.org/wp-content/uploads/2019/07/Preparing-for-Surgery.pdf

Cooper DC, Peterson EC, Grellner CG, et al. Cleft and Craniofacial Multidisciplinary Team Clinic: A Look at Attrition Rates for Patients With Complete Cleft Lip and Palate and Nonsyndromic Single-Suture Craniosynostosis. *Cleft Palate-Craniofacial J Off Publ Am Cleft Palate-Craniofacial Assoc.* 2019; 56(10):1287-1294. doi:10.1177/1055665619856245

Crerand CE, Heppner C, Hansen-Moore J, Sandberg DE. Shared Decision Making in Craniofacial Care. In: Vol 58(4S). The Cleft Palate-Craniofacial Journal; 2021:83.

Donations. Mia Moo. Accessed July 8, 2021. https://miamoo.org/collections/donations

Fox LM. Fundamentals of Team Care. In: Losee JE, Kirschner RE, Smith DM, Lawrence CR, Straub A, eds. *Comprehensive Cleft Care: Family Edition.* Family Edition. CRC Press/Taylor & Francis Group; 2015.

Globe TB. Clash in the name of care - A Boston Globe Spotlight Team Report. BostonGlobe.com. Accessed July 1, 2021. http://bo.st/1MLWmPp

How Many Years of Postgraduate Training do Surgical Residents Undergo? American College of Surgeons. Accessed April 14, 2020. https://www.facs.org/education/resources/medical-students/faq/training

Lee J, Skolnick G, Naidoo S, Snyder-Warwick A, Patel K. Cost of Cleft-Craniofacial Team Care. In: Vol 58(4S). The Cleft Palate-Craniofacial Journal; 2021:87.

Livingston EH. Overlapping Surgery and Perioperative Outcomes. *JAMA.* 2019;321(8):772. doi:10.1001/jama.2019. 1123

Standards of Approval for Team Care. ACPA. Accessed April 20, 2020. https://acpa-cpf.org/team-care/standardscat/standards-of-approval-for-team-care/

Theriault B, Pazniokas J, Mittal A, et al. What Does it Mean for a Surgeon to "Run Two Rooms"? A Comprehensive Literature Review of Overlapping and Concurrent Surgery Policies. *Am Surg*. 2019;85(4):420-430.

Weidler E, Britto M, Sitzman T. Barriers and Facilitators to Implementation of Standardized Outcome Measurements for Children with Cleft Lip and Palate. In: Vol 58(4S). The Cleft Palate-Craniofacial Journal; 2021:65-66.

Chapter 9. Birth! What's Next? A Hospital Reference

Chibbaro PD, Breen M. Nursing and Perioperative Care of the Child With Cleft Lip and Palate. In: Losee JE, Kirschner RE, Smith DM, Lawrence CR, Straub A, eds. *Comprehensive Cleft Care: Family Edition*. Family Edition. CRC Press/Taylor & Francis Group; 2015.

Chibbaro PD, Breen M. Nursing and Perioperative Care of the Child with Cleft Lip and Palate. In: Losee JE, Kirschner RE, eds. *Comprehensive Cleft Care*. Second Edition. Thieme Medical Publishers, Incorporated; 2015:57-82.

Philadelphia TCH of. Feeding Your Baby with Cleft Palate. Published May 5, 2014. Accessed May 9, 2020. https://www.chop.edu/health-resources/feeding-your-baby-cleft-palate

Chapter 10. Birth and the NICU: Speaking Up for Appropriate Care

ACPA Family Services Tips-for-Hospital-Nurseries-2017.pdf. Accessed April 26, 2022. https://acpa-cpf.org/wp-content/uploads/2018/05/Tips-for-Hospital-Nurseries-2017.pdf

Chibbaro P, Barzilai J, Breen M. Nursing Care of the Patient with Cleft Lip and Palate. In: Losee JE, Kirschner RE, eds. *Comprehensive Cleft Care*. McGraw-Hill Medical; 2009.

Chibbaro PD, Breen M. Nursing and Perioperative Care of the Child with Cleft Lip and Palate. In: Losee JE, Kirschner RE, eds. *Comprehensive Cleft Care*. Second Edition. Thieme Medical Publishers, Incorporated; 2015:57-82.

Chibbaro PD, Breen M. Nursing and Perioperative Care of the Child With Cleft Lip and Palate. In: Losee JE, Kirschner RE, Smith DM, Lawrence CR, Straub A, eds. *Comprehensive Cleft Care: Family Edition*. Family Edition. CRC Press/Taylor & Francis Group; 2015.

Chapter 11. Birth and Bonding

CDC. Real Stories: Living With Cleft Lip and Palate | CDC. Centers for Disease Control and Prevention. Published May 16, 2017. Accessed May 13, 2020. https://www.cdc.gov/ncbddd/birthdefects/stories/cleftlip.html

Collett BR, Speltz ML. Social-Emotional Development of Infants and Young Children With Orofacial Clefts: *Infants Young Child*. 2006; 19(4):262-291. doi:10.1097/00001163-200610000-00002

Crerand CE, Heppner CE. Psychological and Behavioral Considerations. In: Losee JE, Kirschner RE, Smith DM, Lawrence CR, Straub A, eds. *Comprehensive Cleft Care: Family Edition*. CRC Press/Taylor & Francis Group; 2015:95-104.

Deramo P, Biaggi-Ondina A, Cepeda A, Nguyen P, Greives M. Survey of Maternal Post-Partum Depression in Infants with Cleft Lip and/or Palate. In: Vol 58(4S). The Cleft Palate-Craniofacial Journal; 2021:20.

Grollemund B, Dissaux C, Gavelle P, et al. The impact of having a baby with cleft lip and palate on parents and on parent-baby relationship: the first French prospective multicentre study. *BMC Pediatr*. 2020; 20(1):230. doi:10.1186/s12887-020-02118-5

Habersaat S, Monnier M, Peter C, et al. Early Mother-Child Interaction and Later Quality of Attachment in Infants With an Orofacial Cleft Compared to Infants Without Cleft. *Cleft Palate-Craniofacial J Off Publ Am Cleft Palate-Craniofacial Assoc*. 2013; 50:704-712. doi:10.1597/12-094.1

HelpGuide.org. Creating Secure Infant Attachment - HelpGuide.org. https://www.helpguide.org. Published November 2, 2018. Accessed May 13, 2020. https://www.helpguide.org/articles/parenting-family/creating-secure-infant-attachment-video.htm

Hrdy SB. *Mother Nature: Maternal Instincts and How They Shape the Human Species*. 1st Ballantine Books ed. Ballantine Books; 2000.

Rumsey N, Stock NM. Living With a Cleft: Psychological Challenges, Support and Intervention. In: Berkowitz S, ed. *Cleft Lip and Palate: Diagnosis and Management.* Third Edition. Springer Science & Business Media; 2013.

Solomon A. *Far From The Tree: Parents, Children, and The Search For Identity.* 1st Scribner hardcover ed. Scribner; 2012.

Chapter 13. The Bottles: A Tour of Cleft-Palate Feeders

ACPA Family Services Feeding Your Baby_2018.pdf. Accessed May 20, 2020. https://cleftline.org/wp-content/uploads/2019/03/Feeding-Your-Baby-Online-2018.pdf

Cleft Advocate - Feeders. Accessed May 20, 2020. http://www.cleftadvocate.org/feeders.html

Cleftopedia Cleft Lip Bottles. Accessed May 20, 2020. http://www.cleftopedia.com/special-feeders/cleftbottles/

Dr. Brown's Medical: Specialty Feeding System Assembly and Cleaning Instructions and Other Info. Accessed May 20, 2020. https://images-na.ssl-images-amazon.com/images/I/71hJLoGF5NL.pdf

Mead Johnson Cleft Lip/Palate Nurser | Anyone have tips for caps? - *BabyCenter.* Accessed May 20, 2020. https://community.babycenter.com/post/a27935789/mead_johnson_cleft_lippalate_nurser_anyone_have_tips_for_caps

Thaete K, Fetter B, Chesser C, Huff H, Kaye A. Nutritional Challenges in Oral Clefting: A Multidisciplinary Approach to Support Growth and Avoid Malnutrition in the Neonatal and Perioperative Periods. In: Vol 58(4S). The Cleft Palate-Craniofacial Journal; 2021:90.

Chapter 14. Lunch Is On: How to Feed This Baby

ACPA Family Services Feeding-Your-Baby-Online-2018.pdf. Accessed May 23, 2020. https://cleftline.org/wp-content/uploads/2019/03/Feeding-Your-Baby-Online-2018.pdf

Baby's Hunger Cues | WIC Breastfeeding. Accessed May 20, 2020. https://wicbreastfeeding.fns.usda.gov/babys-hunger-cues

Chibbaro P, Barzilai J, Breen M. Nursing Care of the Patient with Cleft Lip and Palate. In: Losee JE, Kirschner RE, eds. *Comprehensive Cleft Care*. McGraw-Hill Medical; 2009.

Cleft Feeding Instructions. Seattle Children's Hospital. Accessed July 20, 2021. https://www.seattlechildrens.org/clinics/craniofacial/patient-family-resources/cleft-feeding-instructions/

Goodwyn-Craine A. Bottle-Feeding Strategies for Infants with Cleft Lip and/or Palate. *Lead Live*. Published online January 27, 2021. Accessed July 21, 2021. https://leader.pubs.asha.org/do/10.1044/2021-0127-cleft-palate-bottle-feeding/full/

HopkinsMedicine.Org: Feeding Guide for the First Year. Accessed May 23, 2020. https://www.hopkinsmedicine.org/health/wellness-and-prevention/feeding-guide-for-the-first-year

Infant reflux - Symptoms and causes. Mayo Clinic. Accessed May 23, 2020. https://www.mayoclinic.org/diseases-conditions/infant-acid-reflux/symptoms-causes/syc-20351408

Koltz PF, Albino FP, Hyatt B, Fargione RA, Katzel E, Girotto JA. Incidence of use of acid suppression medications in infants with oral clefting. *Cleft Palate-Craniofacial J Off Publ Am Cleft Palate-Craniofacial Assoc*. 2010;47(5):530-533. doi:10.1597/09-165

Symptoms & Causes of GER & GERD in Infants | NIDDK. National Institute of Diabetes and Digestive and Kidney Diseases. Accessed May 23, 2020. https://www.niddk.nih.gov/health-information/digestive-diseases/acid-reflux-ger-gerd-infants/symptoms-causes

Syndrome TF on SID. SIDS and Other Sleep-Related Infant Deaths: Updated 2016 Recommendations for a Safe Infant Sleeping Environment. *Pediatrics*. 2016;138(5). doi:10.1542/peds.2016-2938

Chapter 15. But I Had Planned to Breast-Feed!

ACPA Family Services Feeding Your Baby_2018.pdf. Accessed May 20, 2020. https://cleftline.org/wp-content/uploads/2019/03/Feeding-Your-Baby-Online-2018.pdf

Collett BR, Speltz ML. Social-Emotional Development of Infants and Young Children With Orofacial Clefts: *Infants Young Child*. 2006; 19(4):262-291. doi:10.1097/00001163-200610000-00002

Despars DJ, Peter DC, Borghini DA, et al. Impact of a Cleft Lip and/ or Palate on Maternal Stress and Attachment Representations: *Cleft Palate Craniofac J.* Published online July 1, 2011. doi:10.1597/08-190

Grollemund B, Dissaux C, Gavelle P, et al. The impact of having a baby with cleft lip and palate on parents and on parent-baby relationship: the first French prospective multicentre study. *BMC Pediatr.* 2020; 20(1):230. doi:10.1186/s12887-020-02118-5

Jessica Burfield. No More Crying Over Spilled Milk. Madison Mom. Published April 30, 2014. Accessed June 25, 2020. https://madisonmom. com/no-more-crying-over-spilled-milk/

Rumsey N, Stock NM. Living With a Cleft: Psychological Challenges, Support, and Intervention. In: Berkowitz S, ed. *Cleft Lip and Palate: Diagnosis and Management.* Third Edition. Springer Science & Business Media; 2013.

Chapter 16. What's for Dinner?

Baker, R. D. & Baker, S. S. Need for Infant Formula : Journal of Pediatric Gastroenterology and Nutrition. *Journal of Pediatric Gastroenterology and Nutrition* 62, 2–4 (2016).

Barrera CM, Kawwass JF, Boulet SL, Nelson JM, Perrine CG. Fertility treatment use and breastfeeding outcomes. *Am J Obstet Gynecol.* 2019; 220(3):261.e1-261.e7. doi:10.1016/j.ajog.2018.11.1100

Colen CG, Ramey DM. Is Breast Truly Best? Estimating the Effects of Breastfeeding on Long-Term Child Health and Wellbeing in the United States Using Sibling Comparisons. *Soc Sci Med.* 2014; 109:55-65. doi:10.1016/j.socscimed.2014.01.027

Eckhardt KW, Hendershot GE. Analysis of the reversal in breast feeding trends in the early 1970s. *Public Health Rep Wash DC 1974.* 1984;99(4):410-415.

Edwards J. Tips and Tricks Guide to Exclusively Pumping by Sylvia Noyes. The Global Big Latch On. Accessed June 30, 2020. https://biglatchon. org/a-tips-and-tricks-guide-to-exclusively-pumping-by-sylvia-noyes/

Girard L-C, Doyle O, Tremblay RE. Breastfeeding, Cognitive and Noncognitive Development in Early Childhood: A Population Study. *Pediatrics.* 2017; 139(4):e20161848. doi:10.1542/peds.2016-1848

Jacobson M. The Rise of the "Fed Is Best" Campaign. *ParentMap*. Published online May 30, 2019. Accessed with_mean_people July 1, 2020. https://www.parentmap.com/article/rise-fed-best-campaign

Kaye A, Cattaneo C, Huff HM, Staggs VS. A Pilot Study of Mothers' Breastfeeding Experiences in Infants With Cleft Lip and/or Palate. *Adv Neonatal Care Off J Natl Assoc Neonatal Nurses*. 2019; 19(2):127-137. doi:10.1097/ANC.0000000000000551

Kounang, N. Study shows no long-term cognitive benefit to breastfeeding - CNN. *CNN Health* https://www.cnn.com/2017/03/27/health/breastfeeding-hyperactivity/index.html.

Moossavi S, Sepehri S, Robertson B, et al. Composition and Variation of the Human Milk Microbiota Are Influenced by Maternal and Early-Life Factors. *Cell Host Microbe*. 2019; 25(2):324-335.e4. doi:10.1016/j.chom.2019.01.011

Nommsen-Rivers LA, Chantry CJ, Peerson JM, Cohen RJ, Dewey KG. Delayed Onset of Lactogenesis Among First-Time Mothers is Related to Maternal Obesity and Factors Associated With Ineffective Breastfeeding. *Am J Clin Nutr*. 2010; 92(3):574-584. doi:10.3945/ajcn.2010.29192

Office of the Surgeon General AS for H (ASH). Breastfeeding Reports And Publications. HHS.gov. Published March 29, 2019. Accessed June 30, 2020. https://www.hhs.gov/surgeongeneral/reports-and-publications/breastfeeding/index.html

Radzyminski S, Callister LC. Health Professionals' Attitudes and Beliefs About Breastfeeding. *J Perinat Educ*. 2015; 24(2):102-109. doi:10.1891/1058-1243.24.2.102

Sample Pumping Schedules. Exclusive Pumping. Published September 15, 2019. Accessed June 30, 2020. https://exclusivepumping.com/sample-pumping-schedules/

Shaffer A, Ford M, Choi S, Jabbour N. The Impact of Breast Milk on Tympanostomy Tube Sequelae in Children with Cleft Palate. In: *2017 Oral Presentations Abstracts*. Vol 54(3). The Cleft Palate-Craniofacial Journal; 2017:e67.

Shaffer A, Ford M, Tobey A, et al. Impact of Breast Milk Feeding on Early Otologic Outcomes in Children with Cleft Palate. In: Vol 58(4S). The Cleft Palate-Craniofacial Journal; 2021:27.

Stanway P, Stanway A. *Breast Is Best: A Common Sense Approach to Breastfeeding*. Pan Books; 1978.

Thaete K, Fetter B, Chesser C, Huff H, Kaye A. Nutritional Challenges in Oral Clefting: A Multidisciplinary Approach to Support Growth and Avoid Malnutrition in the Neonatal and Perioperative Periods. In: Vol 58(4S). The Cleft Palate-Craniofacial Journal; 2021:90.

Stortz, A. Why Choosing to Formula Feed Was The Best Decision I Made As A New Mom. https://medium.com/@xoxoadrienne/why-choosing-to-formula-feed-was-the-best-decision-i-made-as-a-new-mom-9b220803ea4f.

Chapter 17. What to Say?

ACPA Family Services For Parents of Newborns_2017.pdf. Accessed July 21, 2020. https://cleftline.org/wp-content/uploads/2018/05/For-Parents-of-Newborns-2017.pdf

Blitz A, Chibbaro P, Russell J, Zuckerberg D. Panel Workshop for Parents/Caregivers: Advocacy for School Age Children with Craniofacial Conditions. In: Vol 58(4S). The Cleft Palate-Craniofacial Journal; 2021:93.

Deramo P, Biaggi-Ondina A, Cepeda A, Nguyen P, Greives M. Survey of Maternal Post-Partum Depression in Infants with Cleft Lip and/or Palate. In: Vol 58(4S). The Cleft Palate-Craniofacial Journal; 2021:20.

Foster L. Mental Health America of Central Carolinas. Suicide Prevention/Mental Health Crisis Resource Guide. https://www.healthycharlottealliance.org/wp-content/uploads/2019/10/mh-resourceguide.pdf

Huitt, W. (2009). Empathetic listening. Educational Psychology Interactive. Valdosta, GA: Valdosta State University. Accessed July 17, 2020. http://www.edpsycinteractive.org/topics/process/listen.html

Lun J, Kesebir S, Oishi S. On Feeling Understood and Feeling Well: The Role of Interdependence. *J Res Personal*. 2008; 42(6):1623-1628. doi:10.1016/j.jrp.2008.06.009

Morelli SA, Torre JB, Eisenberger NI. The Neural Bases of Feeling Understood and Not Understood. *Soc Cogn Affect Neurosci*. 2014; 9(12):1890-1896. doi:10.1093/scan/nst191

Plante Ph.D., ABPP TG. Giving People Advice Rarely Works, This Does. Psychology Today. Accessed July 20, 2020. http://www.psychologytoday. com/blog/do-the-right-thing/201407/giving-people-advice-rarely-works-does

Silk S, Goldman B. Ring Theory: How Not to Say the Wrong Thing - Los Angeles Times. Accessed July 20, 2020. https://www.latimes.com/opinion/ op-ed/la-xpm-2013-apr-07-la-oe-0407-silk-ring-theory-20130407-story.html

Steindl C, Jonas E, Sittenthaler S, Traut-Mattausch E, Greenberg J. Understanding Psychological Reactance. *Z Psychol*. 2015;223(4):205-214. doi:10.1027/2151-2604/a000222

Video: Foundation for the Faces of Children. Foundation for the Faces of Children. Accessed May 23, 2020. https://facesofchildren.org/ resources/videos/

Chapter 18. Why Photos?

Calder's Smile Story | Cleft Lip & Palate Foundation of Smiles. Accessed July 15, 2020. http://www.cleftsmile.org/calders-smile/

Foundation for the Faces of Children. Videos. Understanding Cleft Lip and Palate: A Guide for New Parents. Foundation for the Faces of Children. Accessed February 26, 2020. https://facesofchildren.org/ resources/videos/

Oswalt, MSW A. Early Childhood Emotional and Social Development: Identity and Self-Esteem. GulfBendCenter.org. Accessed July 17, 2020. https://www.gulfbend.org/poc/view_doc.php?type=doc&id=12766

Reschke K. Who am I? Developing a Sense of Self and Belonging. *ZERO THREE J*. Published online January 2019. https://www.zerotothree.org/ resources/2648-who-am-i-developing-a-sense-of-self-and-belonging

Wide Smiles. Pre-Surgical Photos: Yes or No. Published 1996. Accessed July 15, 2020. http://www.widesmiles2.org/cleftlinks/WS-339.html

Chapter 19. Supermarket Stories: Baby in Public

Blitz A, Chibbaro P, Russell J, Zuckerberg D. Panel Workshop for Parents/ Caregivers: Advocacy for School Age Children with Craniofacial Conditions. In: Vol 58(4S). The Cleft Palate-Craniofacial Journal; 2021:93.

Carter, Ph.D. C. How to Deal with Mean People | Greater Good. Accessed July 10, 2020. https://greatergood.berkeley.edu/article/item/how_to_deal_

Center for Adoption Support and Education. C.A.S.E. - Nurture, Inspire, Empower. https://adoptionsupport.org/

Dealing with Insensitive Comments about Your Child | Parent Companion | For parents of children with disabilities in Texas. Parent Companion. Accessed July 9, 2020. http://www.parentcompanion.org/article/dealing-with-insensitive-comments-about-your-child

Ebert, M.A., Ed.M, Ph.D candidate M. Strategies for Responding to Rude Comments About Your Child's Behavior. Stages Learning. Accessed July 9, 2020. http://blog.stageslearning.com/blog/strategies-for-responding-to-rude-comments-about-your-childs-behavior

Foulk, Ph.D. candidate TA. Rudeness on the Brain: Why Rudeness Is So Pervasive, and How One Rude Event Can Have Long Lasting Effects. Published 2017. Accessed July 13, 2020. https://ufdc.ufl.edu/UFE0050836/00001

Gray DE. 'Everybody Just Freezes. Everybody is Just Embarrassed:' Felt and Enacted Stigma Among Parents of Children With High Functioning Autism. *Sociol Health Illn.* 2002;24(6):734-749. doi:10.1111/1467-9566.00316

Konnikova M. The Psychology of Online Comments | The New Yorker. Accessed July 13, 2020. https://www.newyorker.com/tech/annals-of-technology/the-psychology-of-online-comments

Singer E. The "W.I.S.E. Up!" tool: empowering adopted children to cope with questions and comments about adoption. *Pediatr Nurs.* 2010;36(4):209-212.

W.I.S.E. Up! Center for Adoption Support and Education C.A.S.E. - Nurture, Inspire, Empower. https://adoptionsupport.org/w-s-e-giving-adopted-kids-simple-tools-answer-tough-questions/

Whitson LSW,C-SSWS S. Is It Rude, Is It Mean, Or Is It Bullying? Psychology Today. Accessed July 13, 2020. http://www.psychologytoday.com/blog/passive-aggressive-diaries/201211/is-it-rude-is-it-mean-or-is-it-bullying

Chapter 20. The Clinic Visit

Children's Craniofacial Association: Parents: You Are the Official Care Manager! Accessed July 9, 2020. http://www.ccakids.com/assets/one-sheet_parentscaremgr.pdf

Dell'Antonia K. Your Face Is Beautiful -- Do You Want It to Change? Well.NYTimes.com. Published May 30, 2016. Accessed July 9, 2020. https://well.blogs.nytimes.com/2016/05/30/your-face-is-beautiful-do-you-want-it-to-change/

Myhre A, Agai M, Dundas I, Feragen KB. "All Eyes on Me": A Qualitative Study of Parent and Patient Experiences of Multidisciplinary Care in Craniofacial Conditions. *Cleft Palate Craniofac J.* 2019; 56(9):1187-1194. doi:10.1177/1055665619842730

Chapter 21. Early Hearing and Speech

16-Gestures-x16-Months Developed by the FIRST WORDS® Project 2014 Florida State University.pdf. Accessed October 22, 2021. https://firstwordsproject.com/wp-content/uploads/2018/02/16-Gestures-x16-Months.pdf

AAP Schedule of Well-Child Care Visits. HealthyChildren.org. Accessed March 17, 2021. https://www.healthychildren.org/English/family-life/health-management/Pages/Well-Child-Care-A-Check-Up-for-Success.aspx

ACPA Family Services For Parents of Newborns_2017.pdf. Accessed July 21, 2020. https://cleftline.org/wp-content/uploads/2018/05/For-Parents-of-Newborns-2017.pdf

ACPA Family Services Help With Hearing 2018.pdf. Accessed April 20, 2020. https://cleftline.org/wp-content/uploads/2018/12/ACPA_booklet_helpwithhearing_web.pdf

ACPA Family Services SchoolAgedChild-2018.pdf. Accessed April 10, 2021. https://acpa-cpf.org/wp-content/uploads/2018/08/ACPA_booklet_SchoolAgedChild-2018.pdf

ACPA Family Services Speech Development_2017.pdf. Accessed May 6, 2020. https://cleftline.org/wp-content/uploads/2018/05/Speech-2017.pdf

ACPA Family Services Your Baby's First Year.pdf.

American Academy of Otolaryngology Head and Neck Surgery Foundation: Understanding Ear Fluid. Accessed February 26, 2021. https://www.entnet.org/sites/default/files/uploads/PracticeManagement/Resources/_files/patient_info_sheet_-_understanding_ear_fluid-3_0.pdf

Birth to One Year. American Speech-Language-Hearing Association. Accessed March 29, 2021. https://www.asha.org/public/speech/development/01/

Carey B. Talking directly to toddlers strengthens their language skills, Stanford research shows. Stanford University. Published October 15, 2013. Accessed April 2, 2021. http://news.stanford.edu/news/2013/october/fernald-vocab-development-101513.html

CDC. Newborn Hearing Screening | Parent's Guide to Hearing Loss | CDC. Centers for Disease Control and Prevention. Published May 26, 2020. Accessed March 3, 2021. https://www.cdc.gov/ncbddd/hearingloss/parentsguide/understanding/newbornhearingscreening.html

Cleft Lip and Palate. CHLA. Published May 13, 2015. Accessed March 21, 2020. https://www.chla.org/cleft-lip-and-palate

Cohen, SLP S. Better Hearing and Speech Month. myFace. Published May 18, 2017. Accessed January 8, 2021. https://www.myface.org/better-hearing-and-speech-month/

Cwir J. *I Wish I'd Known…How Much I'd Love You*.; 2018.

Daniel A, Duncan F, Fitzsimons D. Hearing Outcomes in Children with Orofacial Clefting: Implications for Management. In: Vol 58(4S). The Cleft Palate-Craniofacial Journal; 2021:1-2.

DeLuca K. Involving All Adults in Treatment After a Toddler's Cleft Palate Surgery. The ASHA Leader. doi:10.1044/leader.OTP.25032020.36

Early Speech Development in Children With a Cleft Palate. Seattle Children's Hospital Patient and Family Education. Aug2019.pdf. Accessed March 31, 2021. https://www.seattlechildrens.org/globalassets/documents/for-patients-and-families/pfe/pe1706.pdf

Grames LM. Speech Therapy for Children with Cleft Palate. In: *Comprehensive Cleft Care: Family Edition*. Family Edition. CRC Press/Taylor & Francis Group; 2015.

Hardin-Jones M, Chapman K, Scherer NJ. Early Intervention in Children with Cleft Palate. The ASHA Leader. shorturl.at/qvyV1

Hardin-Jones MA, Chapman KL, Scherer NJ. *Children with Cleft Lip and Palate: A Parents' Guide to Early Speech-Language Development and Treatment*. Woodbine House; 2015.

Jabbour N. Hearing Disorders. In: Losee JE, Kirschner RE, Smith DM, Lawrence CR, Straub A, eds. *Comprehensive Cleft Care: Family Edition*. Family Edition. CRC Press/Taylor & Francis Group; 2015.

Kummer AW, Baylis AL, Bartley CK. Speech Assessment for Children With Cleft Lip and Palate. In: Losee JE, Kirschner RE, Smith DM, Lawrence CR, Straub A, eds. *Comprehensive Cleft Care: Family Edition.* Family Edition. CRC Press/Taylor & Francis Group; 2015.

Kummer AW. A Pediatrician's Guide to Communication Disorders Secondary to Cleft Lip/Palate. *Pediatr Clin North Am.* 2018; 65(1):31-46. doi:10.1016/j.pcl.2017.08.019

Kummer, PhD, CCC-SLP AW. Cleft Lip and Palate: Effects on Communication Development. Presented at the: Cincinnati, OH. https://cchmcstream.cchmc.org/mediasiteex/Play/0d39c24d-d16c-4826-a8f6-58a364171dde

Kuo C-L. Glue Ear in Children with Cleft Lip and Palate: An Update. *CMT.* 2018;1(1). doi:10.24983/scitemed.cmt.2018.00062

Lous J, Burton MJ, Felding J, Ovesen T, Rovers M, Williamson I. Grommets (ventilation tubes) for hearing loss associated with otitis media with effusion in children. *Cochrane Database of Systematic Reviews.* 2005;(1). doi:10.1002/14651858.CD001801.pub2

Lucille Packard Children's Hospital. Handout: Tips for Early Speech Stimulation. 2014.

McAndrew L. Parental Judgement of Hearing Loss in Infants With Cleft Palate. *The Cleft Palate-Craniofacial Journal.* 2020; 57(7):886-894. doi:10.1177/1055665619899743

Parameters For Evaluation and Treatment of Patients With Cleft Lip/Palate or Other Craniofacial Differences. *The Cleft Palate-Craniofacial Journal.* 2018; 55(1):137-156. doi:10.1177/1055665617739564

Philadelphia TCH of. Ear Tubes. Published June 16, 2015. Accessed March 8, 2021. https://www.chop.edu/conditions-diseases/ear-tubes

Publishing HH. Hearing Loss in Children. Harvard Health. Accessed March 11, 2021. https://www.health.harvard.edu/a_to_z/hearing-loss-in-children-a-to-z

Resonance Disorders. American Speech-Language-Hearing Association. Accessed April 10, 2021. /practice-portal/clinical-topics/resonance-disorders/

Rosenfeld RM. Tympanostomy Tube Controversies and Issues: State-of-the-Art Review. *Ear Nose Throat J.* 2020; 99(1_suppl):15S-21S. doi:10.1177/0145561320919656

Sabo DL. Diagnostic Audiology. In: Losee JE, Kirschner RE, Smith DM, Lawrence CR, Straub A, eds. *Comprehensive Cleft Care: Family Edition.* Family Edition. CRC Press/Taylor & Francis Group; 2015.

Shaffer AD, Ford MD, Choi SS, Jabbour N. The Impact of Timing of Tympanostomy Tube Placement on Sequelae in Children With Cleft Palate. *The Cleft Palate-Craniofacial Journal.* 2019; 56(6):720-728. doi:10.1177/1055665618809228

Skuladottir H, Sivertsen A, Assmus J, Remme AR, Dahlen M, Vindenes H. Hearing Outcomes in Patients with Cleft Lip/Palate. *The Cleft Palate-Craniofacial Journal.* 2015; 52(2):23-31. doi:10.1597/13-009

Speech and Language Birth to 3 years | Cleft Lip & Palate Foundation of Smiles. Accessed April 2, 2021. http://www.cleftsmile.org/speech-and-language-birth-to-3-years/

Stanford Children's Health. Accessed May 12, 2020. https://www.stanfordchildrens.org/en/topic/default?id=the-neonatal-intensive-care-unit-nicu-90-P02389

The Washington State Department of Health Children and Youth with Special Health Care Needs Program, Seattle Children's Hospital Craniofacial Center Seattle, Washington. Cleft Lip and Palate CRITICAL ELEMENTS OF CARE. Published online Sixth Edition, Revised 2018. https://www.seattlechildrens.org/globalassets/documents/clinics/craniofacial/cleft-lip-and-palate-critical-elements-of-care.pdf

Viswanathan N, Vidler M, Richard B. Hearing Thresholds in Newborns with a Cleft Palate Assessed by Auditory Brain Stem Response. *The Cleft Palate-Craniofacial Journal.* 2008; 45(2):187-192. doi:10.1597/06-078.1

What Is Speech? What Is Language? American Speech-Language-Hearing Association. Accessed April 2, 2021. Httpa://asha.org/public/speech/development/speech-and-language/

Chapter 22. My Story, Part 3

Henderson A. Understanding the Breast Crawl: Implications for Nursing Practice. *Nursing for Women's Health.* 2011; 15(4):296-307. doi:10.1111/j.1751-486X.2011.01650.x

Chapter 23. YIPPEE-I-O: Presurgical Infant Orthopedics

ACPA Approved Teams – ACPA Family Services. Accessed July 27, 2020. https://cleftline.org/find-a-team/acpa-approved-teams-in-the-us-and-canada/?country=US

Alfonso AR, Ramly EP, Kantar RS, et al. What Is the Burden of Care of Nasoalveolar Molding? *Cleft Palate Craniofac J.* 2020; 57(9):1078-1092. Doi:10.1177/1055665620929224

Basri OA, Schuster LA. Presurgical Infant Orthopedics and Nasoalveolar Molding. In: Losee JE, Kirschner RE, Smith DM, Lawrence CR, Straub A, eds. *Comprehensive Cleft Care: Family Edition.* Family Edition. CRC Press/Taylor & Francis Group; 2015:263-274.

Beals S, Glick P, Long Jr. R, et al. Comparison of CUCLP dental arch relationships between five centers with varied infant management protocols (NAM, GPP, primary grafting, infant orthopedics). *The Cleft Palate-Craniofacial Journal.* 2015; 52(4):103-159. Doi:10.1597/1545-1569-52.4.e103

Cleft Taping. Cleftopedia. Accessed July 27, 2020. http://www.cleftopedia.com/pre-surgical-techniques/taping/

DynaCleft® + Nasal Elevator | CJ Medical: Agency for Medical Innovations. Accessed July 27, 2020. https://www.cjmedical.com/products/specialties/dynamic-tissue-systems/cleft-palate

Foundation for the Faces of Children. Videos. Understanding Cleft Lip and Palate: A Guide For New Parents. Foundation for the Faces of Children. Accessed February 26, 2020. https://facesofchildren.org/resources/videos/

Ganske I, Sanchez K, Le E, et al. Costing Analysis of Pre-Surgical Infant Orthopedics (PSIO): A Critical Component of Establishing Value for NAM and Latham. In: Vol 58(4S). The Cleft Palate-Craniofacial Journal; 2021:69.

Garland K, McNeely B, Dubois L, Matic D. Systematic Review of the Long-Term Effects of Presurgical Orthopedic Devices on Patient Outcomes. *The Cleft Palate-Craniofacial Journal.* 2022; 59(2):156-165. Doi:10.1177/1055665621998176

Khavanin N, Jenny H, Jodeh DS, Scott MA, Rottgers SA, Steinberg JP. Cleft and Craniofacial Team Orthodontic Care in the United States:

A Survey of the ACPA. *The Cleft Palate-Craniofacial Journal*. 2019; 56(7):860-866. Doi:10.1177/1055665618822235

Kornbluth M, Campbell RE, Daskalogiannakis J, et al. Active Presurgical Infant Orthopedics for Unilateral Cleft Lip and Palate: Inter-Center Outcome Comparison of Latham, Modified McNeil, and Nasoalveolar Molding. *Cleft Palate Craniofac J*. 2018;55(5):639-648. Doi:10.1177/1055665618757367

Mancini L, Gibson TL, Grayson BH, Flores RL, Staffenberg D, Shetye PR. Three-Dimensional Soft Tissue Nasal Changes After Nasoalveolar Molding and Primary Cheilorhinoplasty in Infants With Unilateral Cleft Lip and Palate: *The Cleft Palate-Craniofacial Journal*. Published online April 26, 2018. Doi:10.1177/1055665618771427

Mulliken JB. Mulliken Repair of Bilateral Cleft Lip and Nasal Deformity. In: Losee JE, Kirschner RE, eds. *Comprehensive Cleft Care*. McGraw-Hill Companies, Inc.; 2009:343-360.

Patel PA, Rubin MS, Clouston S, et al. Comparative Study of Early Secondary Nasal Revisions and Costs in Patients With Clefts Treated With and Without Nasoalveolar Molding: *Journal of Craniofacial Surgery*. 2015; 26(4):1229-1233. Doi:10.1097/SCS.0000000000001729

Sischo L, Clouston SAP, Phillips C, Broder HL. Caregiver responses to early cleft palate care: A mixed method approach. *Health Psychology*. 2016;35(5):474-482. Accessed February 21, 2021. /doiLanding?doi=10.1037%2Fhea0000262

Varman R, Demke J. Cleft Team Care Distribution and Subjective Deficiencies by ACPA Member Survey. In: Vol 58 (4S). The Cleft Palate-Craniofacial Journal; 2021:85.

Chapter 24. Tips for NAM Treatment and Lip Taping

Amazon.com : 500PCS Disposable Micro Applicators Brush for Makeup and Personal Care (Head Diameter: 2.0mm)- 5 X 100 PCS : Beauty. Accessed July 31, 2020. https://rb.gy/kmwyor

NAM Taping Tips. Cleftopedia. Accessed July 31, 2020. http://www.cleftopedia.com/pre-surgical-techniques/nam/nam-taping-tips/

Chapter 25. A Second Smile

Bushnell IWR. Mother's Face Recognition in Newborn Infants: Learning and Memory. *Infant and Child Development.* 2001;10:67-74. doi:10.1002/icd.248

Grollemund B, Dissaux C, Gavelle P, et al. The impact of having a baby with cleft lip and palate on parents and on parent-baby relationship: the first French prospective multicentre study. *BMC Pediatr.* 2020; 20(1):230. doi:10.1186/s12887-020-02118-5

Lorenz K. The Comparative Method in Studying Innate Behavior Patterns. *Physiological Mechanisms in Animal Behavior.* Published online 1950:221-254. http://klha.at/papers/1950-InnateBehavior.pdf

Lorenz KZ. The Companion in the Bird's World. *The Auk.* 1937; 54(3):245-273. doi:10.2307/4078077

Mobbs EJ, Mobbs GA, Mobbs AED. Imprinting, latchment and displacement: a mini review of early instinctual behaviour in newborn infants influencing breastfeeding success. *Acta Paediatr.* 2016; 105(1):24-30. doi:10.1111/apa.13034

Nelson PA, Caress A-L, Glenny A-M, Kirk SA. 'Doing the "Right" Thing': How parents experience and manage decision-making for children's 'Normalising' surgeries - ScienceDirect. *Social Science & Medicine.* 2012;74:796-804. Accessed February 21, 2021. https://www.sciencedirect.com/science/article/abs/pii/S0277953612000202?via%3Dihub

Sullivan R, Perry R, Sloan A, Kleinhaus K, Burtchen N. Infant Bonding and Attachment to the Caregiver: Insights From Basic and Clinical Science. *Clin Perinatol.* 2011; 38(4):643-655. doi:10.1016/j.clp.2011.08.011

Chapter 26. Lip-Repair Basics

ACPA Family Services Preparing for Surgery_2019.pdf. Accessed May 6, 2020. https://cleftline.org/wp-content/uploads/2019/07/Preparing-for-Surgery.pdf

Adetayo OA, Kirschner RE, Losee JE. Cleft Lip and Nose Adhesion. In: Losee JE, Kirschner RE, Smith DM, Lawrence CR, Straub A, eds. *Comprehensive Cleft Care: Family Edition.* Family Edition. CRC Press/Taylor & Francis Group; 2015.

Berkowitz S. The Influence of Conservative Surgery on Growth and Occlusion. In: *Cleft Lip and Palate: Diagnosis and Management.* Springer; 2013:347-387. doi:10.1007/978-3-642-30770-6_16

Charkins H. *Children With Facial Difference: A Parents' Guide.* Woodbine House; 1996.

Chen PK-T. Bilateral Cleft Lip and Nose Repair. In: Losee JE, Kirschner RE, Smith DM, Lawrence CR, Straub A, eds. *Comprehensive Cleft Care: Family Edition.* Family Edition. CRC Press/Taylor & Francis Group; 2015:209-216.

Cleft Lip and Palate Repair Surgery | Children's Hospital of Philadelphia. Accessed August 3, 2020. https://www.chop.edu/treatments/surgical-repair-cleft-lip-and-palate

Common Cold in Babies - Diagnosis and Treatment - Mayo Clinic. Accessed August 6, 2020. https://www.mayoclinic.org/diseases-conditions/common-cold-in-babies/diagnosis-treatment/drc-20351657

Crerand CE, Rosenberg J, Magee L, Stein MB, Wilson-Genderson M, Broder HL. Parent-Reported Family Functioning Among Children With Cleft Lip/Palate. *Cleft Palate Craniofac J.* 2015; 52(6):651-659. doi:10.1597/14-050

Cuddles for Clefts. Cuddles for Clefts. Accessed August 21, 2020. https://www.cuddlesforclefts.com/

King K. Cutest Little Cleftie: Lip Repair Surgery. Cutest Little Cleftie. Published May 27, 2017. Accessed August 3, 2020. http://cutestlittlecleftie.blogspot.com/2017/05/lip-repair-surgery.html

Massachusetts Department of Early Education and Care. Best Practices in Early Childhood Transition: A Guide for Families.pdf. Accessed August 21, 2020. https://www.mass.gov/doc/best-practices-in-early-childhood-transition-english/download

Nelson DPA, Kirk DSA. Parents' Perspectives of Cleft Lip and/or Palate Services: A Qualitative Interview: *The Cleft Palate-Craniofacial Journal.* Published online May 1, 2013. doi:10.1597/11-293

Pediatric Anesthesia | Howard County General Hospital | Johns Hopkins Medicine. Accessed August 5, 2020. https://www.hopkinsmedicine.org/howard_county_general_hospital/services/surgery/anesthesiology/pediatric_anesthesia.html

Perspective-Taking: Considering Different Points of View | Bing Nursery School. Accessed August 21, 2020. https://bingschool.stanford.edu/news/perspective-taking-considering-different-points-view

Philadelphia TCH of. Preparing Your Child for Surgery. Published May 12, 2014. Accessed August 22, 2020. https://www.chop.edu/patients-and-visitors/guide-your-childs-surgery/preparing-your-child-surgery

Preparing the Infant for Surgery - Health Encyclopedia - University of Rochester Medical Center. Accessed August 6, 2020. https://www.urmc.rochester.edu/encyclopedia/content.aspx?contenttypeid=90&contentid=P03033

Ronald McDonald Family Room®. RMHC of Greater Washington, DC. Accessed August 5, 2020. https://rmhcdc.org/what-we-do/ronald-mcdonald-family-room/

Salyer A, Green A, Salyer KE. Unilateral Cleft Lip and Nose Repair. In: Losee JE, Kirschner RE, Smith DM, Lawrence CR, Straub A, eds. *Comprehensive Cleft Care: Family Edition*. Family Edition. CRC Press/Taylor & Francis Group; 2015.

The Hospital for Sick Children (SickKids): Preparing for Surgery. Accessed August 6, 2020. http://www.sickkids.ca/VisitingSickKids/Coming-for-surgery/Preparing-for-my-childs-surgery/index.html

Chapter 27. The Handoff

Hrdy SB. Interview. July 21, 2016.

Information NC for B, Pike USNL of M 8600 R, MD B, Usa 20894. *What Can Help Relieve Anxiety Before Surgery?* Institute for Quality and Efficiency in Health Care (IQWiG); 2018. Accessed September 28, 2020. https://www.ncbi.nlm.nih.gov/books/NBK279557/

Noriuchi M, Kikuchi Y, Senoo A. The Functional Neuroanatomy of Maternal Love: Mother's Response to Infant's Attachment Behaviors. *Biol Psychiatry*. 2008;63(4):415-423. doi:10.1016/j.biopsych.2007.05.018

Ofri D. We Doctors Need to Talk to Patients About Raw Fear. Slate Magazine. Published September 22, 2013. Accessed August 25, 2020. https://slate.com/technology/2013/09/fear-of-medical-procedures-doctors-need-to-acknowledge-emotions.html

Chapter 28. Lip Repair: Recovery in the Hospital

ACPA Family Services Preparing for Surgery_2019.pdf. Accessed May 6, 2020. https://cleftline.org/wp-content/uploads/2019/07/Preparing-for-Surgery.pdf

After Your Child's Surgery | UCLA Mattel Children's Hospital | UCLA Health. Accessed September 2, 2020. https://www.uclahealth.org/mattel/after-surgery

Children TH for S. Treating my Child's Pain. Accessed September 7, 2020. http://www.sickkids.ca/VisitingSickKids/Coming-for-surgery/Pain/index.html

Cleft Lip Repair | Children's Hospital Pittsburgh. Accessed September 2, 2020. https://www.chp.edu/our-services/plastic-surgery/patient-procedures/cleft-lip-repair

Cleft Lip Surgery | Children's Minnesota. Accessed September 3, 2020. https://www.childrensmn.org/services/care-specialties-departments/cleft-craniofacial-program/conditions-and-services/cleft-lip/

Dehydration - Symptoms and Causes. Mayo Clinic. Accessed September 8, 2020. https://www.mayoclinic.org/diseases-conditions/dehydration/symptoms-causes/syc-20354086

FDA-Consumer Health Information-Guide-to-Safe-Use-of-Pain-Medicine.pdf. Accessed January 12, 2022. https://portal.ct.gov/-/media/Departments-and-Agencies/DPH/dph/environmental_health/occupationalhealth/Opioid-Symposium-March-2017/FDA-Guide-to-Safe-Use-of-Pain-Medicine.pdf

Helping Your Child Manage Pain | UCLA Mattel Children's Hospital | UCLA Health. Accessed September 7, 2020. https://www.uclahealth.org/mattel/pain-management

Kids with Clefts Utah: How do I Deal With the Emotions of my Child's Surgery? Accessed September 8, 2020. http://kidswithcleftsutah.blogspot.com/2009/11/how-do-i-deal-with-emotions-of-my.html

King K. Cutest Little Cleftie: Lip Repair Surgery. Cutest Little Cleftie. Published May 27, 2017. Accessed August 3, 2020. http://cutestlittlecleftie.blogspot.com/2017/05/lip-repair-surgery.html

Klass P, M.D. Managing Children's Pain After Surgery. *The New York Times*. https://www.nytimes.com/2019/01/07/well/family/managing-childrens-pain-after-surgery.html. Published January 7, 2019. Accessed September 7, 2020.

Managing Cancer Pain at Home. Accessed September 7, 2020. https://www.cancer.org/treatment/treatments-and-side-effects/physical-side-effects/pain/pain.html

Managing Your Child's Pain at Home After Surgery | Gillette Children's Specialty Healthcare. Accessed September 7, 2020. https://www.gillettechildrens.org/your-visit/patient-education/managing-your-childs-pain-at-home-after-surgery

Pain Control After Your Child's Surgery | Children's Hospital of Philadelphia. Accessed September 7, 2020. https://www.chop.edu/patients-and-visitors/guide-your-childs-surgery/pain-control-after-surgery

Pfaff M, Nolan I, Bertrand A, et al. Perioperative Pain Management for Cleft Lip and Palate Surgery: A Systematic Review and Meta-Analysis of Randomized Controlled Studies. In: Vol 58(4S). The Cleft Palate-Craniofacial Journal; 2021:39.

Philadelphia TCH of. Narcotic Pain Medicines. Published May 12, 2014. Accessed September 7, 2020. https://www.chop.edu/patients-and-visitors/guide-your-childs-surgery/pain-control-after-surgery/narcotic-pain-medicines

Shaffer EG, Cladis FP. Anesthesia for Cleft Patients. In: Losee JE, Kirschner RE, Smith DM, Lawrence CR, Straub A, eds. *Comprehensive Cleft Care: Family Edition*. Family Edition. CRC Press/Taylor & Francis Group; 2015.

The Jennings' Jabber: Surgery. Accessed September 8, 2020. http://jenningsjabber.blogspot.com/search/label/surgery

Vega RM, Avva U. Pediatric Dehydration. In: *StatPearls*. StatPearls Publishing; 2020. Accessed September 8, 2020. http://www.ncbi.nlm.nih.gov/books/NBK436022/

Waking Up to Anesthesia. NIH News in Health. Published July 6, 2017. Accessed September 2, 2020. https://newsinhealth.nih.gov/2011/04/waking-up-anesthesia

Chapter 29. Lip Repair: Recovery at Home

ACPA Family Services. Factsheet: Surgical Scars. https://cleftline.org/wp-content/uploads/2019/03/ACPA_factsheet_surgicalscars.pdf

Chen PK-T. Bilateral Cleft Lip and Nose Repair. In: Losee JE, Kirschner RE, Smith DM, Lawrence CR, Straub A, eds. *Comprehensive Cleft Care: Family Edition*. Family Edition. CRC Press/Taylor & Francis Group; 2015:209-216.

Cleft Palate Repair Recovery Tips. Elizabeth From Scratch. Published February 6, 2020. Accessed September 9, 2020. https://www.elizabethfromscratch.com/cleft-palate-repair-recovery-tips/

Flynn, Bohns V. If You Need Help, Just Ask: Underestimating Compliance With Direct Requests for Help. *Journal of Personality and Social Psychology*. 2008; 95. doi:10.1037/0022-3514.95.1.128

Klass P, M.D. Managing Children's Pain After Surgery. *The New York Times*. https://www.nytimes.com/2019/01/07/well/family/managing-childrens-pain-after-surgery.html. Published January 7, 2019. Accessed September 7, 2020.

Koven M, Marsac M, Tran S, Rosenberg J. An Innovative Approach to Supporting Children with Craniofacial Conditions from Diverse Backgrounds. In: Vol 58(4S). The Cleft Palate-Craniofacial Journal; 2021:77.

Recovery and Aftercare: Repair Surgery. CLAPA. Accessed September 9, 2020. https://www.clapa.com/treatment/repair-surgery/recovery-aftercare/

Seattle Children's: Scar Care. Patient and Family Education.pdf. Accessed September 9, 2020. https://www.seattlechildrens.org/pdf/PE2043.pdf

Stock NM, Costa B, White P, Rumsey N. Risk and Protective Factors for Psychological Distress in Families Following a Diagnosis of Cleft Lip and/or Palate. *The Cleft Palate-Craniofacial Journal*. 2020;57(1):88-98. doi:10.1177/1055665619862457

Chapter 30. A New Challenge: Cups!

Aspiration in Babies and Children. Cedars-Sinai.org. Accessed May 18, 2021. https://www.cedars-sinai.org/health-library/articles.html

CDC. When, What, and How to Introduce Solid Foods. Centers for Disease Control and Prevention. Published February 24, 2020. Accessed September 16, 2020. https://www.cdc.gov/nutrition/infantandtoddlernutrition/foods-and-drinks/when-to-introduce-solid-foods.html

Cleft Palate Sippy Cup Transition. Elizabeth From Scratch. Published January 27, 2020. Accessed September 15, 2020. https://www.elizabethfromscratch.com/cleft-palate-sippy-cup-transition/

Coulthard H, Harris G, Emmett P. Delayed introduction of lumpy foods to children during the complementary feeding period affects child's food acceptance and feeding at 7 years of age. *Matern Child Nutr.* 2009; 5(1):75-85. doi:10.1111/j.1740-8709.2008.00153.

Feeding - Common Problems and Solutions. CLAPA.com. CLAPA. Accessed September 16, 2020. https://www.clapa.com/treatment/feeding/

Goodwyn-Craine A. Insights on Feeding and Swallowing Differences for Infants with Cleft Lip and/or Palate. *Leader Live.* Published online December 22, 2019. Accessed May 18, 2021. https://leader.pubs.asha.org/do/10.1044/insights-on-feeding-and-swallowing-differences-for-infants-with-cleft-palate-cleft-lip-and-palate/full/

Madhoun L, Baylis A. A National Survey of Solid Food Introduction for Infants with Cleft Lip and/or Palate. In: *ACPA Annual Meeting 2021.* Vol 58(4s). The Cleft Palate-Craniofacial Journal; 2021:64.

Seattle Children's: Patient and Family Education. Starting Solid Foods-For Babies With Cleft Palate.pdf. Accessed September 16, 2020. https://www.seattlechildrens.org/pdf/PE2389.pdf

Silbert S, Gingrich M, Haynes K, Leatham M. Introduction of Solids for Infants with Unrepaired Clefts. In: Vol 58(4S). The Cleft Palate-Craniofacial Journal; 2021:65.

Sippy Cups - *BabyCenter.* Accessed September 14, 2020. https://community.babycenter.com/post/a22568115/sippy_cups

Sippy Cups and Upcoming Palate Surgery. *BabyCenter* Community. Accessed September 14, 2020. https://community.babycenter.com/post/a27140023/sippy_cups_and_upcomming_palate_surgery

Thaete K, Fetter B, Chesser C, Huff H, Kaye A. Nutritional Challenges in Oral Clefting: A Multidisciplinary Approach to Support Growth and Avoid Malnutrition in the Neonatal and Perioperative Periods. In: Vol 58(4S). The Cleft Palate-Craniofacial Journal; 2021:90.

Chapter 31. Palate-Repair Surgery

Cleft Palate Repair: Instructions After Surgery. Accessed September 7, 2020. https://www.nationwidechildrens.org/family-resources-education/health-wellness-and-safety-resources/helping-hands/cleft-palate-repair-instructions-after-surgery

de Martino M, Chiarugi A, Boner A, Montini G, de' Angelis GL. Working Towards an Appropriate Use of Ibuprofen in Children: An Evidence-Based Appraisal. *Drugs*. 2017; 77(12):1295-1311. doi:10.1007/s40265-017-0751-z

Klass P, M.D. Managing Children's Pain After Surgery. *The New York Times*. https://www.nytimes.com/2019/01/07/well/family/managing-childrens-pain-after-surgery.html. Published January 7, 2019. Accessed September 7, 2020.

Pearson GD, Kirschner RE. Cleft Palate Repair. In: Losee JE, Kirschner RE, Smith DM, Lawrence CR, Straub A, eds. *Comprehensive Cleft Care: Family Edition*. Family Edition. CRC Press/Taylor & Francis Group; 2015.

Seattle Children's: Patient and Family Education. Pain Medicine After Surgery.pdf. Accessed September 18, 2020. https://www.seattlechildrens.org/pdf/PE1251.pdf

Verghese ST, Hannallah RS. Acute Pain Management in Children. *J Pain Res*. 2010;3:105-123. Accessed September 17, 2020. https://www.ncbi.nlm.nih.gov/pmc/articles/PMC3004641/

Well Child, Edge Hill University, University of Central Lancashire, Royal College of Nursing, OCB Media. "My Child is in Pain." Accessed September 17, 2020. http://mychildisinpain.org.uk/

Chapter 32. Conclusion: Now What?

ACPA Family Services: Preparing for Surgery_2019.pdf. Accessed May 6, 2020. https://cleftline.org/wp-content/uploads/2019/07/Preparing-for-Surgery.pdf

ACPA Family Services: Your Baby's First Year_2021.pdf.

Crerand CE, Heppner C, Hansen-Moore J, Sandberg DE. Shared Decision Making in Craniofacial Care. In: Vol 58(4S). The Cleft Palate-Craniofacial Journal; 2021:83.

Crerand CE, Rosenberg J, Magee L, Stein MB, Wilson-Genderson M, Broder HL. Parent-Reported Family Functioning Among Children With Cleft Lip/Palate. *Cleft Palate Craniofac J.* 2015; 52(6):651-659. doi:10.1597/14-050

Fleming V, Cukor G. *The Wizard of Oz.*; 1939.

Gallagher R. An Exploration of Carers' Perceptions of Children's Well-Being During Treatment for Cleft Lip and/or Palate in the United Kingdom. In: Vol 58(4S). The Cleft Palate-Craniofacial Journal; 2021:86-87.

Rosoff M. You Can't Protect Children by Lying to Them—The Truth Will Hurt Less. The Guardian. Published September 21, 2013. Accessed October 15, 2020. http://www.theguardian.com/lifeandstyle/2013/sep/21/cant-protect-children-by-lying

Strauss RP, Watkins SE, Ramsey BL. The Power of Difference: Social and Cultural Issues Associated With Cleft And Craniofacial Conditions. In: *Comprehensive Cleft Care: Family Edition.* Family Edition. CRC Press/Taylor & Francis Group; 2015.

Appendix

Tables: How Much Time for Cleft Care?

HOW MUCH TIME FOR CLEFT CARE? Age Newborn to Lip-Repair Surgery (around 6 months) Cleft Lip and Palate		
Activity	**Time Required**	**What to Expect**
Feeding the Baby	Newborn: 30-45 minutes per session, every two hours, plus time for trial-and-error with special-needs bottles (modifying the bottle or switching to a new bottle) and washing bottle parts.	Feeding a baby with cleft palate may require more concentration and energy than feeding an unaffected baby, especially early on, as you learn to read the baby's signals and make adjustments. "You can't feed the baby and watch Oprah," said one cleft team nurse.
Pumping Breast Milk (if applicable)	30-40 minutes per session, with a hospital-grade breast pump, up to 8 times per day, plus time to wash components and store milk (if applicable).	Mothers who have pumped exclusively have described devoting tremendous time and energy to this activity. It may be helpful to plan to pump milk and feed the baby in separate sessions—at least at first. Some mothers are able to pump while doing other activities, but oftentimes only after gaining some experience. One mother said she pumped while she drove to work (proceed with caution!). See Chapter 16 for more information.

Activity	Time Required	What to Expect
Visits with the Members of the Cleft Team	Presurgical appointments and postsurgical appointments: at least 30 minutes (often longer) for the visit itself. Note that a "clinic visit" may require a half-day or longer (see Ch. 20 for more.)	You'll learn a lot about how your baby is doing overall, how she is doing specifically in terms of CLP, and what is to come. Many parents find these visits emotionally taxing, but also reassuring (See Chapter 20 for tips).
Presurgical Appliance (NAM/ Latham/ face taping): Home Care	NAM and Face Taping: Constant monitoring plus several five-to-ten-minute sessions per day to change the tapes and check the appliance. Fine motor skills are helpful! Latham: 10 minutes, nightly, to turn the screw.	Some babies undergo a treatment called *presurgical infant orthopedics* prior to lip-repair surgery. There are several types. Nasoalveolar Molding (NAM) is a retainer-like orthodontic device held in place with face tapes and rubber bands. A Latham appliance is inserted surgically and needs to be adjusted nightly by parents and regularly by members of the team. Face taping involves taping a baby's face (there is no retainer-like appliance). If the tapes get wet after a bath or a big spit-up, they'll need to be changed. The tapes may loosen over time, as well, or after crying or straining the face. See Chapter 23 for more information.

Activity	Time Required	What to Expect
Presurgical Appliance (NAM/ Latham/ face taping): Visits with Members of the Team	Weekly appointment with the orthodontist/pediatric dentist on the team, (during business hours): 30-45 minutes for the visit itself, plus travel, parking, etc.	Many parents notice that their baby is cranky, fussy, or sleepless following the visit, typically for about 24 hours, as she adjusts to the new position of the appliance and any soreness in the mouth.
Lip-Repair Surgery	One to two days in the hospital plus a week of intense recovery at home (variable), getting easier over time. Some cleft teams perform this repair in more than one surgical session.	Many parents describe the first week after surgery as emotionally and physically taxing. For 3-to-6 weeks following the operation, the baby may be required to wear special padded arm restraints to prevent her from damaging her mouth with her hands (think: robot arms). Some children require constant parental monitoring, others very little monitoring—it depends on the child. The entire experience can be exhausting. Many parents find, however, that their child is remarkably resilient and acts like her normal self within a few days following the procedure, even while wearing the cuffs.

Activity	Time Required	What to Expect
In-Between Activities		Caring for a baby with CLP can require time and energy above and beyond the activities mentioned above. Some extra tasks are relatively simple and concrete, like taking impromptu trips to the pharmacy or teaching a caregiver to use a special bottle. Others happen at the margins, as a result of the emotional intensity of the baby's first year of treatment. Couples may spend more time planning, rehashing, talking, arguing, and making up than they would otherwise (individual or couples therapy can help). Siblings in the family may need extra attention as they adjust to having a baby in the household—especially one who requires so much attention. Even cleft-related phone calls and late-night internet research sessions take time (not to mention reading books like this one!). Very few new parents have ample time to attend to their own needs, CLP aside. But early cleft treatment can add intensity to the experience. Appointments require time and energy, but so do the very real emotions of feeling excited, anxious, nervous, relieved, exhausted, loving, and proud.

	HOW MUCH TIME FOR CLEFT CARE? AGES SIX MONTHS TO ONE YEAR Cleft Lip and Palate	
Activity	**Time**	**What to Expect**
Bottle Feeding	Approx. 30-40 minutes per session, several times per day (based on weight and MD advice)	Caloric needs go up as the baby grows, but by now, caregivers and baby have probably chosen a favorite special-needs bottle and have developed a pretty good feel for it. Make sure to have spares on hand, as the nipples wear out and need to be replaced.
Transition to Sippy Cup	Add 10 mins. to bottle feeding, plus extra time to assess problems and make adjustments to the cups, plus cleanup.	This task can take time and patience for everyone involved, but it is doable. See Chapter 30 for more information.
Transition to Solid Foods	Add 5-10 mins. beyond bottle-feeding, plus more time with growth, and extra for cleanup and buying/making food.	Most pediatricians and cleft teams recommend starting solids at the same age as babies born without CLP. Look for a special-needs spoon for feeding a baby with a cleft palate. With patience and small improvements, this task, too, is doable.
Visits with the Cleft or Craniofacial Team	Same as Table 1. Presurgical and postsurgical appointments: approx. 30 mins. for the visit itself.	As mentioned above, these visits can be emotionally and physically draining while at the same time useful and reassuring. (See Chapter 20 for tips).

Activity	Time	What to Expect
Pumping Breast Milk Beyond Age 6 Months (if applicable)	Same as Table 1. Approx. 30 mins. per session, with a hospital-grade breast pump, up to 8 times per day, possibly fewer over time. Add time to wash bottles, store milk (if applicable).	Because of the extraordinary demands of exclusive pumping, some of the women who do so tend to stop before age 6 months. Those who continue may need sustained (or extra) support, both logistically and emotionally. According to the site exclusivelypumping.com, "Exclusively pumping can be a lonely journey, and almost every mother who travels this road believes she is a lone traveler—until she discovers a group of other women just like her!" Communicating with others can help ease the burden.
Palate-Repair Surgery	One-to-three days in the hospital plus a week of recovery at home, getting easier over time. This surgery can be more painful than lip repair, so recovery may take longer than before (variable).	Many parents describe the first week after palate repair as more intense than the time following lip repair. For 3-6 weeks following surgery, the baby may be required to wear arm restraints, as with lip-repair surgery (as stated above). Caregivers may need to monitor the child constantly during waking hours (again, it depends on the child). Surgeons may ask parents to be more vigilant with arm cuffs following palate repair than they were for lip repair because the site is more delicate and because an older baby, now stronger and more agile than before, may be more prone to damage the site with their hands (recommendations vary).

Glossary

alveolar bone-graft surgery – An operation to close spaces in the gum ridge by inserting bone, to support the eruption of teeth.

alveolus – The bony ridge of the upper and lower jaw, covered by gums, which contains the teeth.

amniocentesis – A prenatal test performed by drawing and testing a small amount of amniotic fluid (the liquid that surrounds the fetus) to learn genetic information about a fetus.

anesthesiologist – A doctor who uses drugs to induce sleep and loss of feeling during a medical procedure.

articulation – The use of the mouth, lips, and tongue to make speech sounds.

aspiration – The abnormal passage of food, liquid, or other material into the airway.

assisted-delivery bottle – A baby bottle that relies on the caregiver to deliver liquid into a baby's mouth by pulsing a part of the vessel.

audiologist – A health care professional who specializes in the diagnosis and treatment of hearing and balance disorders.

bilateral – Relating to both sides.

cheiloplasty – The surgical closure of a cleft lip.

chromosomes – Structures found in the nucleus of most living cells that carry genetic information in the form of genes.

chromosomal microarray – A genetic test for problems with chromosomes, such as extra or missing chromosomes or parts of chromosomes.

chorionic villus sampling (CVS) – A prenatal test in which a part of the placenta is tested to learn information about the genetic makeup of a fetus.

cleft lip – A birth condition characterized by a split in one or both sides of the upper lip.

cleft palate – A birth condition characterized by a split in the roof of the mouth.

cleft-palate speech – Also called velopharyngeal dysfunction (VPI) or velopharyngeal insufficiency (VPD), a condition that occurs when the back of the soft palate doesn't function the way it should during speech, allowing for the abnormal escape of air through the mouth and nose.

cleft team – Also called cleft palate team or craniofacial team, a group of specialists from different disciplines (e.g., speech, dentistry, surgery) who treat children and young adults born with cleft lip and/or palate and, in the case of a craniofacial team, children with other conditions of the head and face.

columella – The strip of skin located in between the nostrils at the bottom of the nose.

complete cleft lip – An opening that extends completely through the upper lip and into the nose.

conductive hearing loss – A type of hearing loss that occurs when sound is unable to reach the inner ear, usually due to an obstruction.

congenital – Present at birth.

craniofacial – Relating to the head and face.

craniofacial team – A group of specialists from different disciplines (e.g., speech, dentistry, surgery) who treat children and young adults born with cleft lip and/or palate and other craniofacial conditions.

dehydration – The absence of sufficient water in the body.

deviated septum – A condition in which the wall that separates the nostrils is displaced to one side.

DNA, or deoxyribonucleic acid – The chemical name for the long molecule that carries genetic instructions in all living things.

dysphagia – Difficulty swallowing.

ENT surgeon – Also called an otolaryngologist, a physician who specializes in disorders of the ear, nose, and throat.

Early Intervention (EI) – The state-run programs and services available to babies and young children with special needs and their families.

emergence – Also called recovery, the gradual return of consciousness after discontinuing anesthetic at the end of a surgical procedure.

emergence delirium – A temporary state of extreme irritability, combativeness, and inconsolability during the recovery from anesthesia.

esophageal reflux – Also called gastroesophageal reflux or reflux, the abnormal movement of food and liquid from the stomach back into the esophagus.

exclusive pumping – The act of expressing milk from the breast to deliver to a baby through another means (e.g., a bottle).

expanding – In the context of speech therapy, the act of rewording a child's utterance into a complete sentence.

Eustachian tube – The air duct that connects the middle ear to the back of the throat, allowing for the equalization of pressure around the eardrum and the ventilation of the middle ear.

feeding tube – A medical device, usually made of soft plastic, used to feed a person who is unable to take food or drink by mouth.

fellowship – In the context of medical and dental training in the United States and Canada, a period of training that a physician or dentist undertakes after completing a specialty training program (residency).

fetal echocardiogram – Also called a fetal echo, an ultrasound of the heart of a fetus.

fetal MRI – A scan of an unborn offspring using Magnetic Resonance Imaging (MRI).

FISH, or *fluorescence in situ hybridization* – A test that looks for gene changes in cells.

fistula – An abnormal opening, such as in the palate.

forme fruste cleft lip – Also called microform cleft lip, a mild form of cleft lip that appears as a notch or vertical scar on the upper lip.

gastroesophageal reflux disease (GERD) – A digestive disorder that affects the ring of muscle between the esophagus and the stomach.

gene – A molecule made of DNA that functions as the basic unit of heredity. Genes are transferred from biological parents to offspring and determine some characteristics of the offspring.

genetics – The science of heredity (how characteristics are passed down from biological parents to a child).

genetic counselor – A health professional with advanced training in medical genetics who works with patients and families to determine and explain their risk of inherited conditions and/or syndromes.

geneticist – A doctor who studies the science of human genetics.

genetic predisposition – An increased chance that a person will develop a disease or condition based on their genetic makeup.

gingiva – The gums.

gingivoperiosteoplasty, also called GPP – The surgical closure of the gums at the site of a cleft in the alveolus.

hard palate – The bony, front part of the roof of the mouth.

karyotype – A laboratory technique that produces an image of an individual's chromosomes to look for abnormal numbers or structures.

imprinting – In psychology and ethology, a phenomenon that occurs in animals, and theoretically in humans, in the first hours of life when a newborn creature bonds to the type of animals it meets at birth and begins to pattern its behavior after them.

incomplete cleft lip – A separation, present at birth, which extends partway through the upper lip but does not reach all the way to the nose.

infant orthopedics (IO) – Sometimes called presurgical infant orthopedics (PSIO), any of several orthodontic techniques used to reduce the dimensions of a cleft prior to surgery.

inner ear – The innermost part of the ear, containing organs of balance and hearing.

Intensive Care Unit (ICU) – An area in a hospital where patients receive specialized medical care such as intensive monitoring and advanced life support.

isolated clefts – A term used in genetic counseling to indicate that a person is at no greater risk than any other person for having learning problems or birth conditions beyond clefts.

language – The expression and understanding of human communication.

Latham treatment – A presurgical orthodontic method (and device) that decreases the size of a cleft prior to surgery.

levator veli palatini – Also called levitor, a muscle in the roof of the mouth that controls palatal movement during speech.

lip adhesion – The first step of a two-part surgical repair of a cleft lip, sometimes used as an alternative to presurgical infant orthopedics.

lip-repair surgery – An operation, usually performed during infancy, to close the gap in a cleft lip and sometimes reconstruct parts of the nose and/or gums.

lower esophageal sphincter – A valve-like ring of muscle located at the bottom end of the esophagus, where the esophagus meets the stomach.

middle ear – A narrow, air-filled space located between the eardrum and the inner ear that carries sound waves to the inner ear.

narcotic – A drug that produces analgesia (pain relief), narcosis (state of stupor or sleep), and addiction (physical dependence on the drug).

nasal regurgitation – In the context of cleft palate, the usually harmless escape of liquid or food through the nose during eating or drinking.

nasoalveolar molding (NAM) – A nonsurgical method of reshaping the gums, lips, and nostrils of a cleft-affected infant prior to surgery.

Neonatal Intensive Care Unit (NICU) – An area in a hospital where newborn babies receive specialized medical care such as intensive monitoring and advanced life support.

occupational therapist (OT) – A health care professional who helps people recover or maintain their everyday activities.

oral defensiveness – Also called oral aversion, a reluctance or refusal of a person to eat, drink, or accept sensation in or around the mouth.

orthognathic surgery – An operation to align the upper and/or lower jaws.

palate-repair surgery – Also known as palatoplasty, a surgical procedure to close and/or reconstruct an opening in the roof of the mouth.

pediatric dentist – A specialist concerned with the oral health of children.

pediatrician – A doctor who focuses on the health of infants, children, adolescents, and young adults.

philtrum – The vertical groove between the border of the upper lip and the base of the nose.

plastic surgeon – A physician who repairs and reconstructs tissue and skin.

premaxilla – The segment of bone of the upper jaw that typically contains the four front teeth.

prenatal ultrasound – An imaging technique that uses high-frequency sound waves to produce images of a fetus in the uterus.

***presurgical infant orthopedics* (PSIO)** – Sometimes called infant orthopedics (IO), any of several orthodontic techniques used to reduce the dimensions of a cleft prior to surgery.

prolabium – The central area of the upper lip beneath the center of the nose and between the philtral columns.

psychologist – A licensed and/or certified specialist who studies the science of behaviors, emotions, and thoughts.

***recurrence* risk** – In the context of genetics, the chances of a hereditary event happening again in a biological family.

residency – In the context of medical and dental training in the United States and Canada, a period of in-depth training that a physician or dentist undertakes after completing medical or dental school.

resonance – The quality of the vocal sounds created as air vibrates through the facial cavities.

rhinoplasty – A surgical procedure to alter the form and/or function of the nose.

sensorineural hearing loss – A type of hearing loss that is caused by damage to the acoustic nerve or other parts of the inner ear.

septum – The wall of cartilage and bone that divides the left and right sides of the nose.

social worker – A professional who helps children and families through counseling, advocacy, education, and access to resources.

soft palate – The back part of the roof of the mouth, made up of mucous membrane and muscle.

speech – In the context of speech therapy, the manner in which we say sounds and words.

speech-language pathologist (SLP) – A communication expert who assesses, diagnoses, treats, and prevents speech, language, social communication, cognitive communication, and swallowing disorders in children and adults.

Steri-Strips™ – Thin adhesive bandages sometimes placed over an incision after surgery and, in the context of cleft lip and palate, used with presurgical infant orthopedics such as nasoalveolar molding.

submucous cleft palate – A separation of the muscles located underneath the membrane lining of the roof of the mouth.

sutures – In the context of surgery, stitches made with sterile surgical threads to close incisions.

syndrome – A group of differences that appear together and collectively characterize a specific disease or condition.

targeted prenatal ultrasound – A scan of a fetus performed during the second trimester of pregnancy to check growth, development, and the presence of birth defects and certain types of genetic conditions.

teratogen – An agent that causes abnormalities in a developing embryo or fetus upon exposure.

tympanostomy tubes – Also called pressure-equalization tubes, PE tubes, ventilation tubes, or ear tubes, these tiny cylinders are inserted into the eardrum via a short surgical procedure to allow ventilation, drainage, and equalization of pressure in the middle ear.

unilateral cleft lip – An opening, present at birth, which occurs on one side of the upper lip.

uvula – A small piece of tissue that dangles from the soft palate at the back of the mouth.

velopharyngeal insufficiency (VPI) – Also called velopharyngeal dysfunction (VPD) or cleft palate speech, a condition that occurs when the back of the soft palate doesn't function the way it should during speech, allowing for the abnormal escape of air through the mouth and nose.

Index

Abbreviations are as follows:

CLP – cleft lip and/or palate

IO/PSIO – infant orthopedics/presurgical infant orthopedics

. . . .

questions for, 273
autobiographical memory, 233

BabyCenter cleft forum/groups, 32, 407, 411, 412, 415
baby photos, 234–237
    the child's point-of-view, 234–235
    over time as feelings change, 236–237
    parents' points-of-view, 235–236
    reasons for taking them, 235–237
Band-Aids Blister Bandages, 322, 323
    See also face tapes
base tapes, 312, 321, 322–324, 334
Berde, Charles (Dr.), 375
Berkowitz, Samuel (orthodontist), 348
beyond year one
    advocacy and courage, 441
    communicating about clefts to the child, 437–438
    decision making, 438–441
    moving beyond "cleft mode", 435, 436–437
    speech, 278
bilateral cleft lip and palate (bilateral CLP)
    complete vs. incomplete, 1–2, 20
    defined, 485
    and face taping, 311
    and feeding, 160, 208, 421
    and Latham treatment, 307, 308–310
    and NAM treatments, 299, 301, 305
    supermarket story, 252
    and surgery prognosis, 103–104
    vs. unilateral, 20
Biological Psychiatry, 365
birth
    and bonding, 124–130
    and the care team, 60–63, 64, 111–113, 351

Made in the USA
Middletown, DE
02 September 2024

60287708R00324